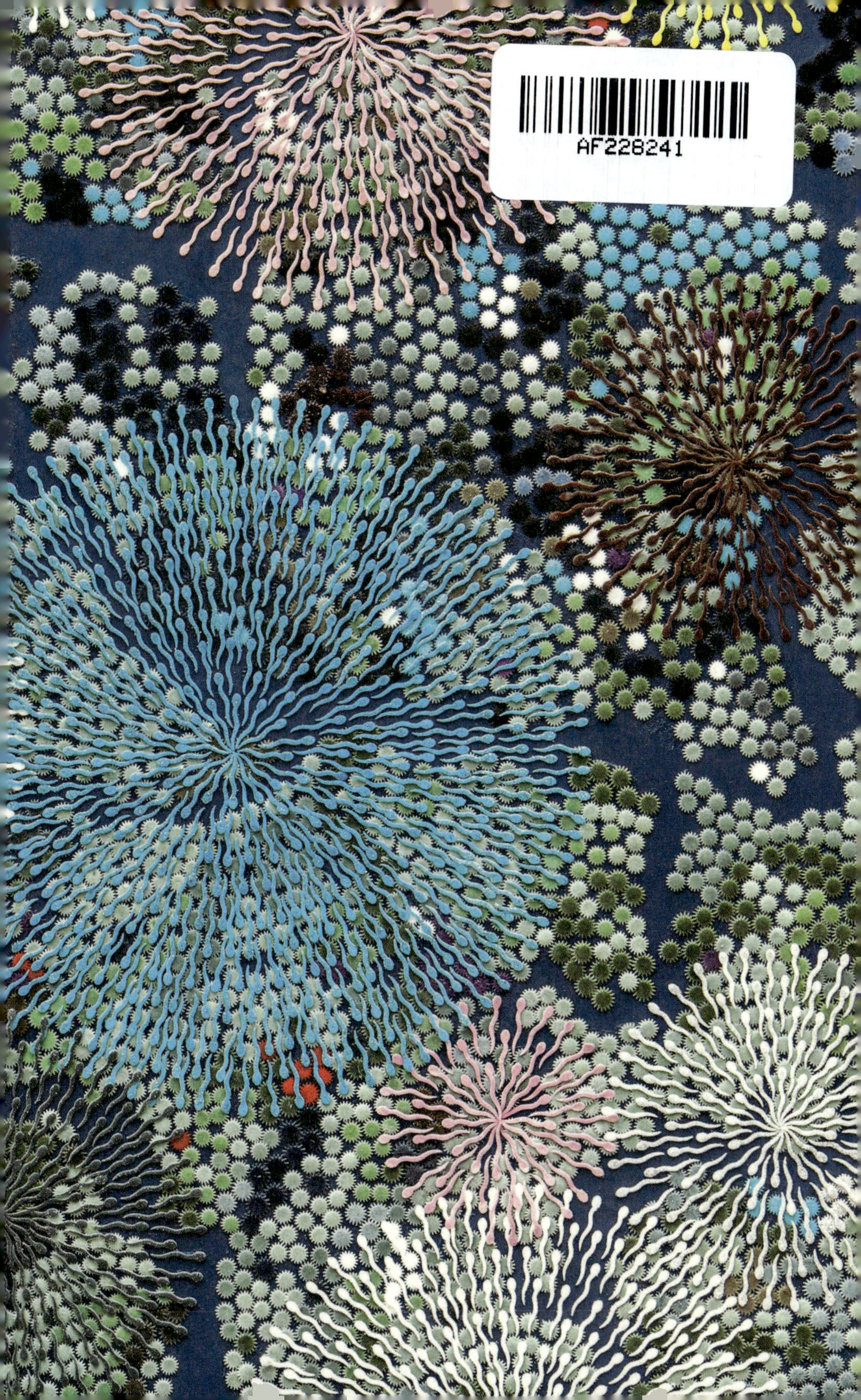

AF228241

Our children are facing more chronic illness, more allergies, and more developmental challenges than ever before—and the root causes often begin before they are even conceived. In this powerful book, Dr. Ann Shippy gives parents a way forward. She brings the science of epigenetics, detox, gut health, and mitochondrial function into a loving, hopeful framework for families. *The Preconception Revolution* is not just a book—it's a gift to every future child and to the parents who are ready to rewrite the story of health.

—Elisa Song, MD, Integrative Pediatrician and *USA Today*
Bestselling Author of *Healthy Kids, Happy Kids*

The single biggest thing you can do to have vibrant energy and live a very long time is to have abundantly healthy parents. It's too late for you to do anything about your parents, but you *can* give that gift to your children and grandchildren. All you have to do is read Dr. Shippy's epic book! The great news is that you'll feel a huge shift in the amount of energy you have for yourself and your family also.

—Dave Asprey, Creator of the Biohacking Movement,
4x *New York Times* Bestselling Author

In *The Preconception Revolution*, Dr. Ann Shippy shines a light on the often-overlooked preconception period, showing how taking the time to detox, nourish, and support both parents' bodies before conceiving can make a world of difference for both mom and baby. Drawing from her own health journey and decades of experience in functional medicine, Dr. Shippy now brings this impact to the next generation in a compelling way. This book is a must-read for anyone wanting to optimize their child's lifelong health and set the stage for an easier, more empowering recovery for moms after birth. It's time to revolutionize how we approach conception—this book will show you how.

—Katie Wells, WellnessMama.com

At thirty-nine, I was told I was infertile—a diagnosis that felt like a life sentence. But I'm living proof that your diagnosis is not your destiny. By detoxing, healing my gut, reducing inflammation, and completely restructuring my lifestyle, I was able to conceive naturally again. Whether you're facing infertility or simply want to give your future baby the healthiest start, *The Preconception Revolution* is the science-backed, empowering road map you need. Dr. Ann Shippy's approach is a game changer for anyone ready to take charge of their fertility and health.

—Anna Cabeca, DO, FACOG, ABAARM,
Triple-Board Certified OB-GYN, Bestselling
Author of *The Hormone Fix* and *MenuPause*

THE
PRECONCEPTION
REVOLUTION

THE
PRECONCEPTION
REVOLUTION

A Science-Backed Path to Your Fertility
and Generational Health

ANN SHIPPY, MD

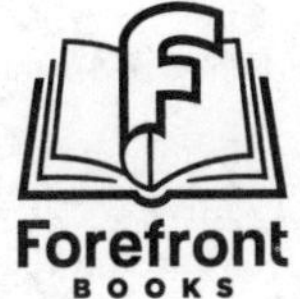

Forefront
BOOKS

Published by Forefront Books, Nashville, Tennessee.
Distributed by Simon & Schuster.

Library of Congress Control Number: 2025912921

Print ISBN: 978-1-63763-329-8
E-book ISBN: 978-1-63763-330-4

Cover Design by Michelle Manley
Interior Design by PerfecType, Nashville, TN

Endsheets © 2025 Bharti Kher. All Rights Reserved, Artists Rights Society (ARS), New York / DACS, London

Printed in the United States of America

25 26 27 28 29 30 RR4 10 9 8 7 6 5 4 3 2 1

To the next generation of souls arriving with a desire for vibrant, healthy bodies—so they may shine their light and bring love into the world. To the loving, resilient parents dedicated to nurturing them. And to my patients, who have taught me the true power of healing and the infinite strength of love.

AUTHOR'S NOTE

This book serves as a guide for navigating the preconception period, a journey often marked by uncertainty but also by hope—hope that is most powerfully conveyed through the stories of patients who have successfully conceived healthy children. The experiences shared within these pages reflect their deep trust, which is central to this type of journey. To safeguard the privacy of those whose stories are told, I have thoughtfully altered identifying details, sometimes merging aspects of different patients' experiences into one. While these changes protect individual confidentiality, they remain faithful to the essence of each journey. If you happen to recognize yourself in these stories, it is both coincidental and purposeful.

CONTENTS

Believe   Introspect   **R**enew   **T**hrive   **H**ope

Thrive

Hope

FOREWORD
Mark Hyman, MD

When we think about creating life, it's easy to get swept up in the joy and magic of the process—the moment you realize you're ready to bring a child into the world, the excitement of imagining their first laugh, their first steps, and the dreams they might one day pursue. It's a journey filled with love, hope, and purpose. Yet as I've learned through my decades of work in functional medicine, the most powerful gift we can offer our future children begins long before their first breath. That gift is a legacy of health and resilience.

The Preconception Revolution, written by the brilliant and compassionate Dr. Ann Shippy, is a profound guide to one of the most important yet overlooked periods in life—the preconception phase. It's a road map not only to improving fertility and preparing for pregnancy but also to shaping the foundation for your child's lifelong health. The wisdom in these pages is rooted in cutting-edge science, evidence-based practices, and the deep humanity that Dr. Shippy brings to her work as a physician and a healer.

We often think of conception as a moment, but it's the culmination of countless factors—genetics, environment, nutrition, and lifestyle—all of which you have the power to influence. As Dr. Shippy so beautifully explains, this phase is a golden opportunity to optimize the health of both parents, ensuring that the "ingredients" you contribute to your child's creation are the best they can be. This isn't about perfection or fear—it's about empowerment and intentionality.

One of the key concepts explored in this book is the science of epigenetics—the idea that our lifestyle choices, from the foods we eat to the toxins we avoid, can influence how our genes are expressed and, ultimately, how our children's genes are expressed too. Imagine the power of knowing that the choices you make today can set your child up for a future of vitality, strength, and resilience. This is the promise of the preconception road map Dr. Shippy has laid out: a chance to rewrite the narrative of health for generations to come.

Dr. Shippy's approach is both deeply practical and profoundly compassionate. She understands the complexities of modern life and the challenges many couples face when it comes to fertility and health. Whether you're navigating infertility, grappling with health conditions, or simply seeking to give your future child the best possible start, *The Preconception Revolution* meets you exactly where you are. With clarity and empathy, Dr. Shippy guides you through actionable steps, from detoxifying your environment to balancing your hormones, enhancing your nutrition, and tuning in to the emotional and spiritual aspects of preparing for parenthood.

As you read through these chapters, you'll find more than just information—you'll find inspiration. You'll discover that the journey to parenthood is not only about creating life but also about transforming your own. It's about becoming the healthiest, most vibrant version of yourself so that you can model that vitality for your child. It's about building a partnership with your coparent that is grounded in love, respect, and shared commitment. It's about recognizing that the choices you make now will ripple out, not just into your child's future, but into the future of our planet.

Dr. Shippy's work resonates deeply with me because it aligns with the principles of functional medicine that I've championed throughout my career: addressing the root causes of disease, embracing a systems-based approach to health, and recognizing the interconnectedness of mind, body, and environment. Her program is a testament to the power of personalized medicine—acknowledging that every individual, every couple, and every family is unique.

I hope you'll approach *The Preconception Revolution* with an open heart and an open mind. Let it inspire you to take ownership of your health, to embrace the preconception phase as a time of preparation and possibility, and to honor the sacred responsibility of creating life. The journey you're embarking on is nothing short of miraculous, and the steps you take now will resonate for generations.

As a parent myself, I can tell you that the love you feel for your child begins long before you meet them. It begins with the choices you make today, the care you invest in your health, and the intention you bring to this process. With Dr. Shippy as your guide, you're in the best possible hands. I have no doubt that this book will become a cherished companion on your journey to parenthood.

So take a deep breath, open these pages, and let the journey begin. The health and happiness of your future child are worth every moment of effort. And I promise you, the rewards will be immeasurable.

Dr. Mark Hyman

MAPPING OUT YOUR PRECONCEPTION JOURNEY

As you and your partner begin this journey together, think of this Preconception Blueprint as a practical guide and checklist—your first glimpse of the intentional path toward the "green light" for conception. These steps are more than a checklist; they're a reminder that the work you do now can shape not only your future child's health, but the legacy you leave for generations to come. With each chapter, you'll find support, clarity, and encouragement to take these steps hand in hand, grounded in both science and hope.

While you won't find a one-size-fits-all timeline here—your journey will unfold at the pace that's right for your unique bodies and test results—you will find a clear, empowering path forward. I encourage and invite you to refer to this blueprint from time to time, so you can feel empowered by your progress and excited by all that you're accomplishing.

Preconception Blueprint

☐ **Set Your Intentions**
This journey truly begins in your heart. Setting your intentions with your partner helps align your mindset with your

mission—to create a healthy, thriving family for generations to come. Create time together to reflect on why this season matters to you. Your intentions will become your compass, guiding your decisions with clarity and purpose.

☐ Choose Your Birth Control

This is essential because the last thing you want to do is get pregnant before you've completed this program together. So, make a specific plan for contraception until you have the "green light!"

☐ Assess Your Starting Point

Before you chart a new course, it's helpful to know exactly where you stand. This step is about honest, compassionate inventory—your current health, lifestyle, habits, stress levels, and even generational patterns. With awareness comes the power to shift and grow.

☐ Testing

Knowledge is power—and precision testing gives you the insights you need to personalize your journey. From nutrient panels and toxin levels to hormone levels and gut health, these tests help uncover hidden imbalances that may be silently affecting your fertility or epigenetics. Choose the tests that your budget will allow, and that your intuition guides you to. The data doesn't define you; it empowers you. While not required, it can give you concrete objectives to work toward. And don't forget to retest at the end! That's how you can see your incredible progress and ultimately get the "green light to baby!"

☐ Maintain Continuously Healthy Blood Sugar Levels

You'll wear a continuous glucose monitor for at least a month so you can learn how to adjust your lifestyle so that your blood sugar consistently stays in a good range. You can verify that you have a good handle on your blood sugar control by checking your hemoglobin A1C.

☐ **Set a Goal for Your Ideal Weight Range**

Determine your healthiest BMI, and make sure you achieve that goal. You can use a full body DEXA scan to follow your progress along the way.

☐ **Clean Up Your Environment**

Your body is affected by the world around it. Reducing your exposure to environmental toxins—found in everything from plastics to personal care products—lightens your body's load and gives your detox systems room to thrive. This is a critically important step toward optimizing your epigenetics prior to conception.

☐ **Detox**

Your body was designed to detox beautifully, but our modern world often overwhelms these pathways. In this phase, we gently support your methylation and other cellular detox pathways as well as your liver, kidneys, skin, lymph, and gut to release what no longer serves you—without harsh cleanses or suffering.

☐ **Dial In Nutrition and Fortify**

Food is more than fuel—it's information for your cells. Here, we reframe nutrition as one of the most sacred ways you can prepare for parenthood. You'll learn to nourish deeply, honoring your body's changing needs with delicious, real, healing foods.

☐ **Mind, Body, Spirit**

Preparing for a child isn't just physical—it's deeply emotional and spiritual too. This part of your journey invites you to slow down, reconnect with each other, and explore what brings you peace, joy, and strength. Part of this is recognizing any habits you'd like to stop (i.e., alcohol, nicotine, THC, etc.) and new ones you'd like to add (i.e., improved sleep hygiene, meditation, exercise, morning sunlight, less screen time, etc.). These practices can help balance your nervous system and enhance your whole-body readiness.

☐ **Smart Supplementing**

While whole foods come first, strategic supplementation helps fill in the gaps—and sometimes, those gaps are more significant than you'd think. In this step, we'll guide you toward evidence-based, personalized supplements that give you and your partner's bodies exactly what they need for conception, pregnancy, and beyond.

☐ **Revitalize Your Gut and Microbiome**

Your gut is your foundation. It's where nutrients are absorbed, immune balance is maintained, and even your mood is influenced. A healthy gut also supports your baby's earliest microbiome. In this step, you'll learn how to nurture this internal ecosystem and heal any hidden imbalances.

☐ **Harmonize Your Hormones**

Hormones are your body's messengers—delicate yet powerful. When they're in sync, everything works more smoothly: mood, energy, cycles, libido, and fertility. Here, we'll help you bring your hormones into harmony through lifestyle changes, targeted support, and deep listening to your body's rhythms.

☐ **Tame Inflammation**

Your lab work will reveal whether your body is fighting inflammation, which can wreak havoc on your reproductive health and if you conceive a child while fighting inflammation, you run a risk of passing that on. Now is your moment to discover the real reason you're inflamed, and to minimize it going forward.

☐ **Support Your Mitochondria**

Because healthy mitochondria are essential on this journey, make sure you're taking the recommended supplements, doing the detox, and eating the foods that support, heal, and optimize your mitochondria since they are your energy powerhouses that allow you to be fertile and to pass on the healthiest possible epigenetics.

☐ **Navigate Fertility**

Whether you're just starting out or have been trying for a while, fertility tracking tools can offer valuable insights. From understanding your ovulation window to exploring sperm health, this step offers practical ways to align your biology with your intentions, increasing your chances of healthy conception.

☐ **Re-testing and Reassessment to Optimize**

One of the most rewarding moments in this journey is seeing measurable progress. Re-testing offers tangible proof that your efforts are working. It's an opportunity to celebrate how far you've come and fine-tune any areas that still need attention before giving yourself the green light.

☐ **Green Light for Conception**

There's a beautiful moment when you know: Your body is ready, your systems are aligned, and your heart is open. This is the green light. It doesn't mean perfection—it means preparedness. With hope, trust, and joy, you can move forward knowing you've done the deep work to welcome your baby well.

Please feel free to add things to this list as you read through the book that relate specifically to what you and your partner want to accomplish before conceiving!

INTRODUCTION

Is there anything more precious than a baby? Holding that tiny human in your arms, gazing into those little eyes, observing the big yawns, seeing the toothless smiles, experiencing the deep and inexplicable desire to watch their every move—it's all a wondrous and even spiritual experience. Author and essayist Elizabeth Stone eloquently wrote, "Making the decision to have a child—it is momentous. It is to decide forever to have your heart go walking around outside your body."[1] Don't those words just ring so true and reflect so beautifully the depth of love we feel for our children?

Love is the reason we are having this conversation. I daresay you wouldn't have picked up this book if you had not been propelled to do so by love—for your partner, for your family, for your future child. If you are dreaming of starting or expanding your family, then you know quite well that *love* is the most important and fundamental ingredient when you are inviting a new life into the world. But here's something you might not yet know—when it comes to conception, you can have an impact on the physical "ingredients" you and your partner contribute to the creation of your future child.

What does that mean? Well, I think most people believe they have no control whatsoever over how their future child will turn out. Whether they will be at higher or lower risk for physical or mental health challenges. Whether they will have a strong or weak immune system. Whether they will be diagnosed with type 1 diabetes, or asthma, or if they'll be on the autism spectrum, and whether they will have a genetic advantage or disadvantage in every area. Most parents think it's all a matter of luck—they're just rolling the dice and hoping for the best. But what I want you to know right up front is this: You have a lot more control than you might realize. In fact, what you do *right now* can set your future child up for success . . . or not. The power is in your hands.

If you are planning to have a child in the somewhat near future, then you are currently in what I refer to as the *preconception phase*. This is an often-overlooked time in our lives—most people just skate right by it, oblivious to its significance. But I am convinced that it is a crucial time—perhaps the weightiest, most meaningful time in our entire lives. So, your first step is to throw away any preconceived notions you might have regarding both preconception and conception itself and replace them with evidence-based, research-backed, transformative information. To that end, there are two main subjects we will be addressing simultaneously throughout this book—*fertility* (your ability to conceive a child and—if you're the mom—to carry it to full term) and the *quality of the genetic materials* both parents contribute to their child.

I'd like to say something very important here: Whether you are the future mom or future dad, it is imperative that you and your partner read this book and go through this program together. If it takes two to tango, then it certainly takes two to make a baby. This is a true 50/50 partnership, and what you both do during preconception matters equally. In this book, I'm going to ask you to have specific lab work completed, to detoxify your body based on those lab results (as well as your lifestyle), to change the way you eat and exercise, possibly to modify your recreation, and much more—but it is a lot more effective if both of you are participating. And more than that, you'll both be more successful if you are keeping each other accountable and encouraging one another along this journey. So if you're reading this on your own, pause, go get your partner, discuss your goal, and then dive into this plan together.

Depending upon your current circumstances, you might be coming into this preconception journey in an emotionally very raw state. When I first meet new patients who have been in a gut-wrenching season of infertility, I know they are often carrying a lot of emotion and fear. There might need to be some healing that occurs first. We are going to create time and space for that healing. I'm also going to help you learn how infertility is just a sign that one or both partner's bodies are imbalanced, and rather than dealing with that symptom in isolation, we are going to discover and heal the root cause. If infertility has been part of your journey, please know you are not alone. Later, I will share with you some shocking statistics about how much infertility has increased in recent years.

Alternatively, you might not have experienced any fertility challenges, but you have a child or multiple children with various types of health-related issues. You want to have another child, but you're worried that there's something "wrong" with your DNA that's causing these problems. Or perhaps you don't have children yet because you've had other priorities up until now, and you think your age might have a negative impact on your child. It could also be that you've heard my message that *everyone* needs to prepare for pregnancy. You might fall into one of those categories, or a different one altogether. Regardless of your situation or your goals, I designed this program to help *you*.

The Preconception Readiness Quiz

On my website, I have a dynamic quiz that can help you gauge your readiness for the preconception journey. It includes some questions you might not expect, but as you read this book, they will all start to make sense! Here's a code you can use to access the quiz.

My Story

As of the writing of this book, I have been practicing functional medicine for twenty years. Just in case that term is new to you, functional medicine treats root causes of disease and restores healthy function through a personalized patient experience.[2] It's different from conventional medicine in many ways, but rather than list those out, I'd like to share the story of my own discovery of this particular lens through which we view health. It all started back when I was a chemical engineer working for IBM.

Well, maybe even a little before that. I got married between my junior and senior year in college. My former husband, David, was a couple years older than me, and he was already in the workforce as an electrical engineer. It was 1985, and the economy was in a slump. I wasn't even sure I'd be able to get a job. But I interviewed with IBM in Endicott, New York, and it went great. They offered me a job, and it just so happened they also had a need for electrical engineers, so David got a great job there too. We were both thriving.

I was often the only woman in the room at that time in the tech industry. There were a handful of other women in similar positions, but I noticed that as soon as they had a child, many of them would quit or only come back to work for a short time. Granted, that was in the '80s and '90s, but even recent research indicates that 42 percent of women in STEM (science, technology, engineering, and mathematics) fields with children leave their full-time jobs or switch to part-time work due to family responsibilities—a much higher rate than the 28 percent of men in similar situations.[3] I do think those kinds of statistics tell a story about why many women hold off on having kids until they reach a certain point in their career, but more on that later.

After about four years at Endicott, though we both loved our jobs and the friends we'd made there, David and I knew we couldn't do another New York winter. So we requested to be transferred. They moved us to the Austin, Texas, plant. There, I had the opportunity to work on some fascinating projects, like leading teams to get the chlorofluorocarbons out of our cleaning processes and coordinating with product development. It was my dream job, and I was truly thriving in my role. I really thought I would stay with IBM until I retired.[4]

In 1992, my journey took a significant turn after I went on a cruise with friends. Upon returning, I became extremely sick with severe gastrointestinal symptoms. My body essentially stopped digesting food. For months, multiple doctors conducted tests, including endoscopes and a barium enema, trying to find possible infections or parasites, but they couldn't discover the cause. So, they gave me medication to treat my symptoms. I got so thin and appeared so sickly that rumors started flying around that I had cancer. And truly, I felt like I was dying. I could barely function or participate in my daily life, and I was beginning to lose hope simply because I didn't have the physical strength I needed to fight whatever was going desperately wrong inside my body.

The Internet was fairly new at that time and didn't have much health information on it yet, so I had to think outside the box. I sought help from an acupuncturist, an herbalist, an allergist, and a nutritionist. I also learned about ayurvedic medicine and the macrobiotic diet. And I began to piece together the knowledge that made sense to me from all the various experts I was seeing, eventually discovering on my own that I had celiac disease, which had been overlooked by my doctors. I dove into endless health research in an attempt to figure out how to heal myself. Gradually, I began to get better.

During this time, I was traveling a lot for work and had to manage my diet very carefully. I remember carrying around a red cooler with my food and a little hot pot to prepare meals while traveling. On one flight from Dallas to Austin, I sat next to a man named Rusty Talley, whose wife was in law school. The loving way in which he spoke of her as he talked about supporting her desire to start a new career path planted a seed in my mind. The next morning, I woke up at 3 a.m.

and just knew something deep in my soul—I wanted to go to medical school. I waited until David, my husband at the time, woke up and then I told him. To this day, I'm so grateful that he supported me in this new quest; it was a defining moment in my life, and I couldn't have done it without him in my corner.

Going from IBM engineer to doctor wasn't exactly an overnight proposition. First, I needed to take some biology courses. Since my original major in college ten years earlier had been in chemical engineering, I already had all the chemistry and physics prerequisites. Once I finished the biology courses, along with a refresher on organic chemistry and physics, I took the MCAT (Medical College Admission Test) six months later. By December, I had gotten into the University of Texas Medical School at Houston. We sold the house we'd built in Austin and moved to Houston, where I started school that fall. My husband had to leave his dream job, which was a huge sacrifice.

Backing up just a bit, prior to starting medical school, we had tried to get pregnant, but it wasn't happening. We opted to try Clomid for a few months, and we did some IUIs (intrauterine insemination), but those didn't work for us. In hindsight, we were taking a big risk by not addressing the issue, but I just felt so strongly compelled to go to medical school that I started to lose sight of my hopes and dreams for a family. It hadn't totally dawned on me that I might be missing out on having kids, and I didn't yet have the skills in my toolbox for addressing the root cause. But because I had been diligent about eating very clean and taking excellent care of myself, I eventually did get pregnant.

We welcomed our first son, Grant, during my first clinical rotations, at the beginning of my third year of medical school. He was born a few weeks early, right at the end of my rotation. Juggling medical school, a new baby, and getting settled into a new house and neighborhood was *a lot*, but we made it work. My mom had just retired and was excited to spend time with her new grandchild, so she moved from Kentucky to Houston to help, which was a lifesaver.

That adage that the days are long but the years are short really came to life for me during that time. I loved every second I had with Grant, and I loved my work too. It's always been a privilege to be able to help people when they are facing serious medical challenges.

Of all the cases I consulted on during residency, I'll never forget a complex case involving a Hispanic woman who had recently undergone a C-section. This patient, a dedicated Jehovah's Witness, faced a life-threatening situation made more complicated by her religious beliefs, which strictly prohibited the use of blood transfusions. As her hemoglobin levels continued to plummet, we knew she was experiencing severe internal bleeding. The inability to provide her with blood products restricted our options, and the constant presence of several Jehovah's Witness elders outside her room was an intimidating reminder of the importance of her adhering to her faith. As a physician and a mother, it was heartbreaking to watch her deteriorate, and I couldn't do anything about it.

Her internal bleeding worsened, but the surgeons were unable to take her back to the operating room for further intervention because they couldn't perform the necessary blood transfusions. In a desperate attempt to find a solution that complied with her religious convictions, her family and the elders asked me to explore the use of an experimental blood substitute. This innovative treatment, although still in its trial phase, appeared to be their only acceptable option.

With the patient and her husband's consent, I navigated the bureaucratic process of obtaining approval from the hospital's Institutional Review Board (IRB). This required me to leave the hospital to present the treatment protocol and secure the necessary permissions. Once approved, we began administering the blood substitute as her condition worsened.

Unfortunately, the experimental treatment led to a series of severe complications. Her body reacted adversely to the blood substitute, and despite our best efforts, she passed away. I was devastated; the whole experience just cut me to the core. I had encountered relatively few deaths during my medical training, and her death in particular just seemed so senseless. Her funeral was the only one I attended during my residency. The unresolved fate of her baby, left to navigate life without a mother, lingered in my thoughts for years.

Concurrently, my husband and I had been grappling with fertility struggles again. After a few months of trying for our second child and not having any luck, my doctor took one look at my labs and informed us that we needed to do in vitro fertilization (IVF). "There's no way you'll get pregnant [without it]" were his words. I was literally in the most stressful period of my entire residency, and our fertility struggles just compounded it. But we knew we wanted another child, partly because my own siblings are so important to me. So, once my next period came, I would start on a prescribed course of birth control pills in preparation for IVF.

Within weeks of that new mom passing away, I was quietly pondering our next steps toward having a second child. We had attended a class on IVF, and we were prepped and ready. But I was wondering why my period had not yet started. Without really thinking, I decided to take a pregnancy test. When I showed my husband the positive result, he suggested I take another one because he didn't believe it. The doctor had been clear—there was no way I could get pregnant naturally, and frankly, our lives had been moving so fast that we couldn't even recall when we'd last had sex. But the second test confirmed it—I was pregnant. It absolutely felt like a God thing. I saw it as such a gift, and I was so grateful.

My second son, Reed, came at the beginning of my third year of residency. When he was around six weeks old, I noticed he'd stopped making eye contact. I'll never forget that feeling. Something was wrong with my baby, and I felt completely helpless to fix it. Our pediatrician urgently referred us to an ophthalmologist, who said nothing seemed wrong with Reed's eyes, so he sent us to a neurologist. There was no specific diagnosis, but it did appear he could be on the autism spectrum or have some kind of serious neurological disorder. Even as a physician, I missed so much about what factors could be at play. We now know that a child's environment and various exposures matter greatly when you're trying to zero in on a diagnosis, but I had not come to realize any of that yet. I did know the vital importance of only giving my sons breast milk rather than formula. But it wasn't until a year later, when one of my cousins had a baby who died after receiving a vaccine, that I began questioning the role vaccines might have played in Reed's condition, since he had been vaccinated the day before his symptoms started. Thankfully, he did eventually snap out of it and went back to making normal eye contact.

Throughout all of this, I was consistently working on building my own strength and resiliency—which had started with getting healthy enough to even have babies—and learning so much about how our decisions shape our health. And then to have had that experience with Reed—it all had a profound impact on my perspective on wellness.

When Reed was around three years old, I'd been in an internal medical practice with two other doctors for just over two years, but I was off my preferred path of doing medicine more holistically. Like countless other medical school graduates, I had fallen right into the typical routine, seeing twenty patients a day. I *wanted* to spend time with each of them to explore their conditions, to dig for clues as to what was affecting their health, yet within five to ten minutes, I was telling my patients what prescription I was going to write. Then my health took another nosedive. I had such severe dry eyes and mouth that I couldn't wear contacts and really couldn't carry on a conversation without a mint or gum or something to stimulate saliva production. In my workup, I discovered I had developed antiphospholipid antibody syndrome, an autoimmune disorder that increased my risk for stroke. I also had Sjögren's syndrome, which was causing the dry eyes and mouth. It was miserable and I was scared. The approach offered by my profession was taking strong medications that suppressed the immune system and had a lot of potential side effects. I'd arrived at a crossroads where I once again needed to solve my own health conundrum. I was determined to make a change. I knew going into medicine had solved part of the puzzle, but I was still missing the training and framework for how to do medicine differently.

Functional medicine was only barely on the map at this time, but fortunately, I came across a functional medicine physician about an hour south of me. That physician helped me learn how to detoxify and get my body into healing mode. And though the mainstream narrative about autoimmune disorders is that they can't be reversed, I learned firsthand that they absolutely can. With the encouragement of that doctor, I discovered the next step in my journey as a physician, and I began training to practice functional and integrative medicine. Not long after completing that training, I got brave enough to open my own practice and began helping people heal from complex health conditions that they'd been told were irreversible. Finally, I was able to truly help patients heal their bodies rather than just masking or band-aiding their symptoms. It felt amazing.

Everything was going great until about five years later. Reed was in third grade at that time, and he was starting to have some challenges at school. He had such a short fuse—he couldn't even sit still in class and would get out of his chair and roll around on the floor whenever the teacher introduced a new topic for him to learn. He frequently disrupted the rest of the students in his class. At the same time, I was experiencing new and devastating symptoms myself. I was losing my hair and feeling terrible pain throughout my body. I lost the grip strength in my right hand and was having a hard time just getting out of bed. Once again, I found myself at a loss as to the cause of my health issues and Reed's challenges.

Enter a sweet patient who had come to see me—Suzanne Stratton. Even though she was the patient and I was her doctor, Suzanne's intuition told her that I was unwell. Because of her loving, empathetic heart, she insisted on coming to my house to see if she could identify the cause. Immediately upon walking into our home, she recognized the presence of mold. She was highly attuned to a specific strain of mold, and her own neurological symptoms were exacerbated upon exposure. I had recently been to a conference in Dallas about the detrimental effects of toxic mold, so it was just beginning to come onto my radar. With a little trial and error, I eventually found a test that did, in fact, reveal that the mold Chaetomium was present in the house we were leasing due to a problem in the chimney that was allowing water to intermittently leak inside. Where there's a water source, mold will grow. And grow it did . . . with reckless abandon, hidden inside our walls and floorboards. Those mycotoxins, the toxins mold makes, were permeating the air in our home and wreaking havoc on our health.

Suzanne explained that with this type of mold, you need to get rid of everything that isn't a hard surface—i.e., anything that wouldn't survive the dishwasher. We moved out of the house, and I had to get rid of almost everything: books, the kids' artwork, clothes, even furniture that had been contaminated with the toxic mold. Getting out of the environment and removing contaminated items was the first step and fortunately, my functional medicine training and experience helped me put together a protocol, a plan, to then help us heal quickly.

I feel blessed to have tapped into deep reserves of strength and resilience throughout my life. (I now realize those reserves are the result of an intersection of genetics, epigenetics, microbiome, mitochondrial function, nutritional status, toxin load, and more—all of which we'll get into later in the book.) This has enabled me to keep a lot of balls in the air even through the most challenging times. My father, who had a profound influence on my life, taught me a lot about the healing power of love. Even after his passing, I still feel his presence and guidance. My mother, who encouraged me to go into engineering, was there for me when my boys were little and I was completing medical school. She and my stepdad even invited us to stay with them for months to heal after the Chaetomium exposure and again a few years later when I had my second run-in with another type of mold, which caused my adult-onset asthma. I am so grateful for their generosity and care.

My sons are now both in their twenties, and they have inspired me in countless ways. When I became a mother, my whole world transformed. It was an indescribable soul shift that ushered in a sense of joy, transcending anything I'd experienced in the physical realm. That's what I desire for my readers and my patients.

The Telemedicine Component

When I first set out to create this program, I knew I wanted to offer a comprehensive version where people would have the option for more customized support and accountability. You can certainly get everything you need by following the plan in this book, but if you desire an approach that includes more assistance in analyzing your data and someone to walk alongside you on this journey, simply go to: www.everybabywell.com learn more. There, you can see what's available and get started right away.

There's no two ways about it: There is a health crisis among our youth in America. Every major illness and condition has been on the rise since the 1990s, including but not limited to diabetes, cancer, autism spectrum disorder (ASD), childhood obesity, attention deficit hyperactivity disorder (ADHD), anxiety, depression, and more.

Let's look at diabetes for a moment. A cross-sectional study looking at the incidence, mortality, and disability-adjusted life-years of childhood diabetes from 1990–2019 found a 39.4 percent increase in childhood diabetes over that period.[5]

According to the CDC, autism spectrum disorder was diagnosed at a rate of 1 in 150 children in the year 2000, then 1 in 110 by 2006, 1 in 68 by 2010, and 1 in 31 by 2022.[6] That's an alarming trend, to say the least. Here's a chart from the CDC website:[7]

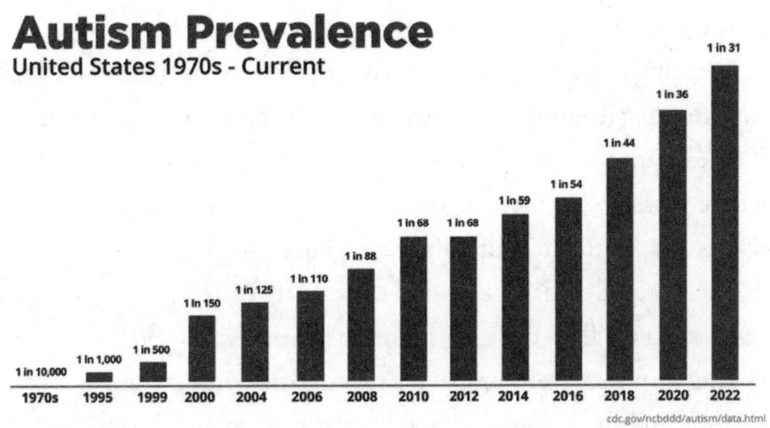

As if that's not unsettling enough, childhood obesity is also on the rise. The World Health Organization reports on its website that, "While just 2% of children and adolescents aged 5–19 were obese in 1990 (31 million young people), by 2022, 8% of children and adolescents were living with obesity (160 million young people)."[8] If you do the math, that's a 300 percent increase over thirty-two years. It's heartbreaking, really.

Another childhood disorder has been experiencing a shocking increase over time, and that's ADHD (attention deficit hyperactivity disorder). National surveys reflect an increase in the prevalence over a 20-year period; it went from 6.1 percent in 1997 to 10.2 percent in 2016.[9] This represents a 67.2 percent increase. Just imagine the challenges that represents for families, not to mention teachers in classrooms. And the trend continues to escalate. During 2020–2022, 14.3 percent of children ages 12–17 were diagnosed with ADHD; interestingly, there is a higher prevalence of boys at 17.9 percent.[10]

I know it's terribly emotional to consider, but the prevalence of childhood cancers is also on the rise. Approximately 1 in 285 children in the US will be diagnosed with cancer before their twentieth birthday.[11] Between 1975–2019, the number of children diagnosed with leukemia increased by about 35 percent.[12] And in America, cancer is the most common cause of death by disease for children.[13] I think this is tragic.

Certainly, one factor in the increase for some of these conditions is improved screening or awareness. But I do not accept that as the whole explanation; I believe there's something more going on here. Despite massive advances across all health sciences over the last few decades, it appears that our kids are getting sicker, not healthier. Why?

There are all kinds of ideas and theories that attempt to answer that question. And I'll be clear—I do not believe we can point to any *one* smoking gun that's responsible for this disaster. I think this is a complex issue and there are multiple factors at play, many of which we will look at closely later in the book. But I do know, without a doubt, that these numbers can be quite intimidating to people who are considering having a baby. They feel like the deck is stacked against their future children before they are even conceived. And I can't blame them for feeling that way. From a statistical standpoint, it just doesn't look good.

I've alluded to *resiliency* a couple of times in this introduction, and I want to zero in on it again because it's really the cornerstone of this entire program. We must build resiliency—first in ourselves, and then in our kids. We are living in an increasingly toxic world. Later in this book, we'll jump right into all the muck, and I'll reveal to you more than you probably wanted to know about the toxic soup we're eating, drinking, breathing, and living in daily. How do we—and more importantly, our children—survive all that without becoming one of those sad statistics? *Resiliency.*

Going back to what I said earlier, you have a lot of power during this preconception phase, and my goal is to help you harness that power to build resiliency for your future child. What you do *before* you conceive has a profound impact on the genetic expression you pass on to your baby and thus the future health and resiliency of that child. In fact, I'd go so far as to say that you can actually change your child's life before your child is even conceived. It's a huge opportunity, and I don't want you to miss it.

You might be wondering, *What could I possibly do right now that will help my not-yet-conceived child be healthier?* The answer is inspiringly simple: Optimize your and your partner's health. Notice I didn't say "improve" your health, or "tweak" your health, or "enhance" your health. I said you need to *optimize* your health, and by that, I mean make it the very best it can possibly be. Optimization is a process that's as unique as you are, and it requires a scientific, methodical approach. But don't worry; I'm going to walk you through it every step of the way.

Based on the latest research in epigenetics (how your genes can be influenced and expressed differently based on external factors, without changing the actual DNA code), I firmly believe that couples need to utilize this preconception window as a time to run key lab work, detoxify, and add in specific supplementation to create the healthiest "ingredients" for their future child. While we can't change our actual DNA, we *can* change how our DNA behaves, and we can pass those epigenetic markers on to the next generation. (Check out chapter 3 for an in-depth look at this topic.)

Maybe that all sounds wonderful, but you're in a hurry to get pregnant because you've waited so long, and the clock is ticking louder every second. I understand, but let me encourage you to find just a little more patience to follow this program step-by-step instead of rushing toward conception. The total length of time required will vary somewhat based on your unique data, but I generally recommend at least six months to experience the best results. Whether it's three months, six months, or even a full year, taking the necessary steps to improve your health can profoundly increase your chances of conceiving easily and having a healthy pregnancy and child. I'll offer several of these reminders through the course of this book, but it's important to use condoms during this preconception period because you might become fertile very quickly and you don't want to get pregnant before we've laid the necessary groundwork. I've had several patients who didn't take this advice seriously, and they got pregnant right away. So let this be your first caution sign—be careful!

As you know, we show our love for each other not only through words but also through actions. It's not what we say, but what we do, that reflects the love in our hearts. The foundation you're laying during this program is the first way you can show love to your future child. You'll be so glad you did.

My hope is that this book becomes a trusted companion for you, one you don't just put on a shelf but keep close at hand, with pages dog-eared, notes in the margins, and passages highlighted that speak to you. May it be a book you can open to any page for a spark of inspiration or a moment of clarity, especially if you're journaling or simply reflecting on your journey. I hope you and your partner will walk through these pages together, sharing the insights, questions, and encouragements. Let this book be a steady source of guidance, always ready to meet you where you are.

Section I Introduction

The sections of this book are built around an acronym using the word *BIRTH*, which is both the ultimate goal—to bring a healthy baby into the world—and a symbol of the new beginning this journey represents. BIRTH stands for Believe, Introspect, Renew, Thrive, Hope. Together, you are not only preparing for the physical birth of a child but also giving birth to a new paradigm in your lives, one that prioritizes health, connection, and intentional living. Through each stage of this program, you're laying the groundwork for a legacy of health, resilience, and love that will impact not only your future child but generations to come. This is where your journey as a family truly begins.

In preparing to become parents, *belief* plays a powerful role—belief in your body, belief in your health, belief in each other, and belief in the life you're creating together. This first section, *Believe*, invites you and your partner to examine the foundation of these beliefs with open minds and a shared sense of purpose, ensuring that your thoughts, intentions, and expectations align as you plan for a healthy beginning to your family. The chapters in this section are designed to help you clarify your motivations, set intentions, and strengthen your joint commitment to this extraordinary path.

To start, you'll both reflect on why you feel drawn to have a child and what hopes you have for their future. Understanding your personal and shared "why" is essential for approaching parenthood with intention and integrity. The chapters in *Believe* will guide you through exploring the values and motivations that matter most to you as a couple, helping ensure that they will nurture and guide both of you, and ultimately your future child.

From there, you will move toward a more introspective look at how your beliefs about health, well-being, and resilience shape the choices you make today. The self-assessment tools and reflections here offer you both insight into your lifestyle, mindset, and even the way you communicate with yourselves and each other. These first steps lay a supportive foundation for you, your partner, and, ultimately, your child.

By embracing this time for shared reflection and intentionality, you are creating a meaningful foundation not just for conception but for a healthy, resilient family life together.

Oh, Baby! Setting Your Intentions Well

The decision to have a baby is a monumental one. If you're reading this book, you're serious about doing whatever is necessary to give your baby the best possible start in life, and that's commendable. In this chapter, we're going to dig a little deeper into the reasons *why* you've decided to have a baby. Whether it's your first child or your fifth, I believe it's critical to understand your and your partner's motivations so that you can align your intentions and then stay aligned every step of the way. The process of setting intentions is as unique as each of us, and we really don't want to rush past this part of the process.

What's Your "Why" for Having a Child?

There are endless reasons why we feel led to have a baby. A lot of influences can play a role in our decision—pressure from our own parents or family, society, culture, religion . . . the list goes on. But when you look deep inside at the heart of your motivation to have this baby, what do you find there?

This is an exercise in brutal honesty, because sometimes the true reasons we discover can surprise us. There could be some deep-seated desire to "right the wrongs" of our own childhood, or to fill a sense of loneliness or lacking. It might even stem from wanting someone to love you, or a sense of obligation, or a need to prove yourself. I'm not necessarily making a value judgment on these types of reasons as much as I'm asking you to first acknowledge them. Don't simply push them aside and try to ignore them.

If this won't be your first child, your reasons for having another one could be multifaceted as well. Perhaps you miss those "baby days" (I know I miss them even though my boys are grown!) and you want to experience them again. Or you are hoping for a different gender this time around. (I have one patient who has six sons, so just remember there are no guarantees!) The reasons for having each child could differ slightly, so even though this isn't your first time, be sure to take the time to explore your motivations.

It's critical that both you and your partner do this work and then come back together for a candid, nonjudgmental discussion. And remember to have grace for each other in your findings.

Once you've both had a chance to acknowledge and digest each other's "why" for having this baby, it's now time to ask yourselves if you feel good about proceeding. Are your reasons realistic? Are they authentically coming from within you rather than from external pressure? Most importantly, do they serve your future child? Remember that you're talking about bringing another human being into this world—someone who will be fully dependent on you to care for them, guide them, teach them, and love them. If you get excited about how fulfilling that will be and feel like you have much love, time, and energy to give to this endeavor, then that's a good sign. On the other hand, if this exercise has revealed to you that this is less about caring for another and more about you or your partner, then it's time to pause and reevaluate.

Hopes and Dreams

Next, I encourage you to take some time to sit down with your partner and daydream about your child's future. What do you envision? Rather than focusing on what this baby might *become*, or in what ways they might contribute to the world, turn your attention to what kind of person they will be. What kinds of values will you model for your child? As you go inward, write down your thoughts, ideas, revelations, discoveries, prayers, desires, beliefs, plans, hopes, dreams, and visions for the future. How will you create space for allowing your child to discover who they genuinely are, what matters to them, and how they receive the world and fit into it?

I'd suggest writing down your answers individually first and then come together and share them with each other. Discuss the differences and similarities in your answers and talk about whether each of them is realistic or if you're setting unrealistic expectations. (If you need more space to write, just use a sheet of paper.)

....

....

....

....

....

....

....

Finally, create a shared vision for your child's future and write it down:

....

....

....

....

If you're feeling extra inspired right now, consider writing a letter to your future child, to be shared with them one day!

What Kind of Parent Do You Aspire to Be?

Often, the ways in which we ourselves were parented will become our default for how we might parent our own children. But if you're intentional about defining what kind of parent you desire to be, then you can exert more control over this than you might realize. However, if you wait until you find yourself in the pressure cooker of an intense parenting moment, then it's harder to overcome that default. That's why *now* is the perfect time to begin shaping the vision for the type of parent you wish to be for your child.

The best time to discover if you and your partner have different parenting styles or grew up in radically different households is before you have a child! This will give you time to co-create a new parenting style that you'll both embrace. I've worked with couples who have intentionally set aside certain aspects of their own upbringing so they could parent in a way that was authentic to their new family unit, and it's worked beautifully.

Questions to ask yourself in this process include: *What do I believe about the various parenting styles? What is my philosophy on discipline? If I have more than one child, how willing am I to adjust my parenting based on each child's personality and characteristics? Thinking about my own parents, what would I do the same and differently? How willing am I to evaluate, learn, research, and adjust my parenting techniques as I go? How would I complete this sentence: "I intend to be the kind of parent who . . ."?*

What Will You Model?

Now I'm going to ask you a question that really gets to the heart of the matter: *Do you love yourself?* The truth is, if you don't love yourself, it's *really* hard to be a good parent. Now is the time to be honest with yourself about your own mental wellness. If you know that you struggle with your own self-perception, I'd suggest taking some time to soul-search and work on your emotional well-being prior to having a child. We all hope that our children will love themselves, and that love comes from modeled behavior. If you don't have it, you can't teach it or model it. Write the thoughts that come to mind when you seriously ponder this question.

....

....

....

....

....

....

....

An Important Message

If either you or your partner are currently struggling with addiction—whether you've admitted it to yourself yet or not—take a pause here. Healing from dependency comes first. It might seem daunting, but it's not nearly as daunting as it will be when you are responsible for another human life. Let this be your wake-up call to seek the help you need.

In addition to AA, counseling, and rehabilitation, another tool for combatting addiction are NAD+ IVs.[14] They're one of the most effective treatments I've seen help patients recover from addiction. I'll talk about NAD+ later in the book, but it is an essential pyridine nucleotide that plays a critical role in cellular energy production and cellular protection against stress, as well as longevity. Though more research is needed, initial findings indicate that components of NAD+ can influence major processes associated with the neurobiology of addiction.[15] I think it's definitely worth looking into if you're battling addiction of any kind. You can find more information on NAD IVs on my website annshippymd.com at https://annshippymd.com/nad-iv-therapy/.

Financial Commitment

As you may already know, it takes significant resources to care for a child. I'm talking about time, energy, and finances. It's important to enter parenting with your eyes wide open so you can devote what's needed to this mission. Of course, if you wait to have the perfect amount of money in the bank, or until you have all kinds of time on your hands, you may never jump in. I'm not suggesting that you just wait forever, but you do need to realize the magnitude of what is required. For instance, how will having a child change your work schedule? Will one of you need to work part-time or stop working altogether? And how will you factor into your budget the cost of high-quality foods as well as nontoxic products for your home? These questions are best addressed beforehand so you can make sure you're on the same page as your partner.

Setting Intentions Together

Entering into the commitment of having a child also means that your relationship with your partner needs to be very strong. Children will test relationships, and any cracks that might exist will really start to show! Are you and your partner in a good place? Or are there areas that need a little TLC before you make this big change? I know some couples think a child will help repair or strengthen their relationship, but that's really just wishful thinking. That precious child is depending on the two of you to be united and give them a strong, safe foundation on which to learn, grow, and develop.

Part of building that strong foundation is deciding *now* how you will divide the labor, address discipline and boundaries, and make parenting decisions. If you're not sure about those specifics yet, then talk them out and do some research together. There are endless parenting books and resources available, so dig into those and see which philosophies fit you as a couple.

Final Thoughts

Allow me to get spiritual for just a moment. I believe when we decide to become parents, we're ushering a soul into existence here on earth. It's so much deeper than just bringing together an egg and a sperm, and forty weeks later a human baby is born. When you sit back and think about your own life and experiences, I'm guessing you can acknowledge the existence of your own soul. You can sense there is something much more going on here than just a body that lives and breathes for a period of time and then passes away. When you're thinking about having a baby, you're really thinking about inviting another soul to come and experience life here with you. It's weighty, right? It's no small thing.

That's why it's so important to truly pour your whole heart into this process. It's not just about checking boxes and getting healthy so your child is healthy—that's part of it, for sure, but that's not the whole of this equation. What kind of environment are you creating for your child's *soul* to exist in? What will the environment of his or her upbringing be like? Will you offer that soul a peaceful, loving, safe place—physically, emotionally, and in every other way?

You'll have an opportunity in the next chapter to answer some specific questions to get you thinking more in-depth about all of these topics. But as you continue down this path, just remember: Becoming a parent (or having another child) is a choice. Despite the pressure you might feel from others, it's *your* choice, not anyone else's. It is sure to become one of the most impactful decisions you'll ever make in your life, so I encourage you to wait until you know in your heart that you have positive, authentic reasons for doing so, and a solid plan in place for showing up as the best possible parent you can be. I hope you will recognize what an honor and a privilege it is, and that you will feel motivated to step up to this challenge. You, your partner, and your child will be so glad you did.

BELIEVE

Q&A

Q: Why is it important to understand my motivations for having a child?

A: The decision to bring a child into the world is one of the most significant choices you will ever make. Understanding your motivations helps ensure that your decision is based on authentic, internal desires rather than external pressures. It also allows you to set realistic expectations and cultivate a parenting mindset that prioritizes the well-being of your future child.

Q: What if my reasons for having a child are complicated?

A: Many people find that their reasons for wanting a baby are layered and complex. Some motivations may stem from childhood experiences, personal insecurities, or societal expectations. The goal is to acknowledge these influences with honesty. Identifying your reasons gives you the opportunity to address any unresolved feelings before becoming a parent.

Q: My partner and I have different reasons for wanting a child. How do we align our intentions?

A: Open and honest communication is key. Set aside time to discuss your motivations without judgment. Acknowledge differences, seek common ground, and create a shared vision that reflects your mutual hopes and values. The stronger your alignment now, the more unified you will be in your parenting journey.

Q: How can I ensure my expectations for my child are realistic?

A: Instead of focusing on who your child might become in terms of achievements or societal contributions, shift your attention to their character and well-being. Consider what values you want to model and how you will support their individuality. Discuss these expectations with your partner to ensure you are both fostering a healthy, flexible outlook.

Q: How can my partner and I strengthen our relationship before having a baby?

A: Children add complexity to relationships, often highlighting any existing cracks. Ensure that your relationship is built on open communication, shared values, and mutual support. Discuss parenting roles, division of labor, and discipline approaches ahead of time to create a unified foundation.

Q: How can I spiritually prepare for parenthood?

A: Recognizing that parenthood is more than just a physical or logistical journey can help you approach it with reverence and intention. Consider what kind of environment—emotionally, spiritually, and physically—you want to provide for your child's soul. Reflection, prayer, and mindfulness can help guide you in creating a peaceful, nurturing home.

CHAPTER TWO

Mirror Focus:
Reflect and Reveal

Now that you have set your intentions for this journey and you're ready to get started, let's take some time to assess your own unique starting point. To do so, we'll focus on several different spheres of your life, including your daily lifestyle (nutrition, exercise, body composition), your emotional life (stress, anxiety, personality type), your relationship (communication, trust, shared vision), your financial life (employment, financial readiness), and your spiritual life.

I realize you might feel tempted to skip over this section and head straight for the medical aspects of conception, especially if you are dealing with the gut-wrenching roller coaster of infertility. But since the topics we'll be covering in this chapter play a significant role in your overall health, and thus your fertility, it's essential to slow down and spend some time on introspection and sharing with your partner.

Nutrition

Many parents opt to feed their kids whatever is easiest, but if you start thinking now about the foods you'll be providing your child, you can lay the important groundwork for their health. So, consider the importance of honing those skills, such as how to grocery shop and prepare nutrient-dense meals, now. Flip to page 223 for some delicious recipes and take a look at my website for even more ideas. Here are some considerations to get you thinking:

Keep a food journal and write down everything you eat or drink over the course of three days. It's smart to include at least one weekend day, especially if you eat slightly differently on the weekends than during the workweek. How would you describe your diet? Here are some common diets:

- **Paleo:** This diet includes fruits, vegetables, lean meats, fish, eggs, nuts, and seeds.
- **Keto:** This diet is very low-carb and high-fat.
- **Vegetarian:** *Lacto-vegetarian* diets exclude meat, fish, poultry, and eggs, and all foods that contain them. Dairy products such as milk, cheese, yogurt, and butter are included. *Ovo-vegetarian* diets exclude meat, poultry, seafood, and dairy products, but do allow eggs. *Lacto-ovo vegetarian* diets exclude meat, fish, and poultry, but allow dairy products and eggs.
- **Pescatarian:** This diet excludes meat, poultry, dairy, and eggs, but allow fish.
- **Vegan:** This diet excludes meat, poultry, fish, eggs, and dairy products, as well as foods that contain these products.
- **Mediterranean:** This diet emphasizes plant-based foods and healthy fats. You eat mostly veggies, fruits, and whole grains. Olive oil is the main source of fat. Meat is included, but it's not the focus of this diet.

- **Raw:** The raw food diet, often called *raw foodism* or *raw veganism*, is an eating plan composed of mostly or entirely raw and unprocessed foods (never heated over 104–118°F, never pasteurized, and never treated with pesticides).

- **SAD (Standard American Diet):** This diet typically consists of a high intake of processed foods, red meat, refined grains, added sugars, and unhealthy fats. Some common components of the SAD include processed foods such as packaged snacks, frozen meals, fried foods, and convenience foods that are high in preservatives, additives, and artificial ingredients; and refined grains, including white bread, white rice, and pasta made from refined flour. Sugary beverages like soda and sweetened juices and desserts are prevalent, as are trans fats and saturated fats found in fried foods, baked goods, and processed snacks. This diet typically lacks sufficient amounts of fruits and vegetables, which are rich in essential vitamins, minerals, and fiber. The SAD has been implicated in the general decline in American health since the 1950s.[16]

Make a list of the foods and drinks that you want to eliminate from or reduce in your diet and those that you want to add or increase your intake of.

Exercise

For the next five days, keep a journal tracking both your cardiovascular and resistance training. Include the type of exercise, duration, and intensity, as well as how you feel before and after exercising. Sometimes people feel drained by exercise, and sometimes it can be a boost. That's important information to have.

General Exercise Routine

How would you describe your overall exercise routine?

- *Frequency*: How often do you exercise each week?
- *Duration*: How long is your typical exercise session?
- *Types*: What types of exercises do you engage in regularly?

How does your exercise routine make you feel?

Pelvic Floor Exercise

Do you incorporate pelvic floor exercises into your routine?

- If yes, please describe your pelvic floor exercise routine.
- If no, are you aware of the benefits of pelvic floor exercises, especially in preparation for pregnancy and childbirth? (Later in this book, I will introduce you to some specific pelvic floor exercises from a renowned expert on the subject. These are game changers.)

Mindful Movement

Do you engage in purposeful movement or mindfulness practices, such as yoga or meditation?

- If yes, how often and what type of mindful movement do you practice?
- If no, have you considered integrating mindfulness practices into your routine for overall well-being?

Support and Modifications

How do you plan to modify your exercise routine, if necessary, during pregnancy or while actively planning to conceive? Are you open to seeking guidance from a healthcare professional or fitness expert for modifications?

Open-Ended Reflection

How would you describe your overall commitment to maintaining a healthy and active lifestyle?

Is there anything else you would like to focus on regarding your current exercise routine and its role in your journey to parenthood?

Hot Tub and Sauna Usage

How often do you use hot tut tubs or saunas? While it's OK to use a sauna, especially an infrared one, during this time, avoid hot tubs due to excess chemicals and heat. For the three months leading up to trying to conceive, also avoid cold plunges to be on the safe side.

Travel

How often do you travel, especially by airplane? If you have to travel a lot for work, if possible, minimize air travel during the three months leading up to trying to conceive. If you're a woman and you're planning a trip abroad, consider traveling before you get pregnant, as it's best to avoid long flights during pregnancy.

For Frequent Flyers

You've probably heard that when we fly in airplanes, we are exposed to some radiation. It's true that in commercial flights at typical cruising altitudes of 30,000–40,000 feet, you will be exposed to cosmic radiation (radiation from space).[17] But exactly how much depends on several factors. A higher altitude means less atmospheric shielding from cosmic rays. Plus, flights near the poles also experience more radiation due to the earth's magnetic shield being weaker at those points. Obviously, a longer flight exposes you to more radiation.

Your exposure is also dependent on solar activity, which can fluctuate. While you can (more or less) control the other factors, depending on your flight, this last one is obviously not within your control. It typically takes about thirty-three hours of flying to reach the same levels of microsieverts (µSv) as a chest X-ray. There is a very helpful online calculator you can use to calculate your exposure (you'll find the web address in the endnotes).[18]

Astronauts can experience short-term radiation sickness due to solar flares, and long-term, high doses of exposure can increase cancer risk or nervous system disorders, memory problems, or cardiovascular disease.[19] While you probably will not experience those effects, you might still want to mitigate your exposure, especially if you are a frequent flyer or are part of an airline crew, as exposure can accumulate over time. You can do this with a combination of antioxidant-rich supplements, a nutrient-dense diet, and healthy lifestyle practices. These strategies focus on supporting the body's natural ability to repair DNA, neutralize oxidative stress, and maintain overall health.

Antioxidants help neutralize free radicals generated by radiation, protecting cells from damage.[20] I suggest taking antioxidant supplements after each flight. Supplements include vitamin C (supports immune health), vitamin E (protects cell membranes from oxidative damage), selenium (enhances antioxidant enzyme systems),[21] glutathione (supports detoxification), and alpha-lipoic acid (ALA) (regenerates other antioxidants).

For additional DNA repair and cell protection, use zinc (repairs DNA and immune function),[22] N-acetylcysteine (boosts glutathione production and supports detox pathways),[23] melatonin (has radioprotective properties).[24] Anti-inflammatory and radioprotective compounds include curcumin (reduces inflammation and oxidative stress—take a liposomal product or one with black pepper to increase absorption), astaxanthin (a carotenoid, which is known for its radioprotective properties),[25] and omega-3 fatty acids (found in fish oil, these reduce inflammation).

Here's your key takeaway: If you log a lot of flight hours, whether it's for work or for fun, you might consider reducing time spent in the air during the preconception period. Though it's unlikely you'd be exposed to enough radiation to have a direct impact on fertility, it's still good to proceed with caution. And when you do fly, you can still mitigate the effects of any accumulated radiation by eating an antioxidant-rich diet of berries, citrus fruits, and pomegranates, as well as leafy greens, cruciferous vegetables, and sweet potatoes. You can also add turmeric, ginger, and garlic to your diet. Remember to hydrate regularly to support detoxification and cellular health.

Lastly, intermittent fasting can enhance DNA repair and reduce oxidative stress.[26] Moderate-intensity exercise can also help. I also recommend limiting other radiation exposure (such as X-rays or CT scans) soon after a flight. Compression socks are also great for flying to improve circulation, and after your flight, get sunlight exposure to help regulate your circadian rhythms.

Body Composition

Now, let's discuss your body composition for a moment. This can be a sensitive subject. We can be so hard on ourselves if we're not in a range that we feel good about, so part of the focus of this book is to help you feel good about yourself.

On a cellular level, how healthy is your body? Epigenetics—the study of how environmental and behavioral factors can impact how genes function—helps us answer that question. As you know, epigenetics isn't about altering the DNA sequence itself; it involves chemical modifications that "turn genes on or off, dial up or down." These modifications can be influenced by various factors, including diet, environment, and lifestyle. Epigenetic changes are reversible, and in some cases, they can be inherited, meaning that parents' life experiences can affect the gene expressions of their children and even grandchildren.

Let's talk about epigenetics and fertility. Men who are underweight or overweight can be less fertile.[27] And both underweight and overweight women are at increased risk of fertility challenges due to hormonal imbalances and irregular ovulation cycles.[28] And both men's and women's nutrition and dietary habits can impact both their chances of conception and their future offspring's health, potentially affecting traits such as body composition, metabolism, and epigenetic markers.

In one recent study, researchers found that paternal high-protein intake led to leaner body composition and better insulin sensitivity in offspring.[29] They also observed changes in epigenetic markers and gut bacteria, suggesting that paternal diet (the father's diet before conception) can influence metabolic health across generations. Other studies have shown that preconception environmental factors—such as diet, stress, lifestyle, and exposure to toxins—can alter sperm epigenetics, which affects gene expression.[30]

So a woman's or man's weight being too high or too low is passed on epigenetically and can set up the child for preprogramming of their metabolism. We'll dive deeper into these topics later in the book, but for now, the goal is for you to become familiar with your starting point so you know which areas will require your attention.

From the woman's perspective, prepregnancy body composition matters a lot. Some women tend not to gain much weight during pregnancy, and some gain easily. Research does indicate that weight gain in the years before conception is linked to excessive weight gain during pregnancy.[31] You'll thank yourself later if you go into pregnancy at a healthy weight. The more optimal your metabolism is prior to pregnancy, the more likely you're going to remain in a more optimal range of weight during pregnancy.

BMI Calculation

Your body mass index (BMI) is the numerical value of your weight in relation to your height. It's often used to place individuals into different weight status categories. You can quickly calculate your BMI using an online calculator. Here is an online BMI calculator you can use: www.nhlbi.nih.gov/calculate-your-bmi.

BMI categories are:

- *Underweight:* BMI less than 18.5
- *Normal weight:* BMI 18.5–24.9
- *Overweight:* BMI 25–29.9
- *Obese:* BMI 30 or greater

Ideally, you're in the normal BMI range, but if you're underweight or overweight, this program can help you get into the "normal weight" category. If you're in the obese category, it could take a bit more time, or you might want to get some personalized functional medicine help.

I understand that seeing your BMI can feel a little triggering, and it's important to approach it with grace and kindness toward yourself. BMI is simply a measure of weight relative to height and serves as a general guide rather than a definitive judgment of your health. If you don't fall within the "normal weight" range right now, remember that this program is designed to support you in moving toward a healthier range over time. If you want a little more information, you can get a full-body DEXA scan to actually find out your body fat, lean muscle, and bone mass.

Give yourself plenty of grace as you define your starting point and focus on the positive changes you're setting in motion.

Body Image

The next important aspect of this physical assessment is about your own *perception* of your body. How we perceive our body is often very different from the physical reality of it. I want to bring your awareness to this because parents play a significant role in shaping their children's body images. Our children can easily perceive our thoughts or judgments about our bodies, and they will translate that to how they perceive their own bodies.[32]

Recently, we've seen messages in our culture and media about how it's OK to be overweight. While I agree we don't want to be shaming one another for our weight, I do not think it's wise from an epigenetic standpoint to be overweight. This is a good time to work on getting to a healthy weight, not for aesthetic reasons, but in order to optimize your overall health prior to conception. I've worked with multiple patients who were overcoming eating disorders, and that's certainly important to have sorted out before having a baby. Eating disorders and poor body image can become family legacies if you don't deal with them now.

While you are in the preconception journey, I hope you will be in awe of your body and what it can do, rather than focusing on any negative viewpoints you may have developed over time. This can be hard to do, but when it's in the context of passing it along to our child as a legacy, it's more motivating and pressing. Here are some important questions about body image to consider:

- How would you describe your body image? Do you feel comfortable in your body and amazed at what it is capable of?
- Would you say you love your body, regardless of its appearance?
- How would you describe your feelings about your body's current appearance?
- Do you feel pressure to conform to certain standards of appearance, either from culture or social media?
- How do you think your body image affects your overall well-being and self-esteem?
- Are there specific aspects of your body that you feel particularly positive or negative about?
- Have you experienced any negative comments or behaviors from others that have impacted your body image?
- Do you engage in any activities or practices that positively or negatively influence your body image?

BELIEVE

- How do you cope with moments of insecurity or dissatisfaction with your body?
- Are there aspects of your body that you would like to change, and if so, why?
- Do you feel comfortable seeking support or discussing your body image concerns with someone you trust?

A Cautionary Tale: Use Condoms During Your Preconception Period

One of my patients, Emma, came to me at age thirty-five, ready to begin her journey toward a healthy pregnancy. She and her husband wanted to optimize their health before conception, and when I saw her for the first time in July, both she and her husband immediately started on the supplement protocol, even though we were still waiting on lab results to fully tailor the plan.

For nearly ten years, Emma had used the "pullout method" of birth control and had never gotten pregnant, so she and her husband were relaxed, almost certain that this was just the beginning of a longer journey. They even had seven embryos stored as a backup, thinking conception might take some time. Yet, by November—just three months into the preconception program—Emma found herself five weeks pregnant.

They went through a wave of emotions—excited but also anxious, as she and her husband hadn't expected this to happen so quickly. Before she even realized she was pregnant, a bodyworker mentioned seeing a child's soul in her "field," and Emma herself told me she could sense a child's soul connecting with her, as if they were ready to begin their journey.

Emma's story is a powerful reminder to anyone beginning this program: With just a few months of intentional preparation, your body can become *very* ready for conception—even if you've never conceived before. So until you have the green light, use caution and protection, because this program truly primes your body for new life.

Your Emotions

There are so many emotions that we experience as parents. You might already know this, but parenthood will provide us with the highest of highs and the lowest of lows—often all in one day! It's important to have a handle on your emotions going in so that your whole world isn't rocked when something goes awry in your child's life. To that end, let's take a moment to ponder your ability to manage your emotions. Because ultimately, how you deal with your emotions is how your child will learn to manage theirs. The questions listed below will get you thinking. (And if you realize you and your partner have some work to do here, that's actually good because now you're both aware of it and can do something about it, helping each other along the way.)

- How do you typically respond to stress or challenging situations?
- What coping mechanisms do you employ to navigate difficult emotions?
- Are you aware of any patterns in how you handle both positive and negative emotions?
- Do you practice mindfulness, prayer, meditation, or other relaxation techniques to manage stress?
- How comfortable are you in expressing your emotions to others?
- How much time do you spend complaining about things, rather than being proactive about the things you can change?
- Do you have specific activities or hobbies that help you regulate your emotions?
- Do you have a support system or network of people you can turn to during emotionally challenging times?
- Can you identify any triggers that tend to affect your emotional well-being (not getting enough sleep, waiting too long

between meals, not setting boundaries, etc.)? If so, how do you address them?

- How do you prioritize self-care in your daily or weekly routine? Have you identified what you need for self-care?

> Incorporate small, consistent self-care practices, such as scheduling alone time, journaling, taking nature walks, and engaging in deep breathing exercises. Consider activities such as volunteering for a cause you're passionate about or spending time with animals as therapeutic outlets. Schedule intentional digital detoxes—disconnecting from screens and social media for a set period can reduce stress and improve mental clarity.

- Are there instances where you feel you struggle to regulate your emotions effectively?
- Do you set clear boundaries in your relationships and daily life to protect your emotional well-being?
- How do you handle and learn from past emotional experiences?
- Are you open to seeking professional support or guidance for emotional response optimization?
- How do you balance addressing your own emotions with supporting others with their emotional needs?
- Have you identified any unhealthy patterns in how you manage your emotions, and if so, what steps are you taking to address them?
- As you navigate life, how do you speak to yourself? Are you kind? Are you curious?

If this feels like an area where you need some extra guidance, I'd love to direct you to a few resources. First, Kristen Neff has a book (and a program) called *Self-Compassion*.[33] It can teach you some tools for recognizing where you lack compassion for yourself, and it also shows you how to become more compassionate. Also, Dr. Elaine N. Aron wrote a book series called *The Highly Sensitive Person*,[34] which I recommend. And finally, Byron Katie's book series *Loving What Is*[35] can be very helpful in this journey by having you ask—and answer—the key question: "Is it true?"

I would be remiss if I didn't also address trauma in this section. I have had many patients work through trauma—specifically childhood trauma—in preparation for becoming a parent. The Adverse Childhood Experiences Questionnaire (ACE-Q) is a detailed set of questions designed to identify and quantify adverse childhood experiences and their potential long-term impacts.[36] If you've suffered trauma in your past, this is one way you can assess the impact, but I'd definitely recommend finding a practitioner you trust to help you find the treatment modality that will be most effective for you in healing and moving forward.

Your Spiritual Life

I believe your spiritual life can be foundational to all other aspects of your life. But often, it can be overlooked in the everyday hustle and bustle. That's why I think taking an objective look at it is so essential. If you feel you don't have a spiritual life, perhaps you can substitute *ethical* for *spiritual*. You can also focus on how you interact with and honor your partner's spiritual life.

Keep in mind that we tend to want people in our family to have our same spiritual beliefs. But I've found that when a child is forced to have the same beliefs as their parents, tension can form, and they might reject that belief system. Think about your child's spiritual life as a seed that you plant and nurture, or as something you encourage them to explore. The following questions will help get you started.

Individual Spiritual Life

- How would you describe your personal spiritual beliefs or philosophy?
- What spiritual practices or rituals bring you a sense of peace and connection?
- Have you experienced any significant spiritual milestones or moments of growth?
- How would you say your spiritual beliefs influence your decision-making and daily life?
- Are there specific values or principles from your spiritual beliefs that strongly guide your actions?

Shared Vision with Your Partner

- How would you describe your partner's spiritual beliefs, and how do they align with or differ from your own?
- Have you and your partner discussed your spiritual values and how they may impact your relationship?
- In what ways do you and your partner support each other's spiritual journeys?
- Are there shared spiritual practices or rituals that strengthen your bond as a couple?
- How do you navigate differences in spiritual beliefs within your relationship?

Envisioning Your Child's Spiritual Life

- What values and spiritual principles would you like to explore with your child?
- Have you and your partner discussed how to introduce spiritual concepts to your child?

- How do you plan to incorporate spiritual practices or rituals into your family life?
- Are there specific religious or spiritual traditions you wish to pass on to your child?
- How open are you to allowing your child to explore and develop their own spiritual beliefs?

Whether you consider yourself a "spiritual" person or not, these are important conversations to have so you know exactly where you and your partner stand, and so you can chart a course for your child's own spiritual growth.

Your Relationship

As we touched on in the last chapter, having a child will expose any cracks in the foundation of your relationship, so now is the time to really look at that bond and see if there's work to be done. Here is a list of questions designed to get you thinking intentionally about your relationship:

Overall Relationship

- **Overall Satisfaction:** How would you describe the overall satisfaction and fulfillment in your relationship?
- **Relationship Evolution:** How has the dynamic between you and your partner evolved over time? Do you feel it's evolving in a positive direction?
- **Expression of Affection:** How effectively do you and your partner express love, affection, and appreciation for each other?
- **Areas for Improvement:** Identify specific areas of your relationship that need improvement or further attention.

Communication

- **Daily Communication:** How well do you and your partner communicate with each other on a daily basis?
- **Comfort in Sharing:** How comfortable are you sharing your thoughts, feelings, and concerns with your partner?
- **Conflict Resolution:** How do you and your partner resolve disagreements and conflicts? How satisfied are you with this aspect of your relationship?

Trust

- **Level of Trust:** How would you rate the level of trust between you and your partner?
- **Trust Issues:** Are there any trust issues or concerns that you feel need to be addressed before starting a family?
- **Building Trust:** In what ways are you and your partner building and maintaining trust in your relationship?

Shared Values and Goals

- **Discussion of Values:** Have you and your partner discussed your individual and shared values, especially in the context of raising a child?
- **Alignment on Goals:** How aligned do you feel with your partner in terms of long-term goals, including parenting styles and family values (e.g., where to live, when to retire, schooling, financial priorities)?

Individual Well-Being

- **Support for Growth:** How well do you and your partner support each other's individual growth and well-being (e.g., specific goals you each want to achieve, areas of self-improvement or spiritual growth you each want to focus on)?

- **Emotional Support:** How would you rate the level of emotional support and understanding in your relationship?

Preparation for Parenthood

- **Discussion of Expectations:** Have you and your partner discussed your expectations, roles, and responsibilities as parents?
- **Confidence in Teamwork:** How confident do you feel in your ability to work together as a team in raising a child?

Your Relationship with Yourself

You've likely heard the saying, "You can't give away what you don't have." This is especially true for self-esteem. If you don't have high self-esteem, it can be challenging for you to instill it in your child. Use these questions to reflect on your relationship with someone crucial—yourself.

Self-Trust

- Do you trust your own instincts and decisions?
- Are you confident in making choices that align with your values?
- Have you shown self-trust in the past, and could you improve it further?

Self-Commitment

- Do you keep commitments to yourself?
- Are there areas where you struggle to follow through on personal goals?

Inner Conversation

- Is your inner dialogue supportive and encouraging?
- How do you handle self-criticism?
- Can you speak your thoughts out loud positively?

Modeling for Children

- How do you talk about yourself around children?
- Are there any ways you'd like to be an even better role model?

Language and Words

- Are you mindful of the language you use around children?
- Do your words to yourself and others reflect positivity?

Positive Affirmations

- Do you use positive affirmations in your daily routine?
- How can affirmations improve your self-image and emotional environment for children?

Reflection on Past Experiences

- How do past experiences of overcoming challenges build your self-confidence as a parent?

Stress Response Optimization

Stress affects all of us, and how we respond to it can significantly impact our health, including our reproductive health. This tool will help you assess your current stress response and identify areas where you may need to optimize it for better resilience (a key element to good parenting!) and well-being. Answer the following questions to gauge your stress response:

Current Stress Level

- How would you describe your current stress level?

Recognizing Patterns

- Do you notice any patterns or triggers that consistently affect your stress response?

Effectiveness of Coping Strategies

- How effective is your current response to stress? Is there room to further optimize your stress response?

Frequency of Stress Symptoms

- How often do physical or emotional symptoms of stress affect your daily life?

Preparation for Pregnancy

When you experience stress while pregnant, your baby will be bathed in those stress hormones. And this applies to your partner too—if your partner is stressed out, you will naturally become more stressed as well. With that said, what steps can you and your partner take to work on reducing stress levels and improving how you cope with stress?

Recognizing the importance of a calm environment for the baby's development, what specific actions can you include in your daily routine to create a more relaxed and stress-free lifestyle? Think about incorporating activities that bring peace and joy into your daily life.

I hope those questions started to guide you toward increased self-awareness about stressors and your strategies for dealing with them. This will serve you well throughout the preconception phase—and for the rest of your life.

Overall Readiness for Parenting

We've covered a lot of ground already! But there's one more crucial aspect I'm going to ask you to carefully consider, and that's your overall readiness for bringing a baby into your little world. We'll touch on finances, your living situation, and childcare considerations. Perhaps you've already got a handle on all these areas! But these questions might open up new lines of thought for you as well, so I urge you to follow those threads.

Parenthood Readiness Assessment

Finances

- How would you describe your current financial stability?
- Have you created a budget that includes potential expenses associated with having a baby?
- Do you have an emergency fund or savings in place?
- Have you considered the financial impact of parental leave or a potential reduction in work hours?
- How comfortable are you with the idea of adjusting your lifestyle to accommodate additional financial responsibilities?

Living Situation

- Do you currently have adequate living space for a growing family?

- Have you considered the safety and childproofing of your home?
- How satisfied are you with your current living situation in relation to raising a child?

Childcare

- If you're planning to work after having a baby, have you explored childcare options?
- Do you have family or close friends nearby who can assist with childcare when needed? Or do you have plans in place for hiring a professional nanny?
- Have you discussed your plans for sharing childcare responsibilities with your partner?
- How confident do you feel about managing childcare responsibilities alongside work commitments?

General Readiness

- How would you describe your overall level of excitement and preparedness for parenthood at this moment?
- Is there anything specific that you feel you need to address or prepare for before starting a family?

Final Thoughts

You did a lot of introspection throughout this chapter, and I know it might have felt overwhelming at times. But the questions you answered are meant to encourage thoughtful reflection on your overall readiness for parenthood. It's much better to ponder and consider these topics now rather than once the baby has already arrived.

The key takeaway is that you now have a strong sense of your unique starting point. I wouldn't expect anyone to have "perfect" answers to all of these questions; that's not realistic. Instead, you've learned which areas require some of your focused attention as we continue this journey. It's not as if you need to tie all those areas up with a bow. Rather, now that you're aware of them, you'll be able to make the shifts needed over time.

This chapter probably also raised a lot of questions about what steps you need to take in order to get yourself into a stronger, healthier state. Don't worry—we'll get there! Later in this book, I will share specific guidance on what to eat, how to move your body, beneficial ways to optimize your stress responses, and many more tools designed specifically to boost your odds of having a healthy child and healthier future generations of your family as well.

Q&A

Q: Why is assessing your relationship and financial stability important in a preconception plan?

A: Starting a family introduces a lot of new responsibilities—financially, emotionally, and even spiritually. Having a strong relationship foundation and being financially prepared can help both partners feel more secure and supported, which is beneficial for both conception and parenting. This chapter encourages open conversations to ensure that both of you are aligned and ready to handle these new responsibilities together.

Q: How does my BMI impact fertility, and is it something to worry about?

A: Research does indicate an increase in the rate of autism and neuro-developmental and psychiatric disorders in children born to mothers with a high BMI.[37] So it's something you'll want to take seriously. With that said, the goal is not to stress over a "perfect" BMI but to aim for a healthier range over time. This program can help guide you there, and any improvements you make in your nutrition and exercise will benefit both you and your future child.

Q: I've struggled with body image for a long time. How can I make sure this doesn't negatively impact my future child's body image?

A: It's natural to have concerns about body image, but recognizing and working on them is already a huge step. I encourage you to appreciate what your body can do, especially during this journey to parenthood. Focusing on the positives, practicing self-compassion, and modeling a healthy mindset about your body will help you set a great example for your child, allowing them to grow up with a strong, positive body image.

Q: I tend to get overwhelmed with stress. Could this impact our chances of conceiving?

A: Yes, stress can impact reproductive health, as high stress levels can disrupt hormonal balance. But remember, the purpose of this assessment is to identify where stress is affecting you. Later in this book, you'll find specific strategies for optimizing your stress response, which will support your fertility and overall health. Knowing your stress triggers and working to address them now will also benefit you as you transition to parenthood.

Q: My partner and I have different spiritual beliefs. How can we make sure this doesn't become a source of conflict as we raise our child?

A: Having different spiritual beliefs doesn't have to be a barrier to parenting together successfully. This chapter's questions encourage both of you to explore and respect each other's spiritual perspectives and to have open conversations about how you'll approach guiding your child's spiritual life.

Believe

Introspect

Renew

Thrive

Hope

Section II Introduction

This section is all about looking inward to understand the critical factors shaping your health and fertility. Together, we'll examine aspects of yourself that often remain below the surface—your genetic inheritance, your body's current health landscape, and how these two factors influence your physical and biological readiness for conception. By gaining these insights, you're equipping yourself with a foundation not only of knowledge but also of responsibility, setting the stage for a healthy, intentional approach to parenthood.

We'll explore two powerful approaches that lay the groundwork for optimal health and fertility: *understanding your genetic blueprint* and *taking inventory of your body's health*. Each chapter guides you toward greater self-awareness, offering actionable insights into how your genes and physical health impact conceiving—and then raising—a healthy child.

Chapter 3: Your Gene Team invites you to see genetics in a new light. Many of us think of our genes as fixed, unchangeable traits, but this chapter reveals how daily choices—what you eat, how you optimize your stress responses, and even how you sleep—can significantly influence which genes are active, creating a ripple effect of health benefits. Nurturing your genetic potential isn't just about enhancing your well-being but also passing on a legacy to your future child—and even the generations after that.

Chapter 4: Taking Your Body Inventory dives into understanding your physical health with clarity and purpose. By examining key lab tests, you'll discover how your body's current state, from inflammation to hormone levels, can affect your fertility. This chapter empowers you to take control of your health, guiding you to optimize each element in preparation for a healthy conception. Together, these chapters offer a practical and profound start on your path toward parenthood, helping you nurture your body—and your future child.

CHAPTER 3

Your Gene Team

I'm two years old, and we're at my mom's best friend's house with my baby sister, Laura. Of course, Laura is getting all the attention, but while everyone else is focused on her, I spot it—a sparkling crystal dish filled with yummy jelly beans that's sitting atop a little wooden cabinet. *Should I? Or shouldn't I?* I know I might get in trouble if I eat them. I'm not usually allowed to have candy. But everyone's so focused on Laura that I decide to take the risk.

Mom and her best friend, Donna, are sitting right there, but they don't know about my special hiding trick. I know that if I can't see them, they can't see me! Shielding my eyes from them with one hand, I scoop up a fistful of the multicolored candies with my other hand and quickly pop them into my mouth. Suddenly, I hear laughter. I peek over the top of my hand and see both grown-ups cracking up, and even though I'm still chewing, I start to giggle too. I guess I'm not as invisible as I thought.

It sounds silly, like a childish fancy, but the truth is, that's exactly how it plays out when we convince ourselves we can get away with certain decisions regarding our health without our bodies taking notice.

We think if we cover our eyes and pretend, we can behave however we like without any consequences. I know, because that's exactly the illusion I was living under—until it resulted in a life-threatening medical scare when I was thirty-one. As you read in the introduction, it was the kind of health scare that left me feeling utterly alone and broken.

After I recovered, I began my journey toward creating a different kind of medical practice, one where I look for the root cause of illness and use the latest technology, testing, and research to help my patients. I'm much like a detective. The testing that I use allows me to look at each patient's unique genetics, the environmental toxin levels, the intricate ecosystem of the gut microbiome, and so much more. One of the things I've learned from helping my patients in this way and diving into the latest research and testing in genetics is this: *We can influence our genes' behavior—meaning that even though we're born with our genes, our daily choices can influence the chemical modifications around the genes to move us toward either a healthy state or a less healthy one.*[38]

It might sound surprising that you can influence how your genes are expressed, but it's based on an impressive and growing body of research called *epigenetics*, which, as a reminder, is how the chemical modifications around the genes can be influenced and determine how active the genes are.

To help illustrate how this works, think of the pixels in a computer monitor. All the pixels have the same potential, yet each pixel acting differently allows the computer monitor to create an infinite array of images, colors, and words. All of this happens because individual pixels are turned on, off, up, or down. Your DNA is regulated in a similar way. A cell from your liver has the same DNA as a cell from your eyeball. Since all the cells in our body have the same DNA, that means other processes determine how individual cells develop, differentiate, and behave. This is how some cells help us filter our blood while others allow us to see. The gene *expression* in every cell is continuously adjusting to adapt to our current situation and environment.

Lifestyle factors unquestionably alter these pixels, and we can dramatically change the trajectory of our health by knowing which dials to turn and levers to switch. Bottom line: *Your DNA is not your destiny.* And that's great news! But it goes even deeper than that, because one extremely important factor makes your DNA very different from a computer monitor: Many of the changes can be stored—like a screenshot—and passed on to your descendants. So that means when you make these changes in your own gene expression, you can pass those changes on to your child.[39] And *that's* the best motivator of all.

As kids, we're taught, "Mind your manners and tell the truth." And even though epigenetics is a complex subject, it can be as simple as teaching a child to follow three simple rules that can help you unlock your genes' highest potential. Here's a brief overview.

Rule 1: Chill Out

Stress has been linked to Alzheimer's, cardiovascular disease, diabetes, and many degenerative diseases.[40] By managing our stress levels with meditation, sleep, and exercise, we can collaborate with our genes. And this is critical because cumulative lifetime stress accelerates epigenetic aging.[41] Extensive research has shown that meditation can help restore telomere length—a protective cap at the ends of chromosomes that shortens with age and stress—influence gene expression involved in inflammation and blood flow, and actually improve the way our bodies respond to stress.[42]

In a study with recent heart attack survivors, those who practiced meditation for six months showed improved blood vessel function and a reduction in the expression of three key inflammatory genes through epigenetic changes.[43] If there was a drug that did this, it would be a billion-dollar drug, and we'd probably all want to take it. But what if every cardiologist and neurologist—and really *every* physician—taught meditation in their office? How much pain and suffering and medical expenses would we save?

Rule 2: Clean Up

We all know we need to clean up our own messes, but most of us don't realize the invisible mess we've created inside our cells and organs. Every day, we're exposed to small amounts of imperceptible toxins that can build up in our bodies, and I can see the consequences in my patients—and in myself. We think a little bit of something won't hurt us, but toxicity is often cumulative. Among other effects, the exposure affects our epigenetics. When I measure these toxin levels in my medical practice, I can see that making lifestyle changes and taking the right nutritional supplements will decrease toxin levels.

To think that things such as pesticides, mold, plastics such as bisphenol A (BPA), and heavy metals, along with other toxins such as tobacco smoke, air pollution, and alcohol, don't have lasting consequences on our health is like covering our eyes and pretending. These toxins are extensively studied for epigenetic effects, and testing often reveals they're present in my patients.

When it comes to creating a healthy environment in which a baby can grow, the mother's toxicity levels are incredibly important to consider. In 2005, the Environmental Working Group (EWG) in collaboration with Commonweal studied umbilical cord blood in ten babies born in US hospitals. Shockingly, researchers found an average of *200 industrial chemicals and pollutants* in the cord and a total of 287 chemicals in those babies who were studied. They discovered that the umbilical cord blood harbored pesticides, consumer product ingredients, and waste products from burning coal, gasoline, and garbage.[44] Since then, multiple cord blood studies have been conducted internationally. One of many learnings from these studies is that per- and polyfluoroalkyl substances (PFAS, otherwise known as "forever chemicals" because they're man-made chemicals that do not break down) are able to "penetrate the placental barrier and reach embryos through cord blood, probably causing adverse birth outcomes."[45] The moral of the story is this: The same toxins that a mother's body is harboring will be shared with the growing fetus.

But going deeper than the impact of toxins on a person's or a fetus's health, let's consider for a moment how toxins can affect us on a genetic level. There's an advanced test that isn't widely available as of the writing of this book, but may become more readily available in the future, and it allows us to see specifically how environmental toxins are affecting certain genes. One of my patients in her sixties was noticing that her memory was declining, and she was often struggling to recall words. When we ran this test, it revealed that she had a toxin from mold that was attached to a gene that increases the risk for Alzheimer's. Eight months later, after implementing the recommended nutritional supplements, IVs, and lifestyle changes, we reran the test. It showed that the toxins had been removed from her body, and she was recalling words more easily.

Every day, we encounter toxic exposures from places and products we wouldn't expect, such as our mattresses, seafood, beverage and food packaging, and even BPA on paper receipts. Instead of being alarmed, we can become informed and take action on the things we can control and help our bodies detoxify what we can't control.

For example, I'm aware of the quality of the air I breathe, and I filter the air in my home to reduce the outgassing that can happen in my environment.

I'm also careful about what I put on my skin. I eat and drink the cleanest food and beverages I can, buying organic, high-quality food, eating lots of cruciferous vegetables such as broccoli, and paying attention to food preparation and packaging. And several days a month,

I restrict my calories to reset important functions, either by intermittent fasting (calorie restricting for a certain period of time) or a new area of research called *fasting mimicking* (a dietary approach that provides minimal calories while mimicking the physiological effects of complete fasting) that's getting excellent results.

We'll discuss all of this and more in detail later in the book. It's becoming an increasingly toxic world that we live and raise our children in, but we are not powerless. There are simple changes you can make and gentle detoxification protocols you can follow to greatly reduce the impact of those toxins on your body and improve the health of your future child.

Rule 3: Play Well with Others

One of our most important relationships is with our own microbiome. It's like a little army of organisms, all of which work either with us or against us. That "army" is made up of parasites, bacteria, viruses, and fungi, which you might automatically think of as a bad thing, but really, they're fighting to keep us healthy. Collectively, they have one hundred to two hundred times more genetic material than we do, and when they're friendly and cared for, they help keep us healthy. Among other roles, the microbiome helps provide the resources we need to control our genes. An imbalanced microbiome can lead to instability in the entire epigenetic process, which in turn affects many functions in our body, including fertility.

Thankfully, recent advances in testing allow us to look more deeply into what's going on in the body and with the microbiome, and because of this, we can measure and correct the imbalances. As a result, my patients often notice improved blood sugar levels, better mood, stronger immune systems, reduced autoimmunity, and more. These organisms are particularly affected by what we ingest and the toxins we're exposed to.

Later, I'll share many different strategies you can adopt in order to properly care for the organisms that benefit you. Getting your microbiome into balance is of the utmost importance for optimizing your epigenetics, improving your overall organ function, and passing down that optimal gene expression to future generations.

Some of the habits I'll be introducing you to may be new, and consistent practice is key. Research with professional musicians showed that practice increased the genetic expression for their auditory aptitude, meaning it helped their genes optimize their hearing.[46] Practice can help you too. Rather than trying the concepts for a few days here or there, commit to being consistent. It will make all the difference in terms of outcomes.

The study of epigenetics reminds us of an important lesson: The future is ours to shape. Three simple rules can build momentum and change the trajectory of your health. But more than that, you can also have a direct impact on the health and vitality of your future child through the power of epigenetic transgenerational inheritance.[47] How exciting is that?

A Deeper Dive into DNA

To help build a foundation for the work we're going to be doing together over this preconception period, let's take a moment to dive a little deeper into the topic of DNA. As you probably know, your DNA (or your genes) predispose you to certain diseases, and if you have a "faulty" gene, this is something you inherited at birth. Two examples of this are cystic fibrosis and Down syndrome. But as we've been discussing, our genes are constantly affected by our environment, and as such, our lifestyles and nutrition can be influenced by these factors to be either more expressive or less active. *Methylation* is one of the important epigenetic processes by which gene activity is turned on or off, up or down, often in response to environmental triggers.

Methylation can accelerate disease or slow it down or stop it. It's important to have the right amount of methylation—not too much and not too little. There are other processes that modify gene expression through epigenetics, such as histone modifications, but for now, I want to drill down specifically on this topic of methylation.

Methylation is the process of joining a methyl group (CH3) (which is a small molecule of one carbon atom bonded to two hydrogen atoms) to DNA, which plays a major role in gene expression. While it is a normal process in regulating gene activity in humans, this process can sometimes go awry. Under certain circumstances, poor methylation can be caused by inherited or acquired genetic mutations (or single nucleotide polymorphisms, which are known as SNPs) that mediate gene activity in such a way that existing diseases are accelerated or new illnesses arise.

For example, methylation has a significant impact on malignant tumor cells in the human body.[48] And it's also known to have an effect in other conditions such as atherosclerosis, diabetic retinopathy, autoimmunity, Parkinson's, cardiac dysfunction, anxiety, trauma, and even schizophrenia.[49]

Proper methylation is essential for reproductive health because it affects hormone production, egg and sperm quality, and early embryonic development. Methylation regulates how genes are expressed in the reproductive tissues for both females and males.[50]

Your DNA is like a library of instructions, and gene expression is what turns those instructions mainly into proteins. Methylation is the process that controls which of those proteins are made, when they are made, and how much is made. All this is done by turning gene expression "down" (essentially, blocking cellular machinery from reading the DNA) or attracting proteins that inhibit gene expression. This is what determines a cell's characteristics and functions.[51]

Methylation occurs during development, helping cells specialize into different types of cells. Abnormal methylation leads to poor egg or sperm quality, impaired embryo development, and subsequently an increased risk of miscarriage or birth defects.[52] Methylation is also responsible for hormone synthesis—in other words, the production and metabolism of estrogen, progesterone, and testosterone. Poor methylation will lead to imbalances in these hormones, disrupting ovulation in females, the production of sperm in males, and sperm implantation.[53]

Methylation relies on the folate cycle,[54] which is also essential for vital functions such as DNA synthesis and repair. You get folate (vitamin B9) from leafy green vegetables, legumes, and fortified foods.[55] Vitamins B12 and B6 are also essential to this process.[56] This cycle plays a crucial role in *remethylation*: the conversion of homocysteine (an amino acid) into methionine (an essential amino acid—in other words, an amino acid the body cannot produce on its own without having the proper diet). If this conversion isn't happening properly, you get elevated homocysteine levels, which is linked to a reduced ovarian reserve, poor implantation rates, and an increased risk of miscarriage.

Environmental and lifestyle factors are key in regulating the methylation process so that it's working properly. Stress, poor diet, and toxins (such as PFAS or endocrine disruptors) can all disrupt and harm methylation, leading to fertility issues.

When I order DNA methylation testing, we screen for SNPs that can affect many significant biochemical processes such as detoxification, hormonal balance, and vitamin D function. The presence or absence of certain SNPs can affect your risk for disease but without causing any obvious symptoms—that is, you may not be experiencing any current symptoms and no family member may previously have displayed the disease for which you're at risk. However, these health risks can be reduced by lifestyle changes, and altered biochemical processes may be alleviated by diet and nutritional supplements. In other words, there's lots of hope!

In working with couples who want to have a baby, there have been many times when we've discovered that one or both partners were not methylating well. But once we addressed the issue with proper supplementation (which we'll dig into a little later in the book), they became highly fertile. Left unchecked, poor methylation can wreak havoc on your health, but addressing it can be a huge game changer.

Problematic Genetic Variations

One of the first methylation SNPs to be identified was *methylenetetrahydrofolate reductase (MTHFR SNP)*. When methylation was becoming a focus of functional health, MTHFR was identified as an important methylation enzyme. The MTHFR enzyme plays a crucial role in folate metabolism by converting 5, 10-Methylenetetrahydrofolate (a form of folate) to 5-Methyltetrahydrofolate (5-MTHF), the biologically active form of folate. One reason this process is essential is because 5-MTHF is integral in converting homocysteine to methionine. Methionine is then used to synthesize proteins and other important molecules. These are crucial processes for proper cellular function in your body. Certain SNPs, or variants of MTHFR, cause a reduced capacity of this enzyme.[57] What does all this mean, exactly? Well, we now know that MTHFR variants are associated with increased risk for many diseases, including depression, fertility issues, insomnia, and thyroid conditions.[58]

Folate (B9) is a naturally occurring nutrient found in many foods, and the body naturally converts it into the methylated form. When an MTHFR SNP is present, that natural conversion is limited, so it can be helpful to take folate that is already methylated, or 5MTHF, so it's in the form the body can use more readily. Changing to the bioavailable (meaning easier for your body to absorb) folate 5MTHF is often a step in the right direction.

The COMT gene (catechol-O-methyltransferase) is a gene that is responsible for producing an enzyme that breaks down neurotransmitters such as dopamine, epinephrine, and norepinephrine, which help regulate mood, cognition, and stress response. Polymorphisms, or variations, within the COMT gene can lead to variations in the enzyme's activity that break down the above-mentioned neurotransmitters. This can result in either too much or too little of these neurotransmitters in the brain, potentially causing issues with mood regulation, cognitive function, and stress response.[59] Individuals with an overactive COMT enzyme may break down these neurotransmitters too quickly, leading to difficulties with attention and motivation, while those with an underactive enzyme may experience heightened stress sensitivity and anxiety.

Eventually, methylation patterns will almost certainly be commonly used as a predictor for your health and your predisposition to disease. This is why it is very important that you understand your methylation so you can get a jump start on optimizing your health. Later in the book, we will discuss more about methylation testing and genetic testing so you can know exactly what to address and which genes/SNPs are present. We'll also peek at your neurotransmitters with testing. Then we'll follow that up by discussing what actions you can take to help improve your methylation and explore some cofactors that help, such as magnesium. Because when Mom and Dad are in better balance and methylating well, their epigenetics will be better. Getting a handle on it all now is helping set up your future baby for success.

To give you a little encouragement, I'd like to share with you what my patient Brianna recently wrote about her experience working with me. It's such an honor to hear stories like this!

"I first reached out to Dr. Shippy about three years ago because I didn't have a primary doctor and wanted someone who aligned with my approach to health. I wasn't dealing with any major issues, but I wanted to optimize my health and work with a doctor who could integrate food, supplements, and holistic tools. What I love about Dr. Shippy is that she goes beyond the basics—she doesn't just check your thyroid or run standard bloodwork. She does a deep dive into things like heavy metal toxicity, gut health, liver function, and how your body is actually using nutrients.

"When I started working with her, I was also thinking about starting a family, so we spent about six months cleaning everything up before I got pregnant. My diet and lifestyle were already really clean, but we took it further—making sure my body was in the absolute best place to conceive and carry a healthy baby. We worked on my thyroid, gut health, and even ran tests to ensure the nutrients I was eating were reaching the placenta. Along the way, she helped me fine-tune my supplements and incorporate stress-management tools. I had an extremely healthy pregnancy—no sickness, no major symptoms, and I felt amazing all the way through. I was walking miles up until the day I gave birth.

"Now, I have a healthy daughter and we're working on preparing for baby number two. Dr. Shippy has been incredible at helping me take stock of where I am post-pregnancy and get my body ready again. She also worked with my husband, which was really important to us because it takes two to create a healthy baby. I truly believe the work we did together made all the difference in my first pregnancy, and I wouldn't do another one without her. She's not just guessing or following trends—she tests and tailors everything specifically to what my body needs, and that level of care is priceless."

Thank you, Brianna! It's so exciting to walk alongside you on your journey!

The Power of Prevention

I know I covered a lot of scientific information in this chapter, and it's a bit like drinking from a fire hose. As you progress through the book, you'll learn more details about how these genes might be affecting you. But let's zoom back out for a moment and discuss another foundational element, which is *prevention*.

So much of modern healthcare is directed at treating conditions. It's focused on diagnosing illness and then managing that illness with medication and (sometimes) lifestyle changes. But in my practice, the focus is on discovering the root cause of existing health conditions and preventing future ones. Prevention can be a tough sell for some people because it doesn't usually offer a clear "before and after" effect. We're conditioned to desire that instant gratification, rather than a slow progression in the direction of optimized health. But there's so much power in seeing around corners and catching issues before they've had a chance to progress. Let's see if this analogy resonates.

Have you ever had a garden? If so, you know that it requires consistent effort and care, from planting seeds to watering, fertilizing, and weeding. While it may not produce immediate, tangible results, over time it leads to flourishing plants and a bountiful harvest. Similarly, prioritizing prevention may not provide instantaneous results, but it nurtures overall health and well-being, leading to a vibrant and thriving life in the long run. The seeds of a healthy lifestyle that you sow now might take a while to sprout, but before long, you'll be amazed at the beauty and vibrancy that will grow.

This analogy is especially impactful when we place it in the context of fertility. If you're reading this book because you've been in a difficult season of infertility or miscarriages, then it's important to understand that fertility is merely a symptom of deeper imbalances in the body. So as you follow the steps in this book to improve your overall health, your fertility will also vastly improve. Your "garden" will begin to thrive like never before.

With that good news comes an important warning. I've seen it time and again in my practice—a couple begins the work on cleaning up their food and environment, detoxifying, managing stress, and improving sleep patterns, and the first big shift they see is improved fertility. The body wants to reproduce; that's how we're wired. So as soon as our health begins to trend toward the better, fertility can skyrocket. But just because you suddenly *can* get pregnant doesn't mean you *should* get pregnant. That's why I ask couples to give this program at least six months, because it takes at least that long (and in many cases, nine to twelve months) for the deeper issues to get fully addressed and the optimized epigenetics outcomes to play out.

Remember, the goal isn't just to have a baby. The goal is to have a baby that has been set up for a long, healthy, vibrant life . . . on an epigenetic level. So, even if your body clicks into "fertile" mode, I'm asking you up front to hold off a while longer. I'll share more details later in terms of how to know when it's "go" time. For now, just know that being fertile is a sign that you're heading in the right direction, but it doesn't mean you've arrived at the destination quite yet. It shows that you're tending your garden well, but it's not yet time for harvest!

Epigenetics: How Sperm and Egg Influence Future Health

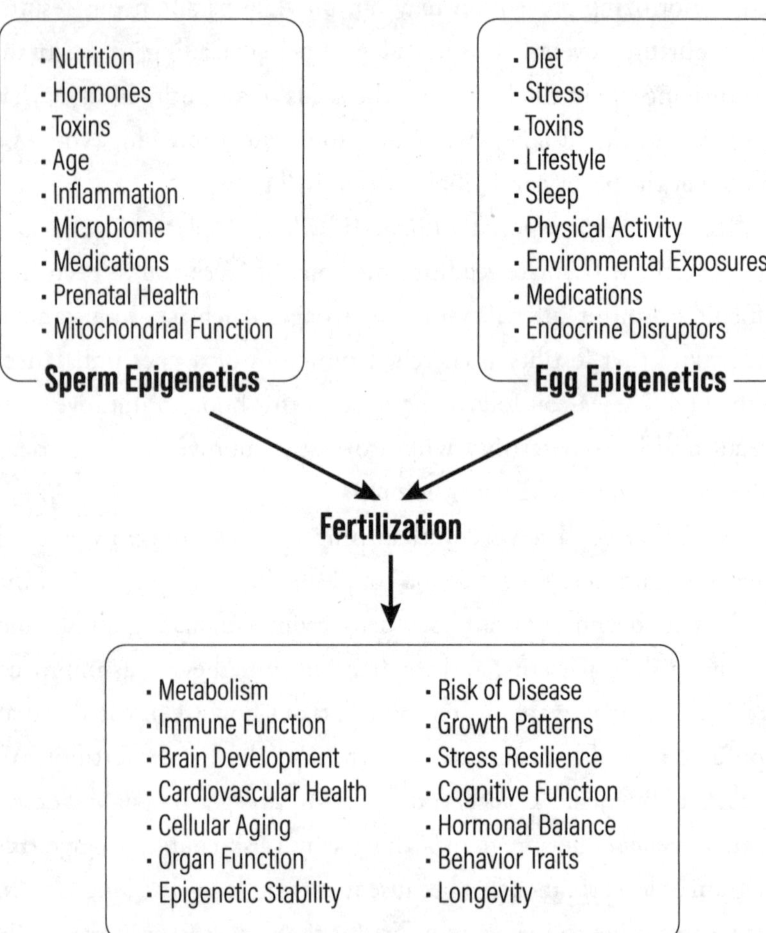

Final Thoughts

I hope this crash course in epigenetics has been enlightening and encouraging rather than daunting. It's a big topic, and an area of rapidly emerging research, but it's also extremely exciting because it takes us out of the mindset that our genes determine our future and puts the control firmly in our own hands. As we continue together on this preconception journey, keep your focus on your future child (or children), because all this groundwork you're laying is really for them. Your choices today have a far-reaching impact on your family legacy.

Oh, and the next time you see a sparkling dish of candy, just remember, your genes can see you!

Q&A

Q: Can I really influence my genes through lifestyle choices?

A: Yes! Factors such as diet, stress management, toxin exposure, and sleep all play significant roles in determining how your genes express themselves. Research shows that positive changes in these areas can lead to healthier outcomes and even improve gene function.

Q: What are some simple ways to reduce stress and its impact on my genes?

A: Optimizing your stress response can slow down epigenetic aging and reduce inflammation in the body. Some evidence-based methods include meditation, deep breathing exercises, regular physical activity, adequate sleep, and engaging in relaxing hobbies. Even small, consistent efforts to reduce stress can have a meaningful impact on your health.

Q: How do environmental toxins affect my genes?

A: Toxins from pesticides, heavy metals, plastics, and pollutants can accumulate in your body and alter gene expression. These changes can contribute to chronic illnesses, fertility issues, and other health concerns. Reducing exposure by choosing organic foods, using nontoxic household products, and filtering air and water can help mitigate these effects.

Q: What is methylation, and why is it important?

A: Methylation is a biochemical process that regulates gene activity by adding or removing methyl groups to DNA. Proper methylation is essential for hormone production, detoxification, and DNA repair. Disruptions in methylation can lead to health issues, but supporting it with nutrients such as methylated folate, B vitamins, and magnesium can improve outcomes.

Q: How does my genetic makeup influence fertility?

A: Genes play a role in hormone production, egg and sperm quality, and early embryonic development. However, lifestyle factors such as diet, stress, and toxin exposure can either support or hinder optimal fertility. Understanding and optimizing these factors can improve reproductive health and increase the chances of a healthy pregnancy.

Q: Why is prevention so crucial when it comes to health and fertility?

A: Many health issues, including fertility challenges, stem from imbalances that develop over time. Addressing these issues proactively through diet, toxin reduction, and stress management can prevent chronic conditions and create the best possible environment for conception and a healthy baby.

INTROSPECT

CHAPTER 4

Taking Your Body Inventory

What you've already accomplished so far is wonderful. You've put energy and thought into your intentions around having a baby, you've started getting more in tune with your intuition, and you've gone through key areas of your life to define your unique starting point. You know which areas require some focused attention and adjustments, and you've committed to making those necessary adjustments throughout this journey. What a great foundation you've begun to build!

In this chapter, we are going to consider your physical starting point—in other words, what your lab work is telling you about your physical health. If you've followed me on social media or seen any of my videos or read some of my blogs, then you know . . . I'm a total data nerd! I love data. Why? Because it paints a super-clear picture of what's going on inside a patient's body. You see, we can put on a façade in our everyday life; we sometimes pretend like everything's just fine even if it's really not. But the data helps us to look beneath the surface and see what is *really* going on. What may feel "normal" to you may not actually be optimal. So I believe collecting data about your body from advanced specific lab tests is the best way to understand the steps you need to take to get your body primed and ready for baby-making.

There's an endless array of advanced medical tests and lab work available these days. And many of these tests and procedures are not covered by insurance. You could very quickly rack up a $20,000 bill just in lab work if you don't know which tests are helpful in this particular quest. I'll admit—it wasn't easy for me to pare down the list because, again . . . I love data! But we want to fit your lab work into your budget and focus on quality versus quantity because not all tests are created equal. I'm going to share with you the key lab tests I recommend for determining—with great specificity—what your body needs to get into tip-top (read: *fertile!*) shape.

Test Brands

I'm always curating the best testing companies that give the most accurate and actionable data available. When I was writing this book, I started putting all my favorite test brands in this chapter, but then I realized that sometimes new, more comprehensive tests come on the market, so I changed my recommendations accordingly. The best way for you to access the latest and greatest list of tests is to join the Every Baby Well program. I'm always updating my recommended lists of lab work and my current favorite testing brands there. But for the purposes of this chapter, I decided to stick with sharing the types of tests I recommend during preconception.

How to Order Tests

Right off the bat, you might be scratching your head wondering how you're going to order lab work without a doctor's prescription. If you're also doing this program on my Every Baby Well platform, then you'll be able to order all the at-home testing kits and download lab orders through your portal. Through the program, you will receive assistance to help interpret your results, which help you develop a customized approach to optimize your fertility and overall health.

Perfection Is Not the Goal

I like to kick off conversations about lab work by setting expectations. First, no one's lab work is "perfect." Something will always show up that could be improved upon. So I don't want you to be surprised when you get your results and spot something that looks out of whack. And be encouraged—if anything *is* off, no matter to what degree, we can work toward improving it. In fact, it can be a big relief when something shows up on a report because it could be an answer to previously unanswered questions. I can't tell you how many patients I've had over the years who came to me out of desperation because they simply had not been getting answers for why they were experiencing certain symptoms. That was exactly why I got into functional medicine in the first place—to solve the mystery of my own devastating symptoms!

I encourage you to look at this like an expedition. We are seeking answers, collecting clues as we go, and then solving issues as we find them. It's nothing to be afraid of or to worry about—quite the contrary, in fact! Allow yourself to feel a little excitement about what you're going to discover along the way. The goal is to optimize, and that's just what we're going to do. These initial lab results represent your physical starting point . . . and they are *filled* with potential.

You might feel like you're just fine and can skip this step, but pretty much everyone I've ever tested had some results that were suboptimal. Especially when it comes to fertility (for both men and women), we want your lab work to be as optimal as possible, because that has a measurable impact on the chances of everything going well with conception and the health of your baby. And here's another thing to keep in mind—there's always the possibility that your test results show something very abnormal, and you might feel like you need more support to fix the problem. If that's the case, I encourage you to join the Every Baby Well program so you can get additional guidance.

Why Blood Sugar Is Key

For both men and women, a key aspect to optimizing health and boosting fertility has to do with controlling your blood sugar levels. For men, high blood sugar can cause damage to sperm because elevated glucose levels can lead to oxidative stress, which can impair sperm quality and motility.[60] In women, high blood sugar levels and glucose spikes can disrupt the hormonal balance necessary for ovulation and menstrual regularity.[61] Plus, you can reduce your risk of gestational diabetes if you control your blood sugar levels before becoming pregnant.[62]

In terms of your future child, the goal is to give them more blood sugar resilience. According to the National Library of Medicine, type 2 diabetes is very much on the rise, with 2021 seeing a large increase of cases.[63] By taking control of your blood sugar now, you can prevent that future for your child.

Even if you aren't aware of having any blood sugar issues, learning how your body reacts to certain foods provides amazing insight. That's why I encourage you to wear a continuous glucose monitor for two weeks while keeping a food journal, so you can see—in real time— which foods and combinations cause your blood sugar to spike and which do not. You might be surprised that certain indulgences don't impact you as much as you'd expect, and you'll be able to identify the ones that do.

There are four options for glucose monitoring systems that I recommend: Theia, Dexcom, Levels, and Freestyle. They are all easy to use, and they all offer real-time data. You can set customizable alerts for high and low glucose levels, allowing for proactive management of blood sugar levels and reducing the risk of hypoglycemia (low blood sugar) and hyperglycemia (high blood sugar). Wearing one of these discreet monitors won't disrupt your lifestyle but will empower you to make informed decisions so you can keep your blood sugar under control.

Cholesterol and Inflammatory Markers: Boston Heart Test

Did you know that our bodies make hormones out of cholesterol? Cholesterol serves as the precursor molecule for the synthesis of steroid hormones. In specialized cells within the adrenal glands, ovaries, testes, and other tissues, cholesterol molecules are converted into specific hormones through a series of enzymatic reactions. So, as you can imagine, having sufficient cholesterol is imperative so your body can make all the hormones necessary for reproduction. Despite the mainstream narrative about cholesterol, I'm actually more concerned about low cholesterol than high cholesterol. Surprising, right?

To accurately assess your cholesterol levels, I recommend the Boston Heart test, which is a comprehensive cardiovascular risk assessment that provides detailed information about your heart health. I like this specific test because it includes a combination of lipid panel testing (including LDL cholesterol, HDL cholesterol, and triglycerides) as well as more advanced lipid markers, including particle sizes, inflammatory markers, genetic markers, and other cardiovascular risk factors. Cleveland HeartLab also offers a multimarker approach and is a wonderful alternative.

Believe it or not, traditional lipid panel testing has very little correlation with who is actually getting cardiovascular disease. That's because it overlooks a key element: particle size. When it comes to

LDL, small particle sizes do more damage and cause more athero-sclerosis (plaque buildup) than larger particle sizes. And for HDL, we want the big particles that are good "garbage trucks" going and picking up all the oxidized cholesterol.

Inflammatory markers are also important to consider because we know that inflammation is highly correlated with infertility.[64] There are many different types of inflammation, and both the Boston Heart test and Cleveland HeartLab look at multiple types. If any are detected, you can get to work reducing your overall inflammation, which directly impacts the quality of both the egg and sperm. Furthermore, when you reduce your inflammation, it can lead to the activation of beneficial genes and the suppression of harmful ones, promoting healthier fetal development.

It's important to find the *source* of the inflammation and address this. Sources of inflammation can be increased gut permeability from dysbiosis (an imbalance in gut bacteria), food allergies, low-grade infections, toxins, and more. Addressing the root cause to lower inflammation can also improve the quality of the egg and sperm at a molecular level. Healthier gametes, or reproductive cells, are less likely to carry epigenetic markers associated with chronic diseases, such as diabetes, heart disease, and obesity. Consequently, your baby has a lower risk of inheriting these predispositions.[65]

Gut Microbiome Test

It's well known in functional medicine that diseases often have root causes in the gut. Improving the microbiome enhances whole-body health and decreases disease risk. More recent evidence on epigenetics helps us understand this connection, and how the microbiome (and genetic material found in the microbiome) influences epigenetics.[66]

One connection we are learning more about is the interaction between the gut microbiome and immune health. Not surprisingly, the epicenter of immune health is in the gut.[67] In fact, 70 to 80 percent of our immune cells are in the gut.[68] The gut is a primary site where the body interacts with the environment. DNA doesn't just exist in our cells; the microbiome accounts for around 90 percent of the total genetic material in the body.[69] Our immune system and microbiome have evolved together—we are forever linked and dependent upon each other.

How Microbes Keep Us Healthy

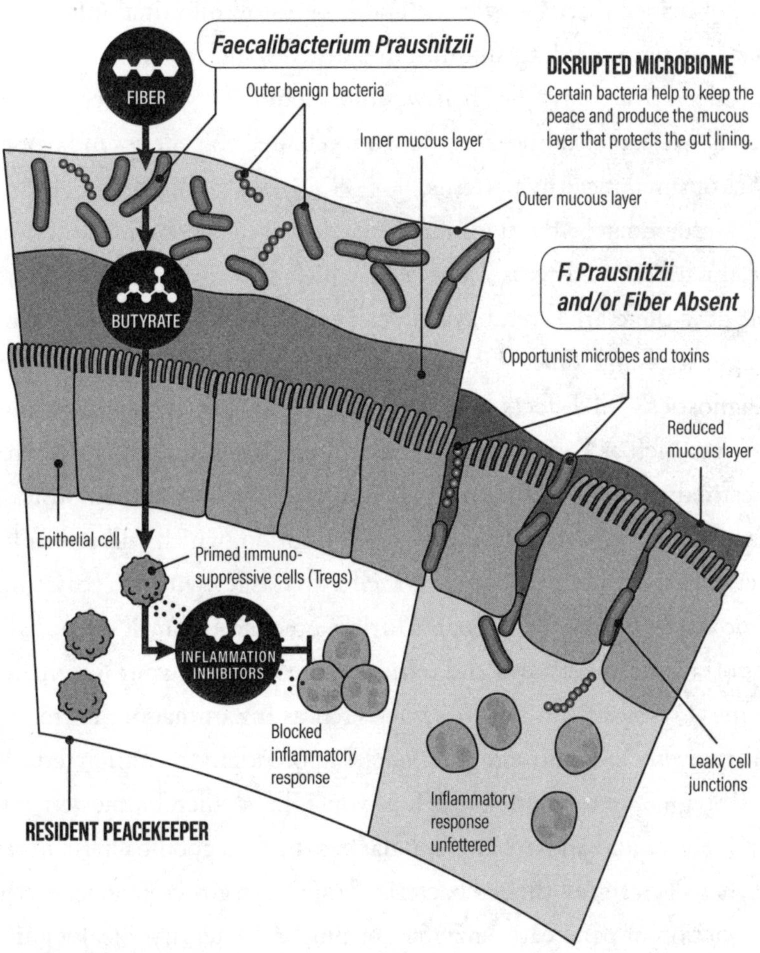

Many immune cells in the GI tract fight pathogens, balance inflammation, and influence epigenetics. The organisms, including bacteria that live in the GI tract, create metabolites, which are substances that are created when the body breaks down food, medications, chemicals, or even its own tissues, which influence immune cells, including helper T cells and other white blood cells. Helper T cells are a critical part of adaptive immunity and produce cytokines, which are inflammatory messengers.

Research suggests epigenetic mechanisms that result in an imbalance of helper T cells may cause and progress to intestinal inflammatory diseases, including autoimmune diseases such as Crohn's disease and ulcerative colitis.[70] When we understand the specific epigenetic drivers, we can also understand how to change epigenetics in favor of more optimal, healthy patterns.

Unfortunately, the traditional labs do not do a good job at testing the microbiome. This is an area in which the advanced labs shine, and now there are several available. Two of my favorites are Genova Diagnostics and GI-MAP. A GI microbiome test, such as Genova Diagnostics's GI Effects test, analyzes the diverse array of microorganisms such as bacteria, parasites, and yeasts residing in the gastrointestinal tract, providing insights into the balance and composition of gut flora.[71] GI-MAP tests are another option, which will screen for over fifty bacterial pathogens, as well as parasites, viruses, yeast, and *Helicobacter pylori* (*H. pylori*). During preconception, it's especially important to understand and optimize the health of your gut microbiome. Dysbiosis can lead to issues such as inflammation, hormonal imbalances, and nutrient deficiencies, potentially affecting fertility and pregnancy outcomes.[72] When you take a microbiome test you can identify and address any imbalances, such as good bacteria insufficiency or overgrowth; bad bacteria; fungal overgrowth; parasites; the production of pancreatic enzymes; or mucosal integrity ("leaky gut"). You can analyze how well the bacteria are doing their job, the strength of your immune system, and any potential sources of inflammation. All of this will assist you in working toward creating a supportive environment for conception and pregnancy.

Hormone Testing

As you might know, hormonal imbalances can impact fertility in both men and women, affecting ovulation, sperm production, and overall reproductive health. Here is a brief overview of why hormone testing is important during the conception process for both men and women, along with specific sex hormones to be assessed.

For Women

- **Ovulation:** Hormonal imbalances, such as irregularities in the menstrual cycle or ovulatory dysfunction, can affect a woman's ability to conceive. Testing hormone levels can help identify issues that may be hindering ovulation. I recommend you track your ovulation using at-home fertility testing kits, which I'll explain further.

- **Progesterone:** Progesterone is a key hormone involved in preparing the uterus for pregnancy and supporting early pregnancy. Low progesterone levels can impact fertility and increase the risk of miscarriage,[73] but the good news is it's an easy fix! One of my patients, Ryan, needed progesterone supplementation throughout her first two pregnancies, but then we worked to get her health optimized, and *voila*—her progesterone levels were perfect in her third pregnancy!

- **Estrogen:** Estrogen plays a crucial role in regulating the menstrual cycle and preparing the uterus for implantation. Imbalances in estrogen levels can affect fertility and reproductive health. A lot of women have low estrogen, but some have estrogen dominance, which is caused by endocrine disruptors. If you've struggled with estrogen dominance, you might consider a pelvic ultrasound or a Prenuvo full-body MRI scan, which can detect polycystic ovary syndrome (PCOS), endometriosis, and more.[74]

- **FSH (follicle-stimulating hormone) and LH (luteinizing hormone):** FSH and LH are important hormones involved in the menstrual cycle and ovulation. Abnormal levels of these hormones can indicate issues with ovarian function and egg maturation.

- **Prolactin:** Your pituitary gland produces prolactin, which is a hormone that primarily regulates lactation. However, high levels of prolactin (hyperprolactinemia) can disrupt ovulation and menstrual cycles, making it more difficult to become pregnant.[75] If it is elevated, further evaluation will be warranted.

- **Androgens:** Androgens are precursors to estrogen synthesis, which is the process of creating estrogen. The enzyme *aromatase* converts androgens like testosterone and androstenedione into estradiol and estrone (forms of estrogen). Estrogen is crucial for follicle growth, ovulation, and endometrial preparation for implantation. Moderate androgen levels support the growth and maturation of ovarian follicles, which house eggs. Androgens enhance:
  - *Follicular recruitment:* The early stages of follicle selection.
  - *Follicular sensitivity:* This is in response to FSH (follicle-stimulating hormone), which is critical for egg maturation. A lack of androgens can impair ovarian responsiveness, leading to poor ovarian reserve or poor-quality eggs.
  - *Sexual health:* Androgens play a role in libido and sexual function, indirectly influencing fertility by promoting intercourse frequency.

However, excess androgens (hyperandrogenism) is a hallmark of conditions like PCOS, which is a leading cause of female infertility. High androgen levels can lead to:

- *Effects on ovulation:* High androgens disrupt the hypothalamic-pituitary-ovarian (HPO) axis, leading to irregular or absent ovulation (anovulation). This occurs because elevated androgens can impair the proper signaling of FSH and LH.

- *Impact on egg quality:* Excess androgens can lead to the accumulation of immature follicles in the ovaries, reducing egg quality.

- *Insulin resistance:* Hyperandrogenism often coincides with insulin resistance, further contributing to ovulatory dysfunction. Insulin resistance increases androgen production in the ovaries, creating a vicious cycle.

- *Endometrial effects:* High androgens can impair endometrial receptivity, making it harder for an embryo to implant.

Low androgen levels can also impair fertility by reducing ovarian function and egg quality in the following ways:

- *Poor follicular development:* Insufficient androgens result in reduced estrogen production, leading to poor follicle maturation. This is common in conditions such as premature ovarian insufficiency (POI) or low ovarian reserve.

- *Decreased libido and energy:* Low androgen levels may reduce sexual activity, indirectly affecting fertility.

Finally, here's a list of conditions linked to androgen imbalance and fertility:

- **Polycystic Ovary Syndrome (PCOS):** Characterized by high androgens, irregular ovulation, and infertility.

Symptoms include acne, hirsutism (excess hair growth), and weight gain.

- **Congenital Adrenal Hyperplasia (CAH):** A genetic condition leading to overproduction of androgens by the adrenal glands. This can cause menstrual irregularities and ovulatory dysfunction.

- **Premature Ovarian Insufficiency (POI):** Low androgen levels are common and contribute to reduced ovarian function.

- **Hypothalamic Amenorrhea:** Low androgens due to stress, excessive exercise, or low body weight can lead to infertility.

For Men

- **Testosterone:** Testosterone is the primary male sex hormone that plays a key role in sperm production and overall reproductive health. Low testosterone levels can impact sperm quality and fertility. I recommend testing for free and total testosterone and sex hormone binding globulin, which equates more to what's happening in the body, in addition to total testosterone.

- **FSH and LH:** In men, FSH and LH are crucial for stimulating sperm production in the testes. Testing levels of these hormones can provide insights into potential issues with sperm quality, production, and fertility.

- **Prolactin:** High levels of prolactin in men can suppress testosterone production and affect sperm production.[76] If prolactin is high, it would be wise to evaluate further to check for tumors and other concerns.

- **Estradiol (Estrogen):** Produced in small amounts in men, estradiol plays a role in sperm maturation and maintaining hormonal balance. High estradiol is common in obese men, as adipose tissue (body fat) converts testosterone to estradiol (via aromatase enzyme). High estradiol can suppress testosterone production and impair sperm quality. On the other hand, low estradiol can disrupt spermatogenesis (the process of sperm cell production) and libido.

- **Inhibin B:** Produced by the Sertoli cells in the testes, inhibin B regulates FSH levels through negative feedback. Low inhibin B indicates Sertoli cell dysfunction, leading to reduced spermatogenesis and fertility.
- **DHEA:** A precursor to testosterone and other androgens, DHEA supports overall hormonal balance and sperm health. Low DHEA levels may contribute to reduced testosterone production.

Cortisol Testing

Often referred to as the "stress hormone," cortisol helps regulate metabolism, reduce inflammation, and control the body's sleep-wake cycle.[77] Cortisol also helps the body respond to stress. To see if you're dealing with chronic stress, check your cortisol levels throughout the day. If you have low cortisol, that can be a marker for adrenal fatigue (or when the adrenal glands have become overworked due to chronic stress and are no longer producing hormones appropriately). A DHEA test will also help ascertain the health of your adrenal glands. The last thing you want to do is attempt to conceive a baby when your body is under stress and your cortisol levels are high. In fact, high levels of cortisol have been correlated to infertility.[78]

Thyroid Hormone Testing

I think of the thyroid as the canary of the body. If something isn't quite right with the thyroid, it can be an indication of nutritional deficiencies, such as being low in iodine, or direct toxicity, such as when a patient still has amalgam fillings releasing mercury into their tissues. And the thyroid is often the first organ to be affected if a patient has an autoimmune process going on (this is when the immune system mistakenly attacks the body's own healthy cells, causing inflammation and disease instead of fighting off harmful invaders). So especially during this preconception period, you want to take a close look at your thyroid labs to detect anything like subclinical hypothyroidism, which is related to sperm and egg quality.[79]

I like to start with bloodwork when it comes to testing all hormones, but depending upon your results, we may also need to consider a saliva and urine test to get a clearer picture. Start with a TSH, Free T4, Free T3, Reverse T3, Thyroid Peroxidase Antibody, Thyroglobulin Antibody, and Thyroid Receptor Antibody.

The Advanced Hormone Test

The DUTCH test (which stands for Dried Urine Test for Comprehensive Hormones) is a type of hormone test that provides a comprehensive assessment of sex and adrenal hormones and their metabolites, as well as daily (diurnal) pattern of free cortisol, along with melatonin (6-OHMS), 8-OHdG, and six organic acids (OAT).[80]

I like to use the DUTCH test for assessing overall hormone balance and finding potential imbalances that may impact fertility and overall reproductive health. Imbalances in hormones such as estrogen, progesterone, testosterone, and cortisol can affect fertility and the ability to conceive. There are also salivary tests that can provide a twenty-eight-day assessment. Genova Diagnostics offers a one-day hormone check salivary test, as well as an Adrenocortex Stress Profile (which measures DHEA and cortisol). Additional tests using serum, urine, or stool samples for gut health, nutritional status, and immune function are also available.[81] By understanding your body's unique interplay between hormones, epigenetics, and reproductive health, you'll be better equipped to make informed decisions about lifestyle changes, nutritional interventions, and other strategies to support fertility and preconception health.

Traditional Fertility Testing

Anti-Müllerian Hormone (AMH)

The anti-müllerian hormone (AMH) is a protein produced by cells in the ovaries and is commonly used as a marker of ovarian reserve. For men, this protein is produced in the testes.

Testing AMH levels is most helpful in couples using assisted reproductive technology (ART) to conceive. Hormone values like AMH and FSH often correlate with how well a woman will respond to fertility medications, how many eggs she'll yield, and her likelihood of getting pregnant with IVF.[82] But if you are trying to conceive naturally, AMH test results may not be particularly helpful to you. In fact, when I was going through infertility myself, this was one test result that led my doctor to conclude that I would be highly unlikely to conceive naturally. So, it can be misleading.

I will use it sometimes to track progress, as it can be an indication of things getting better. But of course, the real indication of improvement is getting pregnant easily and having a healthy baby!

At-home Fertility Test Kits

Earlier, I mentioned that you'll be tracking ovulation during this process. These at-home urine tests measure LH, estrogen, and progesterone, giving insight into hormonal levels crucial for fertility. This is something you can start using right away, but I do want to advise you to take the results with a grain of salt, since it's not a perfect science. Bad results might not be totally accurate, so don't worry. However, if the result does indicate you're fertile, it's likely correct. You can always do a Rhythm saliva test with your physician or the Preconception program to learn generally when you ovulate every month. (And remember . . . just because you *can* get pregnant doesn't mean you *should* get pregnant . . . yet. The goal is to optimize your and your partner's health and epigenetics before you pull the trigger!)

Sperm Testing

The SpermQT test is an innovative diagnostic tool offered by Path Fertility that measures the sperm's ability to locate, bind to, penetrate, and fertilize an egg. Unlike traditional semen analyses that primarily evaluate sperm count and motility, the SpermQT test analyzes DNA methylation patterns of over 1,200 genes essential for sperm function. This test categorizes sperm quality into Excellent, Normal, or Abnormal, and can identify subfertile men who might otherwise be missed by standard semen analyses.[83]

I believe that testing sperm quality with the SpermQT test during the preconception phase is crucial, as it provides a comprehensive evaluation of sperm health. This can be particularly important for couples experiencing unexplained infertility or recurrent IUI failure. By identifying potential issues at the genetic and epigenetic levels, the test helps in tailoring more effective fertility treatments and improving the chances of successful conception, as well as potentially improving the health of the child.[84] Additional in-depth sperm testing is becoming available to help track your progress in optimizing your sperm health and help you know when to get the green light to conceive.

Comprehensive Nutritional Test: NutrEval or ION Profile

The NutrEval® and ION Profile® tests, both offered by Genova Diagnostics, provide comprehensive assessments of your nutritional status. The NutrEval® test evaluates over 125 biomarkers to determine the body's functional need for forty different antioxidants, vitamins, minerals, essential fatty acids, amino acids, and other select nutrients.[85] By analyzing both blood and urine samples, NutrEval® offers personalized nutrient recommendations based on your unique biochemical profile, aiding in the identification of nutritional imbalances that may contribute to various health concerns, including chronic conditions and overall health optimization.

Similarly, the ION Profile® test measures more than 150 biomarkers, providing insight into a patient's health by assessing functional needs for antioxidants, B vitamins, minerals, essential fatty acids, amino acids, and other select nutrients. The ION Profile® combines several test profiles, including amino acid analysis, homocysteine levels, nutrient and toxic element profiles, oxidation markers, fatty acid profiles, and organic acid profiles.[86] This comprehensive evaluation helps identify functional nutritional inadequacies that can contribute to a variety of chronic health conditions.

Gaining a solid understanding of your nutritional status is crucial, since optimal nutrient levels can significantly impact fertility and epigenetics. Both NutrEval® and ION Profile® provide insights into specific nutrient deficiencies or imbalances, allowing prospective parents to tailor their dietary and supplement choices to support reproductive health.

Genetic Testing: A Personalized Approach

Earlier in chapter 1, we explored how our genes were once thought to dictate our health entirely, but we now understand that lifestyle plays a major role in shaping our wellness. The environment we create—through diet, movement, mindset, and daily habits—significantly influences our health and disease risk. This is great news because it means we have more control over our well-being than we once believed, especially when preparing for pregnancy.

That said, genetic testing still provides valuable insights, particularly when it comes to reproductive health. Several testing options can help identify potential risks and guide personalized health strategies:

- **Counsyl** offers extensive recessive gene testing, screening for over one hundred inherited disorders, including cystic fibrosis, sickle cell anemia, and Tay-Sachs disease. Understanding carrier status helps assess the likelihood of passing these conditions to a child.

- **GrowBaby** is designed specifically for mothers-to-be, analyzing genetic variations that impact maternal and fetal health throughout pregnancy. It reports on forty-two key genetic markers linked to biological processes that influence pregnancy outcomes.

- **IntellxxDNA** provides deeper genomic insights into fertility and pregnancy. Founder Sharon Hausman-Cohen has highlighted several key genetic factors, such as variants in the GP6 gene, which may increase miscarriage risk but can often be managed with low-dose aspirin, and Factor 2 and Factor 5 genes, which can contribute to pregnancy complications but may be mitigated with low-dose heparin. Additionally, inflammatory pathways like IL-6, IL-1, and TNF-alpha can play a role in recurrent pregnancy loss, and targeted supplements such as N-acetylcysteine (NAC) and omega-3s may help.

Understanding your genetic profile allows for a more tailored approach to fertility and pregnancy, moving beyond a one-size-fits-all model. Genetic counseling can be an essential next step to explore treatment options that best align with your results.

For a more detailed breakdown of these genetic factors and testing options, please see the appendix, where you can learn more about how you can truly capitalize on the opportunities these tests can offer you and your partner. It might seem daunting to delve deeper into it, but this really is what I think of as your golden chance to make a real difference in your health and your future child's health. So, if you feel that nudge or inspiration, I encourage you to go deeper into this topic!

Part of this overall genetic test can include an analysis of the MTHFR gene and COMT gene. These are two of the most important methylation genes, but there are others. You have the option to do the extensive genetic test, or to add these on to a basic test. Now, let's talk about why testing for these genes is so important.

MTHFR Gene

The MTHFR gene encodes an enzyme involved in folate metabolism, which plays a crucial role in DNA synthesis, repair, and methylation. Variations in the MTHFR gene, such as the C677T and A1298C polymorphisms, can impact the enzyme's activity and affect folate metabolism.[87] Genetic testing for MTHFR variants can reveal whether you have reduced enzyme function, which may impair folate metabolism and increase the risk of conditions such as neural tube defects in children.

Epigenetically, folate metabolism is closely linked to DNA methylation, a process that regulates gene expression. Adequate folate levels are essential for DNA methylation, which in turn influences gene activity and cellular function. Genetic variations in MTHFR may alter folate availability and impact DNA methylation patterns, potentially affecting gene expression and health outcomes in both parents and children.

COMT Gene

The COMT gene encodes an enzyme involved in the breakdown of catecholamines (neurotransmitters and hormones that play an important role in the body's stress response), including dopamine, epinephrine, and norepinephrine. Variations in the COMT gene can affect enzyme activity and neurotransmitter levels. Genetic testing for COMT variants can provide insight into your dopamine metabolism and neurotransmitter balance. Certain COMT variants are associated with differences in cognitive function, stress response, and mood regulation.

Epigenetically, neurotransmitter balance and stress response are influenced by environmental factors such as lifestyle, diet, and stress levels. Genetic variations in COMT may interact with environmental exposures to modulate neurotransmitter levels and stress reactivity, potentially impacting fertility, pregnancy outcomes, and maternal well-being.

I promise I'm not asking you to become a scientist in order to conceive a healthy baby. And I know that this isn't exactly "light reading" at times! But rather than just telling you to go out and get these tests without any explanation, I wanted to give you the "why" behind it. So again, during this preconception period, learning about your own body's unique gene variants through genetic testing empowers you to identify potential risks and take proactive steps to optimize your health and fertility.

Toxic Mold Testing

Mold testing isn't exactly the first thing you think of when you think about the tests needed for preconception, right? But mycotoxins—toxic compounds produced by certain molds—have been shown to impact our epigenetics and potentially have negative effects on fertility and genetic inheritance.[88] Because of that, even if you don't have any symptoms of mold toxicity, it's imperative that you be tested for mycotoxins.

I've shared with you my own journey with toxic mold, and since then, I've worked with countless patients who have had to fight similar battles. But sometimes high mycotoxin levels can lurk beneath the surface without causing a patient to get really sick. So that's why we still want to take a close look to see if you're unknowingly harboring mold.

Exposure to mycotoxins can disrupt normal epigenetic mechanisms, which regulate gene expression without altering the underlying DNA sequence.[89] Changes in epigenetic marks, such as DNA methylation and histone modifications, can cause decreased fertility, problems with fertilization, and have an effect on the ability to carry a baby to term. Plus, mycotoxin exposure has been linked to reproductive disorders, such as menstrual irregularities, infertility, and miscarriage.

Importantly, disruptions in epigenetic regulation caused by mycotoxins can potentially be transmitted across generations. In fact, because men constantly produce new sperm through ongoing cell division, they are more likely than women to collect and keep genetic changes caused by the environment,[90] including exposure to mycotoxins. Thus, understanding the epigenetic effects of mycotoxin exposure is critical for addressing fertility issues and mitigating the risk of passing along genetic issues to your future generations.

In addition to epigenetic changes, mycotoxins can be teratogenic, meaning they can cause birth defects. They can also have immunosuppressive, endocrine-disrupting, and carcinogenic effects. To learn more about how mycotoxins can affect pregnancy, refer to the appendix.

Environmental Toxin Testing

Environmental toxins are a hot topic these days. Depending on how much of a deep dive you've taken into toxin research, it can all start to feel overwhelming—like toxins are everywhere and there's nowhere to hide. I get it! The instinct might be to bury your head in the sand

and simply pretend like toxins don't affect you. But the truth is, toxin exposure *is* a big deal, and it *can* impact you in all kinds of unexpected ways. Toxins can lead to elevated oxidative stress and increase the demand on your body's detoxification pathways, particularly in the liver. And when the liver can't adequately eliminate toxins or infectious by-products, these toxins can clog up normal detox pathways and lead to all kinds of chronic inflammation symptoms. Toxins definitely do not make for the friendliest baby-making or baby-carrying environment!

As if that wasn't bad enough, environmental toxins such as heavy metals, pesticides, air pollutants, and endocrine-disrupting chemicals have been shown to disrupt normal epigenetic processes in various ways.[91] For example, they can alter DNA methylation patterns, histone modifications, and microRNA expression, which can lead to changes in gene expression that may contribute to various health conditions in parents and future children. Furthermore, studies have suggested that these epigenetic changes caused by environmental toxins can potentially be passed on to future generations through transgenerational epigenetic inheritance.[92] As we talked about earlier in the book, this means that the effects of toxin exposure may not only affect you, but also your children and even further descendants. A "toxic legacy," indeed.

In terms of fertility, exposure to environmental toxins can also have negative effects on reproductive health. For example, certain toxins have been linked to reproductive disorders, hormonal imbalances, infertility, and adverse pregnancy outcomes.[93] And we now know that during the crucial weeks when organs, vessels, membranes, and systems are forming, the umbilical cord doesn't just carry essential nutrients but also industrial chemicals, pollutants, and pesticides. This is contrary to what was previously believed—that the placenta protected the cord blood and the developing baby from most environmental chemicals and pollutants.[94]

There is good news here, I promise. You don't have to guess as to whether your body is carrying a toxin overload. And even if you do have an overload, you can significantly improve the situation. As you probably know by now, I believe data-driven knowledge is power. Vibrant Wellness and Mosaic Diagnostics both offer a Total Tox panel test that determines if you've been exposed to many different heavy metals and environmental toxins.[95]

This innovative testing panel can detect a wide range of toxic substances that may be present in the body due to environmental contamination, occupational exposures, or lifestyle factors. The Total Tox test analyzes samples such as blood and urine to provide a detailed profile of your toxic burden. It identifies various heavy metals such as lead, mercury, arsenic, and cadmium, as well as environmental toxins including pesticides, phthalates, PFAS, and volatile organic compounds (VOCs). The whole idea is to track your detoxification success by retesting after several months.[96]

Traditional labs that most doctors have access to do not test for toxins well, other than for acute poisoning. Several advanced laboratory companies are offering tests to assess your toxin levels that have built up in your body. These comprehensive panels are designed to detect and assess toxic exposures and their health impacts. Test panels may include pesticides and glyphosate, phthalates, PFAS, mycotoxins, plastics, heavy metals, and volatile organic compounds. Toxins from food, water, household products, personal care products, and air pollution can be detected. These panels are particularly beneficial for individuals experiencing health issues like ADHD, Alzheimer's disease, anxiety, asthma, autism spectrum disorders, cancer, cardiovascular disease, chronic fatigue, cognitive dysfunction, depression, diabetes, headaches, immune dysfunction, infertility, inflammatory bowel disease, obesity, memory disturbances, mood changes, neurological symptoms, respiratory problems, and sinus/nasal congestion, as well as for anyone interested in prevention.[97] My patients are often shocked at their results and find the importance of learning how to avoid exposures plus improve their detoxification pathways.

Autoimmune Panels

You've probably noticed there's a lot more talk these days about autoimmunity than there was a decade ago. And you might be wondering, *What exactly is an autoimmune process or disease?* To put it simply, when a patient has an autoimmune process going on, it means their immune system is mounting an attack against its own cells.[98] Essentially, it means the immune system has gotten confused because there are enough similarities between the toxin or infection and the body's own cells. Often, there are few or even no obvious symptoms that someone is experiencing autoimmunity, so that's why testing for it is critical.

One of my patients had very high autoimmune markers in her bloodwork, and so we worked to change her diet. When she was meticulous about eating gluten-free for six months, her ANA (antinuclear antibodies—a marker indicating autoimmunity) went to negative for the first time in many years. She still had some other autoimmune markers showing up as positive, but when she became meticulous about going dairy-free, those also normalized. So even if your bloodwork does indicate some autoimmune markers, there's lots of hope, and simple changes can make a huge difference.

Dietary changes are foundational, but some people also need to work on improving detoxification, mitochondrial function, and microbiome balance in addition to making dietary changes to reverse their autoimmune markers.

There's a general autoimmune disorder panel that can be ordered via Quest or Labcorp, and it looks at a range of markers, some of which are directly associated with miscarriage and infertility. During the preconception period, a Vibrant Wellness Autoimmune Zoomer test can also be helpful in assessing and addressing underlying autoimmune conditions that could impact fertility, pregnancy, and the health of your future child. Autoimmune disorders can have long-term effects on reproductive health and may influence epigenetic mechanisms that regulate gene expression and development. Again, I know this can be a little tough to wrap your arms around because many people don't realize they have autoimmune issues when they're going on beneath the surface. In chapter 12, "Taming Inflammation," I'll share a complete breakdown on how autoimmunity can be a serious hurdle to your preconception journey.

For all of these reasons, I recommend the autoimmune panel (a blood test that can be completed at any Labcorp or Quest lab). Here's a list of the autoimmune markers that can be included:

- ANA Screen, IFA, with Reflex to Titer and Pattern
- DNA (ds) Antibody, with Reflex to Titer
- Chromatin (Nucleosomal) Antibody
- Sm Antibody
- Sm/RNP Antibody
- RNP Antibody
- Sjogren's Antibodies (SS-A, SS-B)
- Scleroderma Antibody (Scl-70)
- Jo-1 Antibody
- Centromere B Antibody
- Complement Component C3c and C4c
- Cardiolipin and Phospholipid Antibodies (IgA, IgG, IgM)
- Beta-2-Glycoprotein I Antibodies (IgG, IgA, IgM)
- Rheumatoid Factor (IgA, IgG, IgM)
- Cyclic Citrullinated Peptide (CCP) Antibody (IgG)
- Mutated Citrullinated Vimentin (MCV) Antibody
- Thyroid Peroxidase Antibodies (TPO)[99]
- Thyroglobulin Antibodies
- Thyroid Receptor Antibodies

You can also use the Vibrant Wellness Neural Zoomer Plus.[100] This test measures immune reactivity to structures, tissues, cells, and chemicals in the brain and peripheral nervous system. It detects underlying inflammatory responses that may be causing symptoms related to mood, memory, aging, balance, nervous system function, movement, pain, and more.

Mitochondria Testing

Mitochondria are the powerhouses of the cell, so they are pretty much instrumental in all cellular function, and we need them to work well for optimization. Mitochondrial function is especially important because it clears inflammation, and inflammation is detrimental when it comes to both fertility and epigenetics. A healthy sperm and egg require good mitochondrial function.

An organic acids test gives an indirect view of how well your mito-chondria are making fuel and managing inflammation. I often use this test to get a basic overview of mitochondrial function, and it can be an easy way to assess progress in addressing mitochondrial dysfunction.

The mescreen™ test from Verséa Health, Inc. and MitoSwab allows you to see how your mitochondria are functioning in more detail. It's designed to evaluate mitochondrial efficiency by providing an energetic profile of your cells.[101] By assessing cellular health, we can take steps to improve mitochondrial function, thereby enhancing their fertility and ensuring a healthier environment for conception and pregnancy.

This is an exciting area of research that holds massive opportunity for improving health in general but also for fertility and generational health.

Lower Priority Tests

The tests we've discussed so far are primary tests that I highly recom-mend during preconception, both for women and men. Following are more tests for which the results are nice to have, especially if you are experiencing any specific symptoms described under each test, but I don't consider them absolutely necessary.

Neurotransmitter Test

A neurotransmitter test provides valuable insight into how your body is coping with stress and can predict levels of serotonin and dopamine, correlating these to mood-related symptoms. Neurotransmitters, secreted throughout the body, play crucial roles in both the central and peripheral nervous systems, as well as the gastrointestinal microbiome. Tests such as the Comprehensive Neurotransmitter Profile from Doctor's Data analyze urinary neurotransmitter levels, offering a comprehensive view of the body's neurotransmitter synthesis and breakdown capabilities.[102]

Especially if you are experiencing cognitive and mood concerns, diminished drive, fatigue, sleep difficulties, cravings, addictions, or abnormal gastrointestinal microbiome conditions, assessing urinary neurotransmitter levels can provide important clinical information. These symptoms can potentially be addressed by interpreting neurotransmitter levels to identify any imbalances, which then allows for targeted interventions to improve drive, sleep, and overall mood.

Genetic predispositions to conditions such as depression and anxiety can also be evaluated in conjunction with neurotransmitter levels, guiding specific supplement choices such as fish oil, glycine (an amino acid, which is a building block of protein), and GABA factors (chemical messengers in your brain). Additionally, if you're taking antidepressants, genetic testing can reveal which medications are most effective based on serotonin receptor function and metabolism. Nutritional cofactors, receptor mutations, and lifestyle factors such as diet, age, hormone imbalance, and chronic inflammation can all influence neurotransmitter levels.[103]

From an epigenetics perspective, neurotransmitter levels can impact gene expression and long-term health outcomes. During preconception, ensuring balanced neurotransmitter levels can contribute to a healthier epigenetic environment for the developing embryo. Stress and neurotransmitter imbalances can lead to epigenetic modifications that may affect fertility and the health of your baby.[104] By optimizing neurotransmitter balance through targeted interventions, both partners can enhance the quality of egg and sperm, promoting a healthier conception and pregnancy.

IgG Food Sensitivity Testing

Immunoglobulin G (IgG) food sensitivity tests aim to identify potential food sensitivities or intolerances that could impact overall health and well-being, including fertility and pregnancy outcomes. By assessing IgG-mediated immune responses to specific foods, we can gain insights into potential triggers for inflammation and immune dysregulation. Addressing underlying food sensitivities before conception can help reduce inflammation, support immune function, and create a more favorable environment for conception and pregnancy.

Histamine Intolerance and Mast Cell Activation Testing

Mast cells are immune cells found in all tissues of the body, with the highest levels found in the gut and skin where your body interacts with the environment. The main job of mast cells is to determine if there is a threat, either from an infection or a toxin, and then activate, producing a variety of chemicals that work to neutralize the threat or coordinate the immune system. When activated, mast cells release over two hundred chemicals, depending on the situation. Examples include:

- Inflammatory mediators, such as cytokines (which help the body fight infection or injury)
- Enzymes such as proteases (which break down proteins)
- Biogenic amines, such as histamine, tryptase (chemicals that act like messengers, influencing various bodily functions such as mood, sleep, appetite, and heart rate)
- Chromogranin A (CgA) (which acts like a signal flag in a blood test if a tumor is present)
- Diamine oxidase (DAO) (an enzyme that breaks down histamine). DAO deficiency can lead to histamine intolerance, leading to sickness when eating foods that contain histamine.

Mast cells provide a vital function within the immune system. When mast cells work well, they contribute to a normal immune response. But mast cell activation is when they are overactive, as in the case of extreme swelling from a bug bite or anaphylaxis from a peanut allergy. These allergic symptoms are a result of the release of histamines, powerful immune messengers that are released from mast cells.

Chronic inflammation associated with histamine intolerance and mast cell activation can also have detrimental effects on fetal development and growth. Excessive release of inflammatory mediators, such as histamines and cytokines, may impair placental function, fetal oxygenation (simply referring to how much oxygen the fetus is receiving via the umbilical cord), and nutrient delivery, increasing the risk of adverse pregnancy outcomes. Identifying histamine issues before conception allows for early intervention to minimize fetal exposure to inflammation and optimize fetal development.

I often encourage patients to get lab work done to look at histamine, tryptase, and chromogranin A, which can help indicate whether there is a histamine issue to be addressed.

Lyme Test

If you suspect Lyme disease or another tick-borne illness, check out TLab, which specializes in developing advanced diagnostic methods for detecting vector- and tick-borne pathogens. It's challenging to identify many of these types of pathogens with conventional testing, but TLab's excellent testing methods fill the gap where traditional tests fail. The company's research also helps us understand the role of these pathogens in conditions like neurological Lyme disease and melanoma, which allows for more accurate diagnostics and insights into disease mechanisms.[105]

Of all the different Lyme tests I've used over the years, I've found TLab to be the most reliable because many of the other tests over- or underestimate the presence of organisms.

The Connection Between Autism and the Gut

Researchers are actively investigating the potential links between microorganisms in the human gut and neurodevelopmental disorders, particularly autism spectrum disorder (ASD). Professor Alessio Fasano, a gastroenterologist at Massachusetts General Hospital in the US, leads a research project called GEMMA, which aims to unravel the connections between autism and gut health. Autism is believed to have genetic and environmental influences, with environmental factors potentially acting during the embryonic stage, such as prenatal exposure to infections or toxic chemicals. Fasano suggests that restoring balance to the microbiome, the ecosystem of microorganisms in the gut, could alleviate some autistic behavioral traits.

The GEMMA Study involves tracking five hundred infants who are siblings of children with autism to study microbial contents in their stools and explore potential treatments using probiotics and prebiotics to restore microbiome balance. The ultimate goal is early detection and treatment of autism before the onset of symptoms, through precision medicine approaches.[106]

What can we take away from this research? Creating and maintaining a balanced gastrointestinal microbiome during both the preconception and conception period is mission critical. And the best way to know how to do that is through microbiome testing. It's a significant piece of the epigenetic puzzle.

Methylation Testing

Methylation is a biochemical process that plays a critical role in various physiological functions within the body, including DNA synthesis and repair, gene expression regulation, neurotransmitter metabolism, detoxification pathways, and immune-system function. Proper methylation is essential for maintaining overall health and well-being, and disruptions in methylation pathways have been associated with a wide range of health conditions, including cardiovascular disease, neurodevelopmental disorders, autoimmune diseases, mood disorders, and infertility. In terms of your preconception health, optimal methylation is important for several reasons:

- *Epigenetic regulation*: Methylation plays a crucial role in epigenetic regulation. Epigenetic modifications, including DNA methylation, can influence fertility, embryonic development, and the health of future generations. Testing methylation patterns before conception can provide insights into potential epigenetic factors that may impact fertility and pregnancy outcomes.

- *Fetal development*: Methylation patterns established during preconception and early pregnancy can have lasting effects on fetal development and long-term health outcomes. Disruptions in methylation pathways, such as aberrant DNA methylation patterns, may increase the risk of developmental abnormalities, birth defects, and chronic health conditions in children. Testing methylation status before conception can help identify potential risks and inform preventive strategies to optimize fetal health.

- *Nutrient metabolism*: Methylation processes require adequate levels of certain nutrients, including folate, vitamin B12, betaine, and other methyl donors (which is basically a nutrient that helps regulate various bodily processes by donating a specific chemical unit to other compounds). Deficiencies in these nutrients can impair methylation pathways and increase the risk of fertility problems, pregnancy complications, and adverse maternal and fetal outcomes. Testing methylation status before conception can identify any nutritional deficiencies and help guide supplementation strategies to support optimal methylation and reproductive health.

Genova Diagnostics offers a methylation test called the Methylation Panel, which assesses key markers involved in methylation pathways.[107] This comprehensive panel provides insights into individual methylation status, nutrient requirements, genes, and potential metabolic imbalances that may impact fertility and pregnancy outcomes.

By testing methylation status during preconception, you can spot underlying imbalances, nutritional deficiencies, and genetic factors that may affect reproductive health and fertility. This information can help guide personalized interventions, including lifestyle modifications, targeted supplementation, and dietary changes, to optimize methylation pathways and support a healthy conception and pregnancy journey.

Heavy Metals Testing

Heavy metals are toxic elements that can accumulate in the body over time, primarily through environmental exposure, including air, water, food, and occupational sources. Common heavy metals of concern include mercury, lead, arsenic, cadmium, and aluminum. Here are some of the reasons we want to take potential heavy metal exposure seriously during the preconception period:

- *Impact on fertility*: Heavy metal exposure has been associated with reproductive toxicity and can adversely affect fertility in both men and women. Heavy metals such as lead, mercury, cadmium, and arsenic can disrupt hormone levels, impair sperm and egg quality, and interfere with reproductive processes, potentially leading to infertility or subfertility.

- *Pregnancy risks*: Heavy metal exposure during pregnancy can pose serious risks to maternal and fetal health. Heavy metals can cross the placental barrier and accumulate in fetal tissues, increasing the risk of developmental abnormalities, birth defects, miscarriage, and stillbirth. Identifying and addressing heavy metal exposure before conception can help reduce the risk of adverse pregnancy outcomes.

- *Impact on fetal development*: Heavy metals have been linked to neurodevelopmental disorders, cognitive impairments, and behavioral problems in children exposed during pregnancy. Prenatal exposure to heavy metals, even at low levels, can disrupt fetal brain development and lead to long-term neurobehavioral deficits. Identifying heavy metal exposure before conception can help mitigate these risks and promote healthy fetal development.

- *Optimizing reproductive health*: Addressing heavy metal exposure before conception is crucial for optimizing reproductive health and improving the chances of a successful pregnancy. By identifying and detoxifying heavy metals, we can support optimal fertility, hormonal balance, and overall reproductive function, creating a healthier environment for conception and pregnancy.

INTROSPECT

Since the buildup of heavy metals in the body is so common, I often recommend screening for heavy metals. (An alternative may be a Quicksilver heavy metal test for mercury, but this is not as accurate.) The only way to really know what's stored in the body is to do a heavy metal challenge. I use two different oral chelating agents. These agents form stable complexes that can be excreted via urine or feces. One agent is DMPS (dimercapto-propane sulfonate), and the other is DMSA (dimercaptosuccinic acid):

- *DMPS* has a higher affinity for mercury and is often used in cases of mercury toxicity, including exposure to dental amalgams (mercury fillings) and environmental mercury sources. DMPS forms complexes with mercury ions, facilitating their excretion from the body via urine. DMPS may also have some affinity for other heavy metals, such as arsenic and cadmium, but it is primarily used for mercury detoxification.

- *DMSA* is a chelating agent with a higher affinity for lead and is commonly used in cases of lead toxicity. It forms stable complexes with lead ions, allowing for their removal from the body via urine. DMSA may also have some efficacy in chelating other heavy metals, such as mercury, arsenic, and cadmium, although its affinity for lead is highest.[108]

Quicksilver Scientific's mercury tri-test and blood metals panel doesn't require a chelating agent, so it's not as informative as a test that does use the chelating agent, but it can still be helpful if it is positive. You can order it directly from Quicksilver Scientific.[109]

Testing allows you to assess the levels of heavy metals excreted in the urine before and after chelation therapy, providing valuable information about heavy metal burden and detoxification capacity. Once you know which, if any, heavy metals you're dealing with, you can come up with a specific chelation plan during your detoxification period of the preconception process.

Undiagnosed Celiac and Gluten Sensitivity: Effects on Fertility

Maintaining a gluten-free diet during the preconception period is crucial for women with celiac disease, as gluten exposure can adversely affect fertility and pregnancy outcomes. A study titled "Celiac Disease and Reproductive Disorders: Meta-Analysis of Epidemiologic Associations and Potential Pathogenic Mechanisms" highlights several key points:

- Women with untreated celiac disease may experience reproductive challenges, including delayed menarche, early menopause, and increased rates of infertility. Adhering to a strict gluten-free diet can mitigate these risks and improve fertility prospects.

- Gluten exposure in women with celiac disease is associated with higher incidences of miscarriage, intrauterine growth restriction, low birth weight, and preterm birth. A gluten-free diet helps reduce these risks, promoting healthier pregnancy outcomes.

- The autoimmune reaction triggered by gluten intake in celiac patients can lead to placental damage, adversely affecting fetal development. Eliminating gluten from the diet prevents this immune response, safeguarding both maternal and fetal health.[110]

- I highly recommend avoiding gluten to help lower your overall inflammation, regardless of whether you've identified having a gluten sensitivity.

- Traditional testing often misses gluten sensitivity and celiac. The Wheat Zoomer Test by Vibrant Wellness and the Gluten Sensitivity Stool Test by EnteroLab are examples of testing that are more accurate.

Knowing Your Starting Point

The main areas we want to look closely at during pre-conception are: your mitochondrial function, hormones, gut microbiome, inflammation and autoimmunity markers, nutrient levels, blood sugar and metabolic health, sperm and egg assessment, mycotoxins (mold), genetic testing, neurotransmitters, histamine issues, food allergies, infections, methylation, toxin levels, and gluten issues.

To give you a sense of an order of importance, here's how I like to prioritize the tests. Of course, you'll want to take into account your own, unique set of circumstances and symptoms when deciding which tests to take.

Essential for Any Preconception Patient

- Baseline overall panel
  - CBC (complete blood count)
  - Detailed thyroid test (TSH, tpo ab, tg ab, tr ab, free T3, free T4, reverse T3)
  - Complete metabolic panel
  - GGT
  - HGA1C, insulin
  - Hormones (LH, free testosterone, DHEA, cortisol, fractionated estrogens, prolactin)
  - Iron and TIBC, ferritin
  - General inflammation markers hs-CRP, uric acid
  - Nutrients vitamin D25, B12, B1, homocysteine, folate
  - General autoimmune panel (ANA, phospholipid abs)
- Blood sugar/metabolic health with CGM
- Sperm assessment
- Detailed nutrient levels (CoQ10, vitamin C, vitamin E, zinc, glutathione)
- Toxin levels (plastics, pesticides, PFAS, heavy metals, and other toxins)

Highest Importance: Looking for Big Levers

I recommend these to the vast majority of my preconception patients, as they give such valuable insight.

- Advanced nutrients
- Gut microbiome
- Advanced hormones: DUTCH test or similar
- Methylation
- Mitochondrial function
- Advanced inflammation levels

Important (But Use Your Judgment)

Now that you've read up on these tests, think about your own family history, health history, and any recent symptoms to determine whether you want to invest in these tests. There's no downside to getting more data!

- Mycotoxins
- Heavy metals
- Genetic testing
- Recessive gene testing
- Neurotransmitters
- Histamine issues
- Food allergies (IgG, IgA)
- Chronic infections
- Gluten intolerance or celiac
- Advanced cholesterol
- Autoimmunity, neuroautoimmunity

Final Thoughts

I realize I'm recommending a lot of tests and lab work to be completed. At the beginning of this journey, we talked about the level of commitment required for this process, so I just want to take a moment to remind you of that commitment. You *can* do this, and you'll be so glad to go into the rest of this program armed with specific data about your body.

Q&A

Q: Why should I get lab testing if I feel perfectly healthy?

A: Even if you feel great, your lab work might reveal underlying imbalances that could impact fertility and your future child. Many issues, such as blood sugar irregularities, nutrient deficiencies, and inflammation, don't always show obvious symptoms but can still affect conception and pregnancy. Optimizing your health now can help set you up for success when trying to conceive.

Q: How do I know which tests are actually necessary?

A: There are countless lab tests available, and not all of them are useful for preconception. That's why this chapter focuses on the most essential ones, including metabolic health, hormone balance, inflammation markers, gut health, and genetic risks. To help prioritize, see the test recommendations outlined in this chapter—or refer to the Every Baby Well program for the latest curated list.

Q: I've only ever had standard bloodwork—how is this different?

A: Most routine bloodwork only scratches the surface. In functional medicine, we go deeper, looking at key factors like nutrient levels, hormone balance, and inflammatory markers that standard panels often overlook. This gives you a more complete picture of your overall health and fertility potential.

Q: What if my results aren't "perfect"?

A: No one's lab work is flawless—there's always opportunity for improvement! If something comes back suboptimal, that's actually a good thing—it means you now have actionable information to optimize your body before conception. Small changes based on your data can make a big difference in your fertility and overall health.

Q: How can I get these tests without a doctor's prescription?

A: If you're part of the Every Baby Well program, you can order at-home testing kits and access lab orders directly through your portal. This also includes support for interpreting your results so you can take the right next steps to optimize your fertility.

Want to dive deeper? See the appendix for a full breakdown of recommended tests and the latest advancements in fertility lab work.

Believe

Introspect

Renew

Thrive

Hope

Section III Introduction

Renew is all about giving your body a fresh start—clearing out toxins and nourishing yourself so you and your partner can create the healthiest possible environment for conception. Research shows that exposure to things such as heavy metals, hormone-disrupting chemicals, and even nutrient deficiencies before pregnancy can impact your fertility and the health of your future child's development—affecting everything from IQ to behavior and long-term health. But here's the good news: You have the power to change that!

In this section, you'll learn simple, practical ways to reduce harmful toxins in your daily life, support your body's natural detox processes, and rebuild with the right nutrients. Think of it as hitting the reset button—helping both of you feel your best while optimizing fertility and setting the stage for a thriving, healthy baby.

Chapter 5: Pollution Solutions offers practical guidance on reducing exposure to the most common pollutants in our environment, from household chemicals to dietary toxins. You'll discover how to create a cleaner, healthier environment in which to conceive. You'll also learn to identify and eliminate invisible culprits that may be affecting your body's natural systems.

Chapter 6: Clean Slate: Detox for Baby-Building explores targeted detoxification techniques to support your body's renewal. This chapter provides a step-by-step approach to removing internal toxins, with practical guidance on optimizing nutrition to support your body's natural cleansing processes. You'll leave this chapter with a tool kit for ongoing detoxification and health maintenance, and you'll be equipped to provide a clean and supportive environment for conception.

Chapter 7: You Can't Be "a Little Bit" Nutritious explores how balanced nutrition plays a crucial role in rebuilding and energizing your body. Here, you'll receive guidance on essential nutrients, food choices, and dietary habits that not only support detoxification but also nourish you at a cellular level. With a focus on whole, nutrient-dense foods, you'll learn how to optimize your diet to enhance energy, support fertility, and lay the groundwork for a healthy pregnancy.

Chapter 8: Tuning In: The Art of Balanced Living introduces a vital practice—listening to your body's signals. This chapter encourages you to become more attuned to subtle cues that indicate shifts in energy, stress, and overall wellness. By "tuning in," you gain insight into your body's responses to changes in diet, lifestyle, and environment, helping you make informed adjustments that support renewal. This awareness strengthens your ability to respond to your body's needs, creating a more nurturing and mindful foundation for conception.

As you read these chapters and start making changes, keep your motivation—your love for your future child—in mind, and know that it's not supposed to be easy, but it *is* supposed to be deeply impactful. Gather your inner resources, find your strength, and commit to growing a healthy family.

Pollution Solutions

One of your primary goals during preconception is to minimize variables that could impact not only your own health, but the health of your future child. This means actively reducing your daily exposure to toxins. It helps to think of this like preparing a healthy recipe—using wholesome ingredients is crucial. The same principle applies when preparing your body for conception and pregnancy—creating a healthy environment is essential for making a healthy baby!

Researchers at the University of Texas Health Science Center at San Antonio published a study in 2024 that showed that if prospective parents avoid toxic exposures, it could help prevent autism as well as ADHD in their future children.[111] Further research is needed to fully understand the mechanisms at play, but I think we are on the brink of a scientific revolution, with emerging research confirming what we've seen play out in functional and integrative medicine offices for many years—exposure to toxins plays a key role in the health of future generations.

Cleaning up your environment is an ongoing process throughout this preconception period. It's not something that needs to happen overnight. Instead, aim to make consistent progress each week. Begin by simply becoming more aware of the toxins present in your surroundings. Once you identify them, you can start taking steps to reduce or eliminate these harmful substances.

Your goal is to reduce the overall amount of toxins your body is taking in and accumulating so the work you do later in terms of detoxification, nutrition, and supplementation is even more effective. Here's a visual that might help. Imagine a big sink filled with water, one that has a very slow drain. Your goal is to drain the sink as much as possible so it doesn't overflow, but the faucet is on, and the water coming out of the faucet represents environmental toxins. Before you spend a lot of time and energy unclogging the drain, you first want to drastically slow down the amount of water pouring into the sink. That's what this chapter is all about—slowing down the influx of toxins coming into your body.

Toxins are sneaky. They show up in all kinds of unexpected products that we use or interact with every single day. And since most of us don't have any kind of immediate "reaction" to them, we likely don't realize when we've encountered a toxin. Their effects are silent, but they accumulate in our bodies over time. That's why we need to spend a little time getting educated on how to be on the lookout for toxins.

In the appendix, you'll find a chart of toxins and their potential effects on your reproductive health as well as epigenetics. It's a lot of information to sort through, but it can be a truly valuable tool. For right now, however, I want to draw your attention to some of the most common toxins in our environment and give you some basic tips on how to start avoiding them today.

Common Toxins

Glyphosate

You've possibly heard about the controversies surrounding glyphosate, the active ingredient in many herbicides such as Roundup®.

Toxins' Impact on Male Fertility

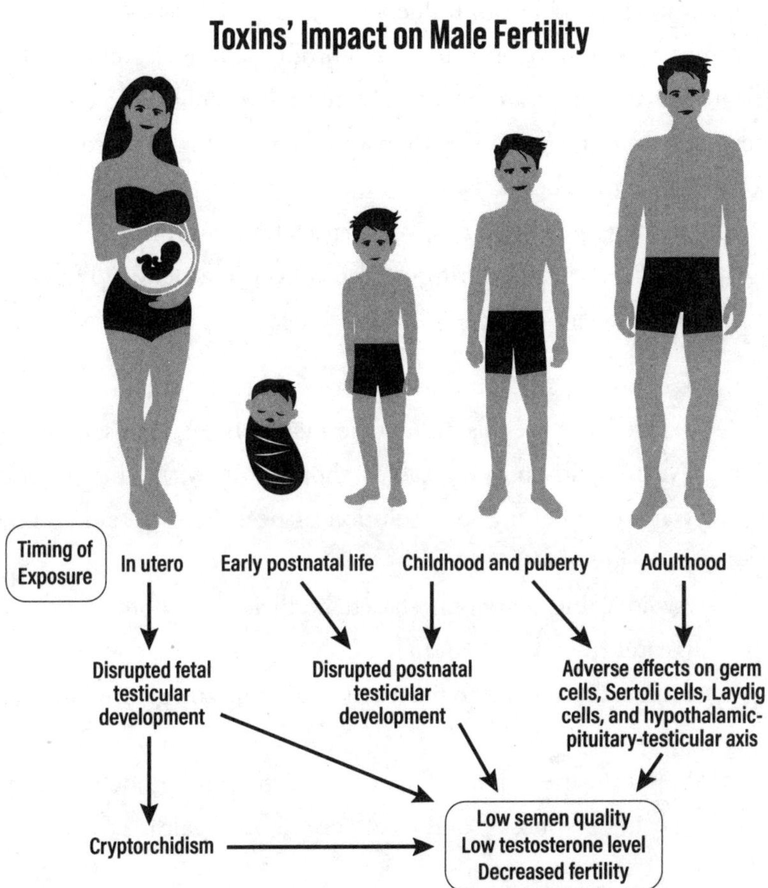

Glyphosate is used extensively in agriculture to control weeds and is one of the most widely used herbicides in the world. According to the Environmental Protection Agency (EPA), glyphosate residues can be found on various crops, including soybeans, corn, and cotton. This toxin is pervasive in our food supply and even in our water sources.[112]

Glyphosate's potential impact on health, particularly its role as an endocrine disruptor, has raised significant concerns. Studies suggest that glyphosate can interfere with hormonal functions by mimicking hormones and binding to hormone receptors,[113] and that this type of endocrine disruption can influence numerous biological processes, including growth, development, and reproduction. Research has also indicated that glyphosate exposure can lead to epigenetic changes, potentially affecting gene expression and contributing to reproductive disorders and other health issues.[114]

Given these potential risks, it's crucial to minimize exposure to glyphosate, especially during the preconception period. Here are some things you can do:

- Choose organic produce when possible, as organic farming restricts the use of synthetic herbicides like glyphosate.
- Wash fruits and vegetables thoroughly with vinegar and water or a baking soda solution or peel them to remove any pesticide residues.
- Avoid using glyphosate-based herbicides in home gardens. (Instead, weed by hand.)
- Support farmers who practice sustainable and glyphosate-free farming methods.
- Stay informed about the latest research and guidelines concerning glyphosate and its effects on our health.

Lead

Lead has its useful place—it's used in various industrial products, such as batteries, paints, pipes, and ceramics—but it is highly toxic to humans, especially when inhaled or ingested through contaminated air, water, soil, or products. Once in the body, lead accumulates in bones, blood, and tissues, where it has been linked to a wide range of health issues, particularly in children. Research shows that lead exposure may contribute to reduced IQ, learning disabilities, and behavioral issues such as impulsivity and attention disorders. It is also associated with disruptions in neural development, potentially affecting memory, learning, and behavior. Physically, lead exposure has been linked to stunted growth, hearing loss, and anemia due to its interference with hemoglobin production.

Lead exposure impacts the hypothalamic-pituitary-adrenal axis, which regulates stress responses and various hormones. In both men and women, lead can affect reproductive hormones, leading to decreased testosterone in men and altered estrogen levels in women. It may also impact thyroid function, potentially disrupting metabolism and growth. And what can all these harmful hormonal disruptions lead to? Reproductive issues, developmental problems, and increased risk for certain diseases.[115]

Studies suggest lead may also weaken the immune system and impair kidney function, increasing susceptibility to infections and ushering in other health challenges. If you've been exposed to lead and you're thinking about getting pregnant, know that lead has been shown to cross the placenta, where it may contribute to low birth weight, premature birth, and developmental delays. So, discovering and dealing with lead exposure *now* is imperative.

Despite all these risks, lead exposure is often incorrectly thought of as just a historical issue, but that's not a safe assumption. Research indicates that up to 30 percent of drinking water may contain lead, often due to aging pipes, and contamination from old paint, soil, and imported products continues to pose risks. I highlighted this in an article on my blog, "Don't Raise Your Glass: It May Be Toxic,"[116] where I explained how families can take proactive steps by using lead test kits, available on Amazon, to detect the amount of lead in their water, air, and household items. Addressing these sources can help mitigate lead exposure and protect against its long-term health effects.

BPA, BPS, and BPB

You've probably noticed "BPA-free" labels on plastic products, and those labels are there for a reason. Bisphenol A (BPA) is a chemical produced in large quantities for use primarily in the production of polycarbonate plastics and epoxy resins.[117] BPA is one of the most common widespread toxins. According to the National Institute of Environmental Health Sciences, "BPA can leach into food from the protective internal epoxy resin coatings of canned foods and from consumer products such as polycarbonate tableware, food storage containers, water bottles, and baby bottles."[118]

When we received results for my patient Catherine, I thought for sure there had been an error. Her BPA levels were off the charts. But when we sat down and talked through every aspect of her day, she mentioned that she loved the clean, organic soups from a local restaurant and ate it for lunch at least three days per week. I asked, "Do you eat in the restaurant or pick it up?"

She answered, "I usually either pick it up or have it delivered to my office."

"What do they put the soup in?" I asked.

Realizing where I was going, she smacked her palm to her forehead, "Oh my gosh. They put that hot soup into a plastic container. That's where I'm getting BPA, isn't it?"

A little detective work goes a long way! I was so happy we were able to find the source of her BPA toxicity. There was no need for her to give up the delicious, healthy soup, so she started going to eat at the restaurant instead, where they served it in a porcelain bowl rather than a plastic container. I put her on my detoxification protocol, and about six months later, we re-tested. There was no sign of BPA. The body is truly amazing!

So it could very well be that you are also unknowingly encountering BPA, so let's talk more about how it can impact your preconception journey. I especially want to draw your attention to how BPA affects hormones. Since it has a structure similar to estrogen, it can interfere with your body's hormone function by binding to estrogen receptors and influencing natural processes such as growth, cellular repair, fetal development, and even reproduction.[119] One scientific review showed that "exposure to BPA has the potential to induce epigenetic modifications in both animal and human cells. Such modifications could in turn play a role in male reproductive disorders and cancer development. An epigenetic transmission to offspring was also demonstrated."[120] As you can see, it's important to avoid contact with BPA during preconception.

BPA has been widely criticized for its endocrine-disrupting effects, and in response, manufacturers have introduced alternatives like bisphenol S (BPS) and bisphenol B (BPB). But BPS and BPB are—you guessed it—structurally similar to BPA, and research shows that both these harmful substitutes pose similar health risks to BPA, potentially disrupting hormone systems and affecting reproductive health. Some studies even suggest BPS may be more resistant to environmental breakdown than BPA, leading to potential longer-term exposure risks in humans and ecosystems.[121]

My strong advice here is to avoid, as much as possible, all plastics that hold or carry substances that enter your body (i.e., food and beverages).

- Avoid microwaving or freezing food in plastic containers.
- Avoid plastic containers marked with recycle codes *3* or *7*. They may be made with BPA. (Also, be aware that new evidence is showing the replacements for BPA may have equally as severe health consequences.)
- Reduce your use of canned foods, as the liner is made of plastic.
- Avoid boxed milks, liquids, and soups, as they are lined with aluminum or polyethylene.
- Use glass, porcelain, or stainless-steel containers, particularly for hot food or liquids.
- Avoid plastic bottles as much as possible.

Effects of BPA on Reproductive Hormones

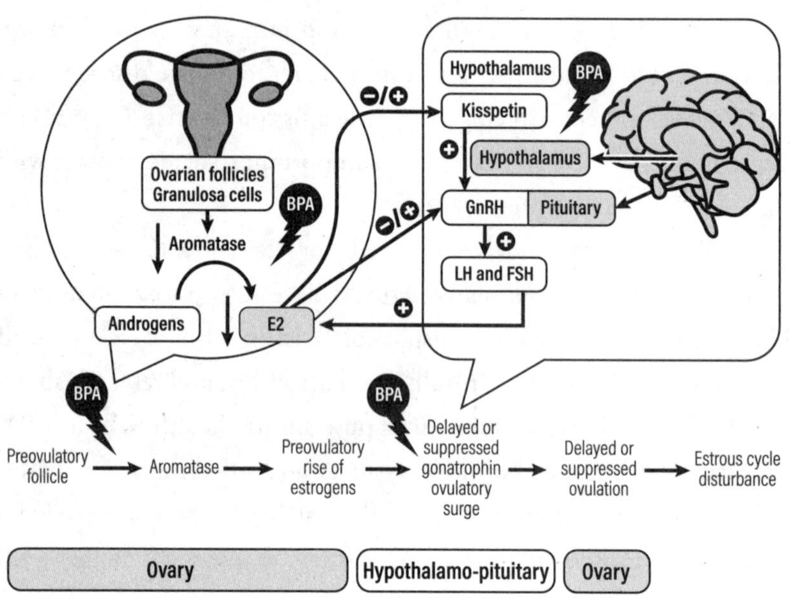

Impact of BPA on Reproduction

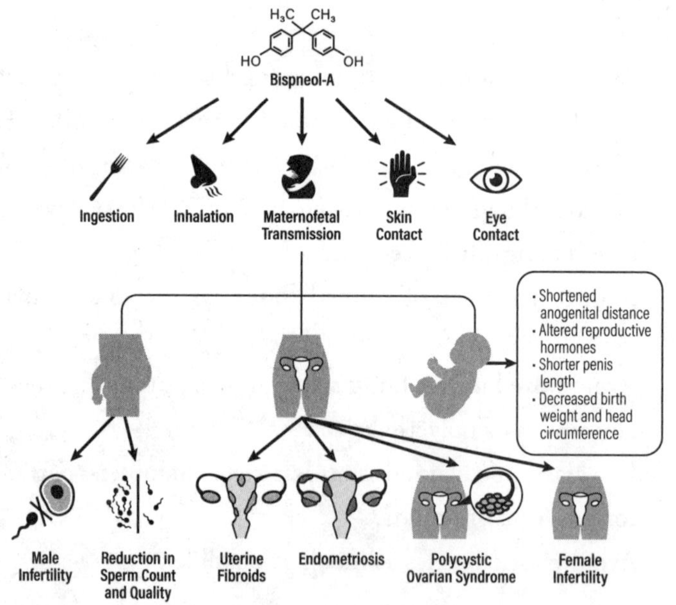

Flame Retardants

If you look closely at labels of mattresses, sofas, toys, rugs, drapes, and other textiles, you may find that most of these items have been sprayed with flame retardant. But here's the problem: The toxins in flame retardants—known as TDCIPP—are known carcinogens, and research has linked them to reproductive and endocrine changes in adult males, as well as damage to immunologic, neurologic, and developmental systems in human cell lines.[122]

Later in this chapter, I'll share some specific resources to help you identify safe textiles to purchase, but for now, read the manufacturer's labels on all your furniture. Be aware of what you have in your home and then consider replacing items over time.

Toxic Mold

As I shared with you earlier in the book, I have fought my own health battles caused by exposure to toxic mold, and it's certainly something I want to bring to your attention during preconception. Mycotoxins are toxic compounds that some strains of mold are known to produce, and they can wreak havoc on your health. A study titled "Mycotoxins: Mechanisms of Toxicity and Methods of Detection" discusses the impact of mycotoxins on fertility, epigenetics, and birth defects. It highlights certain mycotoxins, such as trichothecenes, that can impair fertility and cause birth defects. In animal studies, trichothecenes like T-2 toxin have led to embryo or fetal toxicity, increased postnatal mortality, and intrauterine growth retardation, and fumonisin B1 exposure has been associated with neural tube defects in humans, potentially due to its interference with folate uptake.

When thinking about your environment and possible areas where you could be exposed to mold, there are a couple things to keep in mind. Mold loves to grow in warm, damp areas. In general, preventing mold growth in your home and mitigating its potential health impacts such as respiratory issues and allergic reactions start with controlling humidity.[123] According to the EPA, keeping indoor humidity levels between 30 and 50 percent can significantly reduce the risk of mold development.[124]

If your test results come back positive or you suspect you have hidden or unaddressed mold in your home or work environment, don't ignore it. Get started working on it *now*, because it takes time to get the problem resolved. You can visit annshippymd.com/mold for more resources, but in the meantime, here are a few things you can do to prevent mold:

- Use dehumidifiers; make sure your kitchen, basement, and bathrooms are properly ventilated; and regularly check for condensation.

- Consider buying an inexpensive humidity monitor (available on Amazon and elsewhere), which is a great preventative measure for controlling humidity in your home.

- Promptly address any water leaks. And if there's ever been a leak inside your home (e.g., leaks in a roof, a pipe in the wall, or an air conditioning line, or a bathtub overflow), you need to ensure there was no hidden mold growth in the vicinity. If there was, it needs to be professionally remediated, which means properly removed so it will not grow back.

- If you have central air conditioning, make sure it's properly and routinely maintained, because a common place for mold to grow inside the home is around the condensate drain pan. If it gets clogged and overflows, mold can grow because of the water that leaks.

Mold can also be a problem in your vehicle, school, or workplace, so if your test results reveal mycotoxins but your house doesn't appear to be the source of them, you need to address it with your employer or school. Toxic mold could be a whole book! There's a lot to know about this subject, so I encourage you to go to the appendix to learn more, and you can also visit my website at www.annshippymd.com/mold for more resources.

Chromium-6

Chromium-6 has been at the center of widespread drinking water pollution. Known as the "Erin Brockovich chemical," chromium-6 is in the drinking water of more than 250 million Americans.[125] This toxin is a very deadly carcinogen[126] that is tasteless and odorless. To avoid this dangerous chemical:

- Drink water out of glass bottles.
- Use reverse-osmosis filtration to remove chromium-6 and many other toxins. However, do your research here, as most water filters do not filter out chromium-6, even though they do filter out other toxins.
- Find out what is being tested in the water in your community.
- Do your own water testing. Purchase a hexavalent chromium water test from a company such as Tap Score. They'll send you a test kit, and you'll collect a sample of your tap water and send it back to them for a lab analysis.[127]

Artificial Sweeteners

Artificial sweeteners may be lower in calories than sugar, but research has indicated they are carcinogenic and are linked to type 2 diabetes.[128] Here's how you can still keep things sweet without the use of artificial sweeteners:

- Read labels and avoid all foods and beverages made with artificial sweeteners.
- Use small amounts of organic honey, stevia, or monk fruit in lieu of artificial sweeteners.

- Use recipes that call for fruit or organic honey to sweeten a dish or follow recipes that require no sugar.
- Give your taste buds time to adjust. When you reduce sweeteners of all kinds, your taste buds will recalibrate, and you'll eventually need to use less sweetener in order for things to taste sweet.

Food Coloring

Food coloring has been linked to infertility in animal studies.[129] Dyes including Yellow 5 and Yellow 6 can be found in many processed foods. Read food labels carefully and avoid any products with artificial dyes.

Mercury

Mercury has been identified as a neurotoxicant,[130] meaning it can damage the nervous system. Mercury is particularly harmful during pregnancy and can affect fetal development. To eliminate the chances of mercury affecting you and your future child:

- Avoid eating fish that contain high amounts of mercury. I will go into more detail on fish in the nutrition chapter, but for now, work to reduce your intake of fish in general.
- Avoid vaccines made with thimerosal, which is a mercury-based preservative. Thimerosal is used in some multidose vials of vaccines to prevent bacterial or fungal contamination. Most vaccines for both children and adults often come in thimerosal-free formulations, but always check with your healthcare provider—particularly with seasonal flu vaccines (which may still contain thimerosal in multidose vials; single-dose versions of the flu vaccine do not).[131]

- If you need a filling, ask your dentist about mercury-free options. (We'll talk more about this later in the chapter.)
- Cosmetics and tattoos also contain potentially toxic heavy metals, both as impurities in pigments or as a result of the manufacturing process.[132] Choose cosmetic products that are free from toxic heavy metals, and definitely don't get new tattoos while trying to conceive or while you're pregnant!

Per- and Polyfluoroalkyl Substances (PFAS)

PFAS, known as "forever chemicals," are manufactured chemicals that have been around since the 1940s and are used in many consumer products. According to the EPA:

Current peer-reviewed scientific studies have shown that exposure to certain levels of PFAS may lead to: reproductive effects such as decreased fertility or increased high blood pressure in pregnant women; developmental effects or delays in children, including low birth weight, accelerated puberty, bone variations, or behavioral changes; increased risk of some cancers, including prostate, kidney, and testicular cancers; reduced ability of the body's immune system to fight infections, including reduced vaccine response; interference with the body's natural hormones; and increased cholesterol levels and/or risk of obesity.[133]

PFAS have been found to leach into food during cooking, leading to various health issues.[134] Studies have shown that PFAS can disrupt endocrine function, which is critical for reproductive health, and have been linked to decreased fertility, particularly in men.[135] Additionally, PFAS exposure has been associated with epigenetic changes, including alterations in DNA methylation, which can impact gene expression related to reproductive health and development.[136] To reduce your PFAS exposure:

- Don't use nonstick cookware.
- Avoid using stain-resistant chemicals on furniture and carpets.

- Use safe alternatives (like baking soda and vinegar solutions) for removing stains.
- Don't wear water-repellant clothing.
- Avoid fast-food packaging or anything made to hold greasy foods.
- Stop using paper plates.
- Avoid microwave popcorn.
- Purchase PFAS-free dental floss.
- Use reverse osmosis and charcoal filters to filter your water.

The EWG: An Important Tool

As we go through the various areas of life in which you want to be aware of specific toxin exposures, I will also share with you some specific actions you can take to reduce your overall toxin load. The Environmental Working Group is a wonderful resource that can help guide your decision-making on all kinds of products you use routinely. Their mission is "to empower you with breakthrough research to make informed choices and live a healthy life in a healthy environment."[137] The EWG's robust website has endless research and resources on everything from beauty products to cleaning supplies, textiles to hard goods such as furniture and housewares, foods, and more. I'll refer to specific lists they've curated throughout the chapter to help you along this journey toward cleaning up your environment and getting yourself optimized for baby-making.

In Your Body

Let's begin by looking within your body to see if there are any toxins that need to be removed. And keep in mind, if you do need to have anything currently in your body taken out, allow yourself some extra time for the detoxification process after the removal.

If you have breast implants, I urge you to consider having them removed. There's a growing body of research around something referred to as breast implant illness,[138] which leads me to believe that it's difficult to optimize your health if you currently have breast implants, regardless of if they are silicone or saline.

Amalgam fillings also pose a risk during preconception,[139] so if you have any in your teeth, I encourage you to consider having those removed. Amalgam consists of an alloy of silver, copper, tin, and zinc combined with the heavy metal mercury.[140] And on the topic of teeth, if you've had a root canal in the past, you might want to consult with your dentist about having a 3D CT scan to find out if there's any bone infection lurking where the root canal was performed. I say this because root canals can lead to bacteria and other pathogens that proliferate inside the bone, and this can trigger systemic immune responses due to the inflammation.[141] I always recommend working with a biological dentist when you're addressing these matters.

Many women use vaginal birth control devices such as a NuvaRing or an IUD, and if you're in that category, you'll need to have it removed several months before attempting to conceive. But keep in mind you don't yet have the green light for conception, so you'll want to find another form of contraception such as condoms during this period.

In Your Home

Your home should be a safe, nourishing space—but hidden toxins can lurk in the air, furniture, and everyday products. In this section, we'll walk through each area of your home and simple, practical ways to reduce exposure, creating a cleaner, healthier environment for you and your future baby.

- ***Plastics:*** Especially when it comes to eating and drinking, it's imperative to eliminate plastics from your routine. Opt instead for glass or stainless-steel food storage and beverage containers. Exposure to microplastics is on the rise, and while further research is needed to understand the effects of microplastics on fertility and the transgenerational impacts, there's enough information out there to convince me that we all need to work to reduce our exposure to microplastics and nanoplastics.[142] Keep in mind that if you *do* have plasticware in your kitchen, you'll definitely want to avoid putting it in the dishwasher, because the heat can cause chemicals in the plastic to leach out of the item.[143] But it's even better simply to eliminate all plastics in your kitchen.

- ***Furniture:*** If you're going to be purchasing any new furniture for your home now or leading up to your baby's birth, be sure to opt for nontoxic items. For instance, flame retardants in furniture have been shown to negatively impact the neurobiological development of children and fetuses.[144] Look for furniture that is GOTS (Global Organic Textile Standard)-certified, which means it meets the highest standards for environmental safety.[145] This especially applies to your mattress and bedding, as you're sleeping on it every night and breathing in and absorbing through the skin any toxins that might be emitted.

- ***Indoor Air Pollution:*** Air quality has a direct effect on our overall health, and specifically on our reproductive health.[146] While we can't control the quality of the air we breathe outside, we are able to ensure the air inside our home is well filtered. If you don't already have high-quality air filters in your home, this is a great time to get them and ensure the air in every room—especially your bedroom—is being purified.[147] Also, make sure you are getting regular maintenance on your HVAC system in your home, as well as changing the air filters regularly.

- ***Flooring:*** If you plan to change out the flooring in your home, whether you're going with hardwood, tile, or carpet, investigate nontoxic brands with zero PFAS and VOCs.[148]

- ***Paint***: Paint is another potentially toxic pitfall, so again, I recommending avoiding painting your home during this time.[149] But if a fresh coat is simply a must, then opt for zero-VOC paints, and wear an air-filtering mask when the paint is still wet.

- ***Cleaning Products***: Cleaning products are a huge source of toxins in the home and now is a good time to pull out *all* the products you use to clean your home and check the ingredients. Read cleaning product labels with the same vigilance you'd use when reading food labels. As I mentioned earlier, the Environmental Working Group has some great information on ingredients to avoid, as well as EWG-verified cleaning products that they recommend. Just go to www.ewg.org/cleaners/ to learn more. Here's a list of common household products just to get you thinking about what you're currently using so you can start making some swaps:

  ○ Glass, stainless steel, wood, floor, countertop, and bathroom cleaners (EWG recommends the brands Aspen-Clean, ATTITUDE, ECOS, Dr. Bronner's, Branch Basics, and Babyganics)

  ○ Dish soap and dishwasher detergent (EWG recommends using Dropps dishwasher pods, ECOS dishwasher gel, and Seventh Generation dishwasher pods)

  ○ Laundry detergent (choose fragrance-free, environmentally friendly products such as Aspen, Branch Basics, and Heritage Park)

  ○ Dryer sheets (it's best to avoid these altogether)

  ○ Air fresheners, candles, incense, and other fragrances (also avoid these)

  ○ Dry cleaning (avoid this as much as possible, but, if necessary, use an ecocleaner)

  ○ Pesticides and herbicides (don't use any of these in your yard and garden)

RENEW

Food, Beverages, and Meal Prep

We'll get into much more depth regarding nutrition during the pre-conception period in the Nourishing Yourself Well chapter, but since food and beverages can unfortunately be a major source of toxins, I'd like to spend a little time on the topic here.

- ***Fish***: Research has shown that many fish are contaminated with heavy metals, which are released into the oceans through various types of industry.[150] Epigenetic processes as well as cancer risk have been linked to environmental toxins including heavy metals,[151] so limiting your exposure during preconception is essential. Sadly, freshwater fish are also contaminated, but more often with toxic PFAS,[152] which are manufactured compounds often used in products to make them more resistant to stains, grease, and water.[153] They get released into the water supply and accumulate in the tissues of the fish, which we then ingest. For these reasons, I advise all prospective parents to reduce their consumption of fresh- and saltwater fish during preconception.

- ***Canned Foods***: You might have read that canned food companies have been lining the inside of cans with BPA for decades, but once there was enough evidence to prove the deleterious health effects of BPA on humans, they began phasing out the use of this plastic compound.[154] However, the polymers these companies are using now[155] are not well-researched enough yet to be deemed safe in my opinion, and thus, I strongly encourage you to avoid all canned food products, and to choose fresh or frozen foods instead.

  Research has shown that aluminum exposure, often resulting from the consumption of canned beverages and foods, can negatively affect reproductive health by altering hormone levels and reducing sperm quality.[156] These findings highlight the importance of not only avoiding drinking beverages out of aluminum cans, but avoiding cooking with or storing food in aluminum foil.[157] By doing so, you can reduce your exposure to aluminum.

- ***Processed Foods*:** Preservatives are used in processed foods in order to give them longer shelf lives. But studies have demonstrated that exposure to artificial preservatives such as butylated hydroxyanisole (BHA) and butylated hydroxytoluene (BHT) can impair reproductive health by disrupting hormone balance and affecting sperm quality.[158] Additionally, high-fructose corn syrup (HFCS), commonly found in processed foods, has been linked to epigenetic changes that can influence gene expression related to fertility.[159] These findings are just some of the reasons why I suggest avoiding processed foods and instead choosing whole, natural options. By doing so, you can reduce your exposure to harmful additives and support better reproductive health and overall well-being.

- ***Nonstick Pans*:** In the PFAS section at the beginning of the chapter, I shared that recent research has raised significant concerns about the use of nonstick pans due to the chemicals used in their coatings, particularly PFAS. I highly suggest making the swap from nonstick cookware (even cookware that is free of PFAS, as we just don't know enough about the alternatives that manufacturers are using) and opting for safer alternatives, such as stainless steel, to reduce exposure to harmful chemicals and support better reproductive and overall health.

- ***Microwaves*:** Exposure to the electromagnetic radiation (EMR) emitted by microwave ovens can lead to oxidative stress and DNA damage, which are known to affect sperm quality adversely.[160] Studies have shown that this type of

RENEW

radiation can cause significant disruptions in DNA methylation processes, which are crucial for gene expression and reproductive health.[161] Given these risks, minimizing or, better yet, eliminating the use of microwave ovens during the preconception period can help support reproductive health and prevent potential epigenetic alterations.

Clothing

Yes, even the clothing you wear matters! Keep in mind that your skin is your largest organ! And the clothes you're wearing are rubbing against your skin all day long. Sadly, these days, most clothes are made with thousands of toxins, including fire retardants, dyes, solvents, microplastics, and more.[162] Now, I'm not suggesting you replace all your clothes. But as you add to your wardrobe, consider buying cotton, wool, linen, and silk rather than synthetics. Numerous clothing stores offer 100 percent organic cotton options, and many companies use only natural fibers in their fashions.[163]

Jewelry can also be a potential source of toxin exposure. Lead and cadmium have been found to be common in jewelry for children and adults.[164] Cadmium is especially concerning because it can cause birth defects, reproductive harm, and cancer (because of this, cadmium is listed under Proposition 65 in California).[165] So, avoid low-quality jewelry or go with stainless steel.

Personal Care Products

Toxins found in personal care products have been a hot topic for quite some time, and with good reason. The ingredients found in some mainstream beauty products can be quite shocking—many products include phthalates, parabens, and formaldehyde-releasing preservatives.[166] I encourage you to familiarize yourself with the EWG's database on personal care products. You'll discover a wealth of information there, and you can search for your favorite products and find out what's in them and the potential side effects of those ingredients.[167]

Aim for nontoxic ingredients only in all these personal care products:

- perfume, best to avoid fragrances altogether
- face wash
- makeup remover
- moisturizers, toners, and lotions
- toothpaste and mouthwash
- nail polish (avoid gel nails and nail polish remover)
- deodorant (due to the presence of aluminum)
- shampoo, conditioner, and any other hair-care products
- self-tanners (avoid)
- bug repellent
- sunscreen
- products used at a salon (i.e., hair color) or by an esthetician (i.e., peels or retinol)

Medication/Vaccines

Minimizing medications, including over-the-counter meds and prescription drugs such as antibiotics, during the preconception period is crucial for both men and women. Of course, you'll both want to review your current medications with a healthcare provider before stopping any. If a medication cannot be safely discontinued, work with your doctor to choose the medication that is safest for pregnancy and lactation.

If you're a woman who has been taking oral contraceptives, the longer you're off them before conceiving, the more time you can give your body to get back into its natural ovulation rhythm.

If you're taking antidepressants, talk to your psychiatrist about the possibility of using supplementation and lifestyle factors to improve your mood instead. If that isn't possible or it's recommended that you continue your medication, ask your physician to recommend the medication that is safest for pregnancy and lactation.

Unfortunately, we don't know much about the impact of antidepressants on preconception and pregnancy, as the research is ongoing. But here are some things to consider:

- Some studies have found no significant association between SSRI (selective serotonin reuptake inhibitor) use in pregnancy and birth defects,[168] while other studies suggest that taking SSRIs, especially during the first trimester, may be associated with a slightly higher chance of certain heart defects[169] and may affect fetal brain development.[170]
- Some studies have suggested associations between prenatal exposure to antidepressants and autism spectrum disorder (ASD)[171]; other studies have found no evidence of such an association.[172]
- The American Psychiatric Association, the American College of Obstetrics and Gynecology, and the US Food and Drug Administration (FDA) recommend using antidepressants when the benefits outweigh the risks.[173]

Now is definitely the time to be making any changes regarding antidepressants, as opposed to once you're pregnant. Give yourself time to find the right solution for you, before it can directly impact your child during pregnancy.

Finally, I do not recommend getting any vaccines during this preconception period. We simply do not know the full implications for how various ingredients in vaccines impact fertility and epigenetics. As of November 2024, Merck's M-M-R II vaccine's product insert states, "There are no adequate and well-controlled studies of M-M-R

II vaccine administration to pregnant women."[174] It goes on to say, "M-M-R II vaccine has not been evaluated for carcinogenic or mutagenic potential or impairment of fertility."[175] We just don't know how—or if—vaccines can impact fertility.

As another example, the most common flu vaccine currently being administered to people under the age of sixty-five is the Fluzone Quadrivalant vaccine. Its package insert reads: "Available data with Fluzone Quadrivalent use in pregnant women are insufficient to inform vaccine-associated risk of adverse developmental outcomes."[176] Without clear clinical data supporting its safety in terms of the development of a fetus, why take the risk?

Bottom line: I encourage you to steer away from vaccines during preconception and pregnancy.

Recreation

Ensuring a healthy lifestyle during the preconception period extends to your recreational activities. Here are some essential guidelines to follow:

- ***No Drugs.*** I've seen in my practice that recreational drugs such as marijuana can severely impact fertility by causing hormonal imbalances, reducing sperm quality, and affecting ovulation cycles.[177] Abstaining from drugs is crucial for both partners.

- ***No Alcohol.*** Alcohol can disrupt menstrual cycles in women and reduce sperm count and motility in men.[178]

- ***No Smoking or Vaping.*** Smoking damages eggs and sperm, increasing the risk of miscarriage and birth defects.[179] Plus, there's new research linking paternal smoking during preconception with asthma, low lung function, and obesity in children.[180] Both partners will want to avoid smoking and vaping as well as limit their exposure to secondhand smoke.

- ***Avoid Bodies of Water with Algal Blooms.*** Algal blooms, particularly red algae, produce harmful neurotoxins called *brevetoxins.*[181] Avoid swimming in discolored waters or where algal blooms are known to occur. Always investigate the safety of any body of water before you enter it.

- ***Reduce Frequent Flying.*** If you frequently travel by airplane, consider additional detoxification measures. Frequent air travel exposes you to higher levels of radiation and pollutants, which may require a more intensive detox routine (including vitamin C, CoQ10, vitamin E, liposomal glutathione, EGCG).[182]

- ***Consider Your Hobbies.*** Evaluate your hobbies for potential toxin exposure. Activities such as painting, working with certain crafting products, hunting, flying, golfing, or using industrial chemicals can introduce harmful substances into your system.

- ***Avoid Handling Receipts.*** Thermal receipts contain high levels of BPA, a chemical known to disrupt hormones.[183] Minimize handling these receipts and consider using digital receipts instead.

Self-Care

Taking care of your body during the preconception period is vital, but some common self-care practices can be harmful during this time.

- ***Med Spa Procedures***: Avoid procedures such as Botox, dermal fillers, and chemical peels. These treatments often involve chemicals that can affect your body's natural processes and may have unknown effects on fertility and fetal development.

- ***Hair Coloring***: Chemical hair dyes can contain harmful substances that may be absorbed through the scalp. Opt for natural hair-dye alternatives or avoid coloring your hair altogether during this period to minimize exposure to toxins.

- ***Nail Treatments***: Many nail polishes and treatments contain chemicals such as formaldehyde and toluene, which can be harmful when absorbed through the nails or inhaled.[184] Consider using nontoxic nail products or forgoing nail treatments.
- ***Hot Tubs***: It's especially important for men to avoid hot tubs during preconception, as the wet heat can impair sperm motility and overall production.[185] I suggest avoiding hot tubs during the three months leading up to conception.
- ***Saunas***: Dry heat is also detrimental to sperm production,[186] so I also suggest that men avoid using saunas for at least the three months leading up to conception.
- ***Orthodontic Aligners***: Because X-rays are typically required when using orthodontic aligners, I recommend completing any orthodontic care before beginning this preconception program. It's best to avoid X-rays during this time.

Where You Live

If you're going to be moving to a new residence during this time, and if it's possible to make choices about where you'll live, try to avoid choosing a home near power and gas lines, highways, airports, manufacturing plants, waste disposal facilities, cell phone towers, reservoirs, and water treatment plants. Also, research indicates that living within six miles of oil and gas development can have a negative impact on mental health during preconception.[187]

Employment

Some jobs are higher risk than others based on toxin exposure. Firefighters, morticians, nail and hair salon technicians, agricultural workers, restaurant staff, and healthcare workers are just a few examples of professionals who might be exposed to certain toxins that could impact reproductive health.[188] Some fields that might include chemical exposures are HVAC maintenance and repair, pool cleaning, construction, roofing, pest control, mining, the textile industry, power line repair and installation, and airline jobs. We don't always have an option when it comes to our employment, but if you're in an occupation that routinely exposes you to toxins, wear protective gear and understand that detoxification is going to be an essential step to helping your body reduce its toxic load in order to prepare you for the healthiest possible conception.

Final Thoughts

Talking about toxins can be a bit overwhelming, but hopefully you now feel empowered with information on how to "slow the drip" of toxins that enter your body each and every day. Reducing your exposure is a foundational step in creating a healthier environment for conception and pregnancy. The journey of detoxification, nutrition, and supplementation becomes significantly more effective when the influx of environmental toxins is minimized. Think of this process as an ongoing commitment rather than a one-time task and make consistent efforts to identify and eliminate harmful substances from your surroundings. By doing so, you are taking proactive steps toward a healthier preconception period, setting the stage for a healthier pregnancy and, ultimately, a healthier baby.

Be sure to check the appendix for a table of toxins to avoid.

Q&A

Q: Why is it important to minimize toxin exposure during the preconception period?

A: Minimizing toxin exposure is essential because toxins can be insidious in how they impact your health and your future child's health. Reducing exposure helps create an optimal environment for conception and pregnancy, lowering the risk of developmental issues, reproductive disorders, and epigenetic changes that could affect future generations. I hope you feel empowered by realizing how controllable many of these factors really are!

Q: What are some practical steps to reduce glyphosate exposure?

A: You can reduce glyphosate exposure by choosing organic foods, washing fruits and vegetables thoroughly, avoiding glyphosate-based herbicides in home gardens, and supporting farmers who practice sustainable, glyphosate-free farming methods.

Q: How do BPA and its alternatives, like BPS and BPB, affect reproductive health?

A: BPA and its substitutes mimic estrogen, disrupting hormonal balance, affecting processes such as growth and reproduction, and causing epigenetic changes. These chemicals are found in plastics and canned goods. It's best to avoid plastics for food storage; opt for glass or stainless-steel containers instead and reduce packaged food consumption.

Q: What are some strategies to prevent mold exposure in your home?

A: Prevent mold by controlling humidity (keep it between 30 to 50 percent), addressing water leaks promptly, maintaining HVAC systems, using dehumidifiers, and regularly ventilating bathrooms and kitchens. If mold is suspected, testing and professional remediation may be necessary.

Q: Why is it important to avoid nonstick cookware, and what are some safer alternatives?

A: Nonstick cookware contains PFAS, which are linked to reproductive issues and endocrine disruption. Safer alternatives include stainless steel, cast iron, and glass, which reduce exposure to these harmful chemicals.

CHAPTER 6

Clean Slate: Detox for Baby-Building

You've laid a lot of groundwork, and I hope you're already feeling quite accomplished. Now it's time to turn our attention to detoxification. We just spent a lot of time considering various toxins that we encounter daily, and I know you've already been reducing your exposure to them. That's a huge step in the right direction! Now is the perfect time to start helping your body rid itself of the toxins that are still lurking in your system.

The term *detox* has become a big-time buzzword. It's everywhere! When you hear *detox*, you might immediately think of juice cleanses, hard-to-follow protocols, or even fad products or trendy diets. But detoxification simply refers to the biological processes that eliminate waste. Your body is constantly removing toxic by-products of cellular metabolism and normal functioning, along with environmental toxins. Detoxification starts at a cellular level in every cell in the body. There are six organs that help toxins leave the body: the liver, intestines, kidneys, lungs, lymphatic system, and skin. In this chapter you will learn how to effectively assist those essential organs in doing their jobs even better.

From the epigenetic and fertility perspectives, toxins can impact the quality of both the egg and sperm that come together to form your future child.[189] Now is the time to reduce your toxic load, as once you are pregnant, it will be too late. In a study led by the EWG, researchers at two major laboratories discovered an average of two hundred industrial chemicals and pollutants in the umbilical cord blood of ten babies once they were born, and overall, they identified a total of 287 chemicals in the samples. The umbilical cord blood, collected by the Red Cross after the umbilical cord was cut, contained pesticides, ingredients from consumer products, and residues from burning coal, gasoline, garbage, and more.[190] Many of these toxins are also stored in fatty tissues, the liver, the kidneys, the heart, the brain, muscle, and fluids such as breast milk.[191] In fact, some of these toxins (particularly PFAS) appear to build up in an infant's body by 20–30 percent each month during breastfeeding.[192] It's shocking, right? And if PFAS accumulate in the brain, they "may lead to toxic effects in the central nervous system (CNS), including PFAS-induced behavioral and cognitive disorders."[193] So the more you and your partner can detox now to create a clean slate for baby-making, the better!

IYKYK: Toxin-Free Breast Milk

If you know, you know: Breastfeeding is so important for your baby's health. I'm really glad the tide has turned on this topic and that it's pretty much become common knowledge among mothers that "breast is best!" But there's an aspect that's less commonly known: Toxins in your body can be passed on through breast milk. And *that* is one of the most important reasons to detoxify your body before pregnancy. But it doesn't stop there; I always encourage my patients to be vigilant about avoiding toxins during pregnancy and lactation as well. My sincere hope is you will get so accustomed to this lifestyle that it won't be a challenge once you get to that point!

I know we've been focusing on the various ways that toxins impact your fertility and the health of your little one, so as you enter this detox phase, remember your motivation—to create the healthiest baby possible. The work you'll be doing here will be pivotal when it comes to setting up your child for optimal epigenetics. Isn't it amazing to think about the power you hold to positively influence your child's wellness *before* they are even conceived? It's truly remarkable.

The results of the various lab workups you have completed will help guide you on specific toxins you're targeting in this detoxification process. Some of the supplements and strategies I'm recommending help with general detoxing and are helpful to anyone, while others are more targeted to certain toxins.

When Cassie walked into my office at thirty-seven years old, she was carrying the weight of six years of heartbreak and frustration. Brimming with optimism, she had started trying to conceive at thirty-one, but the journey proved far more challenging than she ever imagined. Years of oral birth control had suppressed her natural cycles, and after discontinuing the pill, her body struggled to recover. She didn't ovulate or have a period for over a year. A reproductive endocrinologist prescribed a course of Lupron and inserted an IUD for six months, followed by two attempts at IVF. The first yielded only two eggs but no viable embryos. The second resulted in an ectopic pregnancy that ruptured, adding physical trauma to her emotional pain. Desperate for answers, Cassie traveled to Chicago to consult with a reproductive immunologist, who uncovered high markers of inflammation and stagnant pelvic blood flow. The consensus from her doctors was grim—her chances of pregnancy were slipping away.

Refusing to give up, Cassie sought a different approach and came in to see me. Together, we addressed root causes and worked to optimize her health. She underwent treatment for parasites and heavy metal toxicity, corrected high homocysteine levels, and supplemented her deficient B12 and vitamin D. With pelvic floor physical therapy and optimized management of her Hashimoto's thyroid condition, she began to regain her health. She adopted a grain-free, gluten-free, and dairy-free diet, which reduced her inflammation and supported her body's healing. Against all odds, Cassie conceived naturally and delivered a healthy baby girl. But her story didn't end there. Six months later, without trying, she became pregnant with twins, who arrived healthy and thriving. And at age forty, Cassie welcomed baby number four into her family.

Cassie's journey is a testament to the power of persistence, faith, and addressing the underlying issues caused by toxin exposure and nutrient deficiencies. Through determination and comprehensive care, she turned what had seemed impossible into a beautiful reality: a house filled with the laughter and love of four children. This can be your story too. It just requires perseverance.

Organs Involved in Detoxification

- **Liver:** The liver is the primary organ responsible for detoxification. It contains a high concentration of Phase I and Phase II enzymes and plays a central role in metabolizing and eliminating toxins.[194]
- **Kidneys:** The kidneys filter blood and excrete water-soluble toxins and their metabolites in urine.[195]
- **Lungs:** The lungs expel volatile toxins and gases, such as carbon dioxide and other inhaled chemicals.[196]
- **Skin:** The skin can eliminate toxins through sweat, a process that also helps regulate body temperature.[197]
- **Intestines:** The intestines, particularly the colon, are involved in the excretion of toxins through feces. The gut microbiota also play a role in metabolizing certain compounds.[198]

Nutritional and Lifestyle Support for Detoxification

Nutritional Factors

Adequate intake of *sulfur-containing amino acids* (e.g., cysteine, methionine) is essential for glutathione synthesis. Foods rich in these amino acids include cruciferous vegetables (broccoli, kale, cauliflower), garlic, onions, and high-quality protein sources.[199] Ultimately, in addition to these factors, most people benefit from taking liposomal glutathione as well.

Consuming a diet rich in *antioxidants* (e.g., vitamins C and E, selenium, flavonoids) supports the neutralization of ROS and reduces the risk of oxidative damage during detoxification. Colorful fruits and vegetables are excellent sources of these antioxidants.[200]

B vitamins, particularly B6, B12, and folate, are crucial cofactors in methylation reactions. Deficiencies in these vitamins can impair detoxification and lead to the accumulation of toxic metabolites, such as homocysteine.[201]

Dietary fiber binds to toxins in the gut and aids their elimination through feces. Soluble fiber helps lower blood cholesterol and stabilize blood glucose levels, while insoluble fiber promotes regular bowel movements and prevents constipation.[202] Many fruits, vegetables, nuts, and seeds are good sources of both types of fiber.

Lifestyle Factors

Adequate *hydration* supports kidney function and promotes the elimination of water-soluble toxins through urine. Drinking enough water also aids in the production of sweat, another route for toxin excretion.[203]

Regular physical activity enhances circulation, supports lymphatic drainage, and promotes sweating, all of which help in the detoxification process.[204] We'll talk a lot more about this in a later chapter.

I want to remind you that *reducing exposure to environmental toxins*, such as pollutants, chemicals, and tobacco smoke, can decrease the burden on the body's detoxification systems. Choosing organic foods, using natural cleaning products, and minimizing the use of plastics are practical steps to reducing toxin exposure.

Chronic stress can impair detoxification by increasing the production of cortisol, a stress hormone that can negatively affect liver function and increase oxidative stress.[205] Stress response optimization techniques, such as mindfulness, meditation, and adequate sleep, are important for maintaining optimal detoxification pathways.

What About a Detox Diet?

Nutrition plays a starring role in the detox process. The truth is that food is often the primary delivery system for toxins entering your system. But looking on the bright side, food can absolutely be your medicine! The right foods, especially ones rich in antioxidants, can help assist your body in its detoxification processes.

Let's take a moment to talk about antioxidants, as this is another buzzword that is often misunderstood. Breaking it down, antioxidants are simply molecules that have an extra electron to give to unstable free radicals that are produced in your body's daily functions.[206] The extra electron is necessary in order to make molecules more stable and neutralize them so they can't cause damage to our cells.[207] Antioxidants are crucial for protecting cell membranes and shielding mitochondria, and they play an important role in detoxification itself.

Because antioxidants are depleted by toxin exposures, stress, poor food choices, and many things that are unavoidable in modern life, your body likely needs more of these incredibly important compounds to work effectively. That's where the detox diet comes in—one that is rich is antioxidants. Detoxification itself produces free radicals that are unstable and highly toxic. The liver turns toxic compounds into water-soluble compounds so they can be excreted from the body, which happens in a two-step process referred to as Phase 1 and Phase 2 detoxification. But the transformation that happens in Phase 1 results in compounds that are often *more toxic* than the original form. That's where antioxidants jump in to save the day and provide protection until Phase 2 is completed.

The Liver Detoxification Pathways graphic shows two of the key steps in the detoxification process and the important nutrients required to support liver detoxification. Hopefully this helps you see that detoxification is a highly nutrient-dependent process. When we have more chemicals to detox, we simply need more nutrition.

This is exactly why some popular restrictive cleanse-and-detox programs don't work: They restrict the nutrients needed for the liver to do its job and can worsen an already risky condition. When we understand how nutrition-dependent detoxification is, it's easy to see how the power of food helps or hinders your detox.

In addition, Nrf2 is a transcription factor (a protein that controls when and how genes get turned on or off) that activates hundreds of genes, including important detoxification pathways. Nrf2 is stimulated by many antioxidants (including phenols and vitamin E) and other compounds (including sulfur compounds, carotenoids, and omega-3 fats), which emphasizes yet another way in which what you eat directly promotes detoxification.[208]

That's a good introduction to the key role your diet plays in the detoxification process. There is a plethora of information in chapter 7, where I delve into the specific foods that can help your body detoxify and give you a clear plan for what to eat during this process.

Doesn't Detoxing = Feeling Miserable?

Contrary to popular belief, detoxifying doesn't mean enduring prolonged periods of low energy or discomfort due to withdrawals or die-off

RENEW

Liver Detoxification Pathways and Supportive Nutrients

The liver has two mechanisms designed to convert fat-soluble chemicals into water soluble chemicals so that they may then be easily excreted from the body through feces, bile and urine.

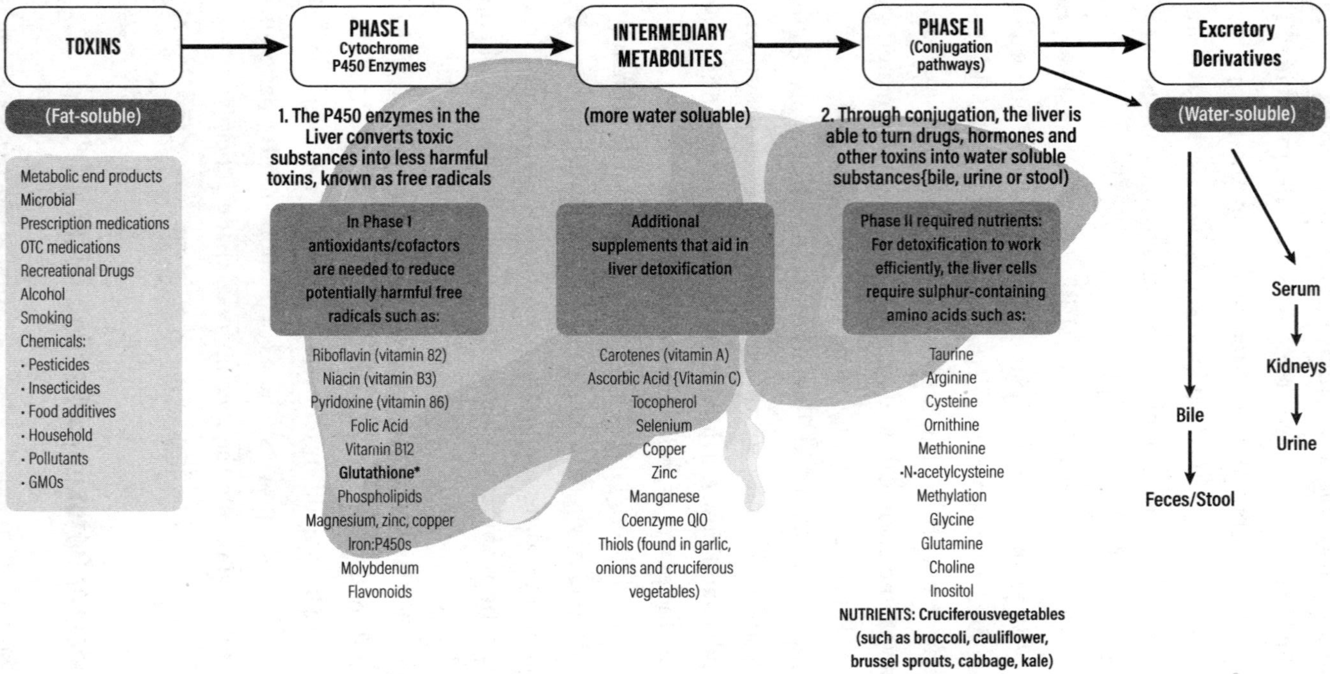

TOXINS → PHASE I — Cytochrome P450 Enzymes → INTERMEDIARY METABOLITES → PHASE II (Conjugation pathways) → Excretory Derivatives

(Fat-soluble)

(more water soluable)

(Water-soluble)

1. The P450 enzymes in the Liver converts toxic substances into less harmful toxins, known as free radicals

2. Through conjugation, the liver is able to turn drugs, hormones and other toxins into water soluble substances{bile, urine or stool)

TOXINS (Fat-soluble):
Metabolic end products
Microbial
Prescription medications
OTC medications
Recreational Drugs
Alcohol
Smoking
Chemicals:
· Pesticides
· Insecticides
· Food additives
· Household
· Pollutants
· GMOs

In Phase I antioxidants/cofactors are needed to reduce potentially harmful free radicals such as:
Riboflavin (vitamin 82)
Niacin (vitamin B3)
Pyridoxine (vitamin 86)
Folic Acid
Vitamin B12
Glutathione*
Phospholipids
Magnesium, zinc, copper
Iron:P450s
Molybdenum
Flavonoids

Additional supplements that aid in liver detoxification
Carotenes (vitamin A)
Ascorbic Acid {Vitamin C)
Tocopherol
Selenium
Copper
Zinc
Manganese
Coenzyme QIO
Thiols (found in garlic, onions and cruciferous vegetables)

Phase II required nutrients: For detoxification to work efficiently, the liver cells require sulphur-containing amino acids such as:
Taurine
Arginine
Cysteine
Ornithine
Methionine
·N·acetylcysteine
Methylation
Glycine
Glutamine
Choline
Inositol

NUTRIENTS: Cruciferousvegetables (such as broccoli, cauliflower, brussel sprouts, cabbage, kale)

Serum → Kidneys → Urine

Bile → Feces/Stool

symptoms. Think of a river with multiple dams, and the water in the river represents the toxins you want to release from your body. Each dam represents a different organ system or "pathway" for the toxins to exit. Now, if you open just one of those dams, many toxins come rushing out and there's a flood. That "flood" is what causes those uncomfortable symptoms like headaches, fatigue, nausea, GI issues, and more. It's no fun at all, and not the most efficient or healthiest way to go about this.

Instead, if you support *multiple* detox pathways at once by gently opening all the dams in synchrony, then there's no flood, and you can actually feel good and maintain your energy levels during detox. And think long game . . . it's not something you accomplish in a weekend or even a week. Think of it in months and then maintain.

In the coming pages, I'll introduce you to supplements and strategies that support each of your detoxification pathways. For instance, glutathione is a supplement made of various amino acids, and it's made in the methylation pathway, but it often gets depleted. We'll also talk about lymphatic work, gut support, and other important methods for gentle effective detoxification.

Methylation Matters

We've talked about methylation, but let's zero in on its vital role in detoxification. In essence, methylation involves the transfer of a methyl group (one carbon atom and three hydrogen atoms—CH3) to a substrate, such as DNA, proteins, or other molecules. This process occurs throughout the body and is necessary for the regulation of gene expression, protein function, and the detoxification of some harmful substances.

Methylation and Detoxification

One of the key roles of methylation in detoxification is its involvement in the metabolism and elimination of toxins. This process primarily occurs in the liver, where toxic substances are made more water-soluble, allowing them to be excreted via urine or bile. Methylation is particularly important in the detoxification of heavy metals, hormones, and some environmental toxins, such as: arsenic, mercury, BPA, pesticides (e.g. atradine, paraquat, organophosphates), PAHs, PCBs (polychlorinated biphenyls), acetaminophen, dioxins, alcohol and ammonia by-products.

Methylation plays a significant role in the breakdown of estrogen. Proper methylation ensures that estrogen is safely metabolized, reducing the risk of hormone-related cancers. Methylation is also involved in DNA repair and protecting the genome from damage caused by toxins and oxidative stress. This process helps maintain genome stability and prevent mutations that could lead to diseases, including cancer.

As you can see, methylation is a cornerstone of the body's detoxification process. Methylation is supported by B vitamins such as B2, B6, B12, folate or 5-MTHF, magnesium, and S-adenosylmethionine. By optimizing methylation through proper nutrition, lifestyle changes, and stress management, you can enhance your body's ability to eliminate toxins and protect against various health issues.

How Long Will Detoxing Take?

The duration and intensity of detoxification depend largely on your individual toxic load and genetics. Some individuals may require a more extended period to cleanse deeply, while others might find a shorter detoxification phase sufficient. The goal is to tailor the detoxification process to your unique needs, fostering a balanced and energized state that supports reproductive health and overall wellness. Plan on six to eighteen months for a successful detox program.

Supporting Cellular Detoxification

There are three steps to supporting your body's cellular detoxification processes: reducing toxin exposures, supporting organs of elimination, and focusing on deeper cellular detoxification.

With the first step, *reducing toxin exposures*, the body has the natural ability to detoxify but hasn't evolved to withstand the level of chemical input found in our modern environment. In the previous chapter, we thoroughly covered this step, but I want to remind you that you can't adequately detoxify if you're simultaneously taking on more toxins.

It's important to not push cellular detoxification in the second step—*supporting organs of elimination*—until the toxins have an easy way out of the body. This means staying hydrated, having daily bowel movements, sweating often (through exercise or infrared sauna), and breathing deeply.

This step may seem simple, but I can't stress its importance enough. If the toxins leave the cells but can't get out of the body, they may simply recirculate, causing further damage. You can support your body's detox pathways by:

- Drinking purified water throughout the day, especially between meals
- Practicing deep breathing exercises, one to three times per day
- Using an infrared sauna, one to three times per week
- Doing exercise that causes you to sweat, three to five times per week for twenty to sixty minutes each session
- Taking supplements to support regular elimination (we'll discuss this in more detail later in the chapter)
- Using IV therapy, if available—intravenous (IV) therapy can deliver key nutrients such as glutathione, vitamin C, and

other detox-supporting compounds directly into your bloodstream for faster absorption and cellular support. This can be especially helpful if you're dealing with heavy metal exposure or high toxin loads.

- Using hyperbaric oxygen therapy (HBOT), if available—hyperbaric therapy involves breathing pure oxygen in a pressurized chamber, which helps increase oxygen delivery to tissues, reduce inflammation, and support detoxification at the cellular level. It can also enhance mitochondrial function, aiding energy production and overall healing.

- Having daily bowel movements (one per day is good; two or three is even better)

With those first two steps now in place, we can focus on the third and final step—*focusing on deeper cellular detoxification*. If you've had the opportunity to test, the results of the testing you completed will point you in the right direction for which specific types of toxins your body is dealing with. If you're using the Every Baby Well program, the practitioners will work alongside you to customize a detox protocol. Either way, if you know what you're dealing with, you can be more specific and effective with treatment.

Overall, here are the detox goals you want to achieve during this process. By supporting your body's natural detox pathways, you'll be clearing out stored toxins, reducing ongoing exposures, and optimizing your ability to absorb key nutrients. This process isn't about perfection—it's about making small, consistent changes that create a cleaner, healthier foundation for fertility and overall well-being.

- **Regenerate membranes:** Toxins damage the membranes of cells and the cell membranes that make up the mitochondria inside cells. When these membranes are impaired, cells lose their integrity. The result is that cellular communication and energy production suffer. Support cell membranes with healthy dietary fats and choline, including phosphatidyl-chloline, EPA and DHA, antioxidant compounds including vitamin C, CoQ10, and curcumin as well as an overall nutrient-dense diet.

- **Boost autophagy:** Autophagy is the cell's inherent cleanup crew that helps to remove waste and damaged parts of the cell, either for removal from the body or recycling into new parts of cells. Autophagy peaks during the sleeping hours, making sleep a critical time for detoxification. In addition, intermittent fasting, the Fasting Mimicking Diet (FMD), or a ketogenic diet, where appropriate, have been shown to improve autophagy and cellular healing. I'll share more details about both of those diets in chapter 7.
- **Optimize methylation:** Optimizing methylation is essential for effective detoxification and overall health. You can do this in a number of ways.

First, you want proper nutrient support. The *B vitamins*—folate (B9), B6, and B12—are critical for methylation. Ensuring adequate intake of them through your diet or supplementation can support the methylation cycle. Use folate as 5-MTHF if you have MTHFR polymorphism (or are unsure if you do). *Magnesium* acts as a cofactor in many biochemical reactions, including methylation. *Zinc* and *riboflavin* (B2) also play supportive roles in the methylation process.

When you're making dietary choices, make sure that you consume methyl donors. Foods rich in methyl donors, such as leafy greens, beets, and cruciferous vegetables (e.g., broccoli and brussels sprouts), can enhance methylation. Also, limit your intake of processed foods, which can introduce toxins and hinder methylation. A diet rich in whole foods supports overall detoxification.

Chronic stress can impair methylation and detoxification. Incorporating stress management techniques such as meditation, yoga, neurofeedback, or regular physical activity can be beneficial.

Reducing your exposure to environmental toxins (e.g., pesticides and heavy metals) and chemicals (e.g., BPA and phthalates) can ease the burden on your detoxification pathways, including methylation.

Finally, pay attention to supplementation. Supporting methylation with liposomal glutathione, a potent antioxidant and detoxifier, can help in handling oxidative stress and toxin elimination. And N-Acetylcysteine (NAC) helps replenish glutathione levels, indirectly supporting methylation.

While many detoxification programs are trendy, the truth is, they may be ineffective and unsafe. Use this road map instead to decrease the toxic burden, open up the pathways of elimination, and support detoxification on the cellular level.

Detox-Specific Supplementation

You can start taking some supplements right away to help your body with its detoxification process. Rather than overload you with dozens of pills to take each day, I recommend you start with these detox-specific supplements, while making ongoing strides toward reducing your exposure to known toxins. This will be simultaneous to changes you'll be making to your diet as well (which you'll read about in the next chapter), since now you know the important role nutrition plays in the detoxification processes.

Magnesium

Magnesium helps facilitate over three hundred chemical reactions in the body. It's no wonder that magnesium supports cardiovascular health, muscles, nerves, bones, mood, brain health, and metabolism. Most people are deficient in magnesium and would benefit from supplementation.[209] They aren't getting enough magnesium from their diet alone, mostly because soil quality has become increasingly depleted over the years.[210] And many people have increased needs for magnesium because of toxin exposures or health issues.

Our bodies are constantly using magnesium and burning it up—we are not absorbing it well. Several factors contribute to depletion of magnesium in our bodies:

- Exercise
- Eating sugar and refined foods
- Environmental toxin exposure
- Foods grown in soil that is low in minerals including magnesium (eat nuts, avocadoes, and bananas to increase your magnesium levels)

Magnesium Supplements

I recommend taking the following supplements to make sure you're not deficient in magnesium:

- **Every Life Well magnesium glycinate 125** contains 250 mg magnesium (as Albion di-magnesium malate and TRAACS magnesium glycinate chelate) and 828 mg malic acid (as Albion di-magnesium malate). Magnesium glycinate and dimagnesium malate are both forms of magnesium that are well absorbed by the body. Glycine (from glycinate) is a calming amino acid that supports brain health, digestion, and joints and promotes sleep. Malic acid (from malate) supports energy metabolism and antioxidant systems in the body. Because magnesium helps so many body functions, you don't want to just be getting by—instead, levels need to be optimal. And almost everyone needs to take magnesium for their levels to be optimal. Plus, there's a dual function to magnesium because it helps keep the stool flowing every day. Take one to four capsules daily in order to keep the bowels working regularly.

RENEW

Liver Detox Protect

This features a powerful blend of ingredients that aid in detoxification, provide antioxidant support, and promote a healthy immune system. Take one capsule twice daily, or as directed. This formula contains:

- *N-Acetylcysteine (NAC)*: an acetylated form of the sulfur-containing amino acid L-cysteine. It aids in the production of glutathione, a tripeptide crucial for detoxification and antioxidant defense. Glutathione also helps protect the body from liver-damaging environmental pollutants, gamma radiation, and other harmful toxins.

- *Alpha-Lipoic Acid (also known as thioctic acid)*: This powerful antioxidant works in both water and fat, making it especially effective at protecting your cells. It helps boost glutathione (your body's master detoxifier), regenerates vitamins C and E, and keeps your mitochondria—your energy powerhouses—running smoothly. ALA also supports liver and kidney health by promoting balanced nitric oxide levels, which are key for detoxification. Plus, it plays a role in maintaining a healthy immune response, giving your body extra support as you prepare for conception.

- *Milk Thistle Seed Extract*: Silymarin, the active compound in milk thistle, promotes liver health by supporting antioxidant activity, neutralizing toxins, and protecting liver cells' genetic material. It boosts glutathione production and helps maintain normal fat oxidation, immune response, and liver tissue regeneration.

- *Selenium (as selenomethionine)*: Selenium is a key coenzyme for glutathione peroxidase, enhancing liver cells' antioxidant defenses by increasing MnSOD expression. It also supports cytokine balance by regulating IL-6 transcription in Kupffer cells, which play a vital role in liver health.

Modified Citrus Pectin Powder or Capsules

These products consist of a clinically proven form of modified citrus pectin, derived from citrus pith and modified for optimal molecular weight and structure. This unique modification enhances its bioavailability, allowing for absorption into the bloodstream and providing broad-spectrum benefits for healthy cell, tissue, and organ function.

Metal Detox Capsules

These are formulated to assist the body in eliminating harmful oxidative elements. They contain targeted ingredients like EDTA, Himalayan shilajit extract, chlorella, and nutrients that boost antioxidant activity. Together, these ingredients support your health when working to eliminate environmental toxins, including heavy metals. Take two to four capsules daily, or as directed.

Liposomal Glutathione

This is the most important antioxidant support nutrient produced by the body and is found in every cell. This molecule is depleted every time you are exposed to environmental toxins, so it's the perfect companion to bring on board while you are reducing controllable toxins in your life. Glutathione is known as the body's master detoxifier because of its ability to neutralize a broad range of free radical compounds and protect your cells from damaged caused by toxins, including pollution in the air.[211] Research has shown that daily supplementation of liposomal glutathione increases glutathione in the body and therefore enhances immune function and reduces markers of oxidative stress.[212] This is one of the supplements I most often recommend to patients, and it's one I personally never want to be without, especially when traveling. Typical glutathione supplements can break down in the digestive system without being absorbed intact, which is why I chose to package the Every Life Well liposomal glutathione in phosphatidyl-choline liposome for optimal absorption, bioavailability, and cell support. Liposomal glutathione provides 500 mg of pure glutathione and activated B vitamin cofactors delivered in phosphatidylcholine liposomes for optimal absorption and bioavailability support. Take one to two teaspoons or one to two capsules every morning.

Every Life Well Zeo Binder

This broad-spectrum binding formula contains natural ingredients from the purest sources to support enhanced clearance of heavy metals, unwanted organisms, and organic compounds from the GI tract. Binders have been used for centuries as a remedy for toxin exposure. They play an important role in many detoxification protocols and have a vital role in protecting the gut lining. Selective binders like Zeo Binder are used to bind and remove specific toxins from the GI tract for a thorough detoxification protocol. I recommend Zeo Binder because it supports elimination to reduce hepatic reabsorption (which is when the liver releases substances into the intestines through bile, and then the body reabsorbs those same substances back into the bloodstream from the intestines, essentially recycling them instead of eliminating them from the body). Zeo Binder also helps relieve the toxic load. If you know you have a highly reactive immune system, Zeo Binder works to limit the effects of die-off reactions and sweep toxins away from the gut lining before they can cause a severe reaction or immune response. The mineral content in Zeo Binder comes from the purest sources across several geographic areas, from rich mineral deposits in Eastern Europe to the vast mountains of Central Asia. Zeo Binder contains Purified Zeolite (G-PUR®), a purified zeolite mineral with a distinctive affinity to ionically bind to and absorb heavy metals and unwanted organisms.[213] G-PUR® is sourced from rich mineral deposits and is thoroughly tested for inorganic impurities.[214] It also contains activated charcoal, which has a long history of use in reducing the harmful effects of a wide variety of toxins. Unlike charcoal from wood or peat, the coconut shell charcoal in Zeo Binder is highly purified, dense, clean, and naturally dust-free, making it a safe and viable binder for toxin removal, especially for unwanted organisms. Its carbon lattice and porous structure is ideal for trapping and removing a variety of toxins, preventing absorption by the gut lining, and safely carrying the toxins bound to its surface out of the body. Purified Shilajit (PrimaVie®) is another ingredient in Zeo Binder. This is a highly purified form of shilajit (a mineral substance found primarily in the rocks of the Himalayas), diverse in many bioactive compounds, containing over forty different minerals, including a rich source of humic and fulvic acids. These types of organic acids have absorbent properties and are best known to bind various agents, including many organic compounds. Due to the unique liposomal structure of Primavie®, it encapsulates such toxins for efficient removal from the body.[215] Take one to two capsules daily, but not within two hours of taking other supplements or medications.

Heavy Metal Chelation

This chemical process refers to the chemical process where a "chelating" agent binds to heavy metals in the bloodstream. *Chelation* is derived from the Latin word *claw*, referring to how the agent "grabs" metal ions. The therapy itself, which incorporates administering chelation agents, should be done by a professional who can administer these properly and monitor the results closely. (I do not recommend IV chelation, as it is too potent and sometimes creates unexpected side effects.) But there are some things you can do at home. Much of this has to do with detoxification—for example, increasing your fiber intake, hydrating well, eating antioxidant-rich foods, supporting your liver health, exercising (sauna use is also recommended, but not within three months of conceiving), and avoiding heavy-metal sources (use water filters and minimize products that use these sources). In terms of supplements, increase your liposomal glutathione plus Zeo Binder and add Every Life Well Metal Detox dosages. Over the years in my practice, I've found that the supplements I'm recommending here in the book often do an excellent job of removing the metals without having to take more aggressive measures.

Candida Cleanse

You should have a Candida Cleanse if your labs show that you have an overgrowth of candida. This means eating no sugar, consuming no alcohol, eating a low-carb, gluten-free, and dairy-free diet, and taking supplements. (Please bear in mind that this condition might also require medication.) I recommend you incorporate these products into your candida cleanse:

Candex

This blend of enzymes breaks down the carbohydrates in yeast cell walls, offering rapid and effective microbiome support with the recommended dietary changes.

Candida Complete

This offers a blend of nutrients, botanicals, and essential oils to support microbial balance and immune health. It includes biotin to prevent yeast from becoming more aggressive and sodium caprylate to disrupt candida metabolism. Additionally, it features botanicals such as berberine HCl, pau d'arco, oregano, rosemary, cinnamon, and ginger to soothe the GI tract, provide antioxidant support, and maintain microbial balance. Sometimes pharmaceutical prescriptions are also helpful.

Daily Probiotics

Probiotics help maintain a healthy gut microbiome, which includes the bacteria, viruses, yeast, and parasites in the intestinal tract. My Daily Probiotics provide four researched strains of beneficial bacteria, including *Bifidobacterium lactis* HN019, *Lactobacillus acidophilus*, *Lactobacilluslantarum* Lp-115, and *Bifidobacterium longum* (*Bifidobacterium longum* Bl-05).

GI Defend or GI Restore Powder

These healing powders contain a blend of ingredients to support optimum GI health and function. These include L-Glutamine, MSM, N-acetyl glucosamine, DGL, slippery elm, marshmallow, chamomile, okra extract, cat's claw, aloe vera, quercetin, mucin, prune powder, and citrus pectin.

Parasite Cleanse

I recommend this basic protocol if your parasite test results come back positive (or abnormal). Start with magnesium to keep the bowels moving. I also recommend a product called Paracid Forte. The plant compounds in Paracid Forte provide strong antioxidant support and help maintain a healthy microbial balance in the GI tract, creating an unfavorable environment for parasites. Each capsule contains 150 mg of sweet wormwood, 100 mg of olive leaf extract, 85 mg of black walnut hulls, and 25 mg of artemisinin. Sometimes pharmaceutical prescriptions are also helpful.

Final Thoughts

As you embark on this detoxification journey, I hope you will take pride in the progress you've already made toward reducing your toxic load. The science is clear: Minimizing exposure to toxins and actively supporting your body's detox pathways can significantly impact not just your health but the health of your future child. The steps you are taking to assist your body with the detoxification processes right now will play a crucial role in optimizing your epigenetic legacy. By following the strategies and supplements tailored to your specific needs, you're setting the stage for a healthier pregnancy, as well as a healthier future for your little one. I encourage you to embrace this empowering process with confidence, knowing that everything you're doing has the potential to positively shape generations to come.

Q&A

Q: What is detoxification, and why is it important during preconception?

A: Detoxification is the biological process by which the body eliminates harmful substances, including environmental toxins and by-products of cellular metabolism. During preconception, detoxification is essential to creating a clean, healthy environment for conception, reducing the risk of passing toxins on to your baby, and supporting optimal egg and sperm quality.

Q: Which organs are involved in detoxification, and what are their roles?

A: The six primary organs of detoxification are the liver, intestines, kidneys, lungs, lymphatic system, and skin. The liver processes toxins for excretion, the intestines and kidneys eliminate waste through feces and urine, the lungs expel volatile toxins, the lymphatic system removes cellular waste, and the skin eliminates toxins through sweat.

Q: How can I support my body's detox pathways effectively?

A: Supporting detox pathways involves staying hydrated, engaging in regular exercise to promote sweating, eating nutrient-dense foods that are rich in antioxidants, using supplements such as glutathione and magnesium, and having daily bowel movements to prevent toxin recirculation.

Q: What role does methylation play in detoxification?

A: Methylation is a biochemical process that neutralizes toxins, supports DNA repair, and helps metabolize hormones and heavy metals. Proper methylation is supported by nutrients such as B vitamins (B6, B12, and folate), magnesium, and foods rich in methyl donors, such as leafy greens and cruciferous vegetables.

RENEW

Q: What are some common misconceptions about detoxing?

A: A common misconception is that detoxing requires extreme diets or juice cleanses, which can be ineffective or even harmful. Effective detoxification involves gradual, balanced approaches that support all detox pathways simultaneously, ensuring the body eliminates toxins without overwhelming its systems or causing discomfort.

CHAPTER 7

You Can't Be
"a Little Bit" Nutritious

In this chapter, I invite you to experience the awe-inspiring impact of preconception nutrition. I encourage you to approach it with a deep willingness to learn just how much power you hold in each of your food choices and how profoundly they can impact the health and vitality of the child you and your partner will be conceiving. In the same way you can't be "a little bit" pregnant, I also believe you can't be "a little bit" nutritious. This is an all-or-nothing proposition.

It's important that you go into this willing to leave behind all your preconceived notions about food. We all have them, but this is the time to set those aside and absorb new information about how to truly nourish your body so it can do its very best work. I realize setting aside your lifelong eating habits and embracing a new nutritional plan can feel monumental; it's like you're changing your very way of life. But I have witnessed incredible transformations in my patients when they've been willing to commit to this nutrition plan, and I am confident you will feel transformed as well.

The food you choose to eat is the single most important decision you can make when it comes to preconception . . . and it's a decision you make multiple times every day, so you've got to get it right. Remember that love is your underlying motivation, and allow that love to fuel you on this journey and inspire you to keep going even when it feels tough.

Your Kitchen Reset: A Fresh Start with Nutrition

Your quest for deep nourishment begins in the kitchen. I encourage you to look at the contents of your refrigerator, freezer, pantry, and cabinets and see what's in there. As you do, ask yourself, *What is my food story?* As you peruse the shelves, what story are those food products telling you? Do they speak of someone who is always in a rush at mealtime? A person who hasn't been prioritizing time for preparing food, but rather just heating it up? Someone who likes the idea of eating healthy but is always looking for a shortcut? No guilt or shame here—this is simply an exercise in storytelling.

Once you've been able to honestly acknowledge what your current food story says about your overall nourishment, I want you to start working on bringing this important truth into your consciousness: *You do not have to purchase or consume prepackaged foods.* Items such as canned goods, frozen meals, bags of chips, boxed mac and cheese—you can absolutely live without them . . . all of them. That might be shocking, and you might be wondering how you'll have time to cook everything from scratch. But let me encourage you— you *can* create time in your life for cooking real, whole foods, not just rehydrating something that's been sitting in a box on a shelf for months, or longer. This process is about more than just organizing your kitchen; it's about making a fresh start, paving the way for healthier choices and reminding you of your commitment to your future baby.

You might be wondering, *OK, how do I actually tackle this?* Here's what I suggest: Set aside a dedicated time—perhaps on a quiet weekend morning or during an evening when you can focus without distractions. Go through every shelf and drawer, examining each item with a discerning eye. Ask yourself: *Does this food align with the goals I've set for myself and my family? Will it deeply nourish this body that is preparing to bring new life into this world? Is it something I would want my future child to eat?* If you answer no to any of those questions, either donate it or throw it out. Take the process one shelf at a time and spread the task out over several weeks if you need to.

This act of clearing out the old will make room for the nourishing, whole foods that will support you on your health journey. After all, the sooner you adopt this new way of feeding yourself, the easier it will be to model that behavior when you're parenting your future child! As you transition to a cleaner, more intentional way of eating, remember that fresh, whole ingredients will become the foundation of all your meals. To make this shift easier, I've compiled a base grocery list of essentials that will support you now and continue to be invaluable once you become a parent. By having these staples on hand, you'll find it easier to prepare nutritious meals, even on busy days.

Your "New Essentials" Grocery List (choose all organic items)

- **Oils:** Olive oil, avocado oil, coconut oil
- **Vegetables:** Broccoli, cauliflower and cauliflower rice, onions, garlic, cabbage, carrots, celery
- **Fruits:** Blueberries, raspberries, avocados, lemons, limes, apples
- **Beverages:** Black cherry juice, sparkling water (unflavored, in glass bottles)

- **Proteins:** Organic free-range eggs, grass-fed beef and turkey (from the meat counter, not prepackaged), organic chicken, bone broth (stored in glass)
- **Nuts and Seeds:** Cashews, almonds (store in the fridge or freezer), walnuts, pumpkin seeds, chia seeds
- **Spreads and Condiments:** SunButter, cinnamon, garlic salt, garlic powder, sea salt from Spain (such as Mallorca) or Premier Research salt
- **Minimally Processed Foods:** Grain-free granola (Paleonola, Purely Elizabeth, Thrive Market, Wildway), turkey or grass-fed beef jerky (Chomps, Thrive Market, Epic, Paleovalley), plantain chips, guacamole, bars (Paleovalley superfood bars, Paleo Bars by Universal Bakery, Thunderbird Bars, N!ck's protein bars), Thrive Market Paleo Snack Mix
- **Dairy and Alternatives:** Miyoko's Creamery salted cultured vegan butter, applesauce (in a glass jar, not plastic)
- **Snacks and Sweeteners:** Seaweed snacks, honey (for immunity and flavor)
- **Smoothie Ingredients:** Frozen blueberries, mangos, cherries, bananas

Remember, by making time for this reset, you're not just organizing your kitchen and stocking it with new foods—you're laying the foundation for a healthier lifestyle. The effort you put in now will make healthy eating easier later, especially when you're a parent and your time is even more limited.

Making Nut Milk at Home

When you make nut milk at home, you gain the peace of mind that comes with knowing exactly what's in your drink. Unlike store-bought options that may have been sitting in a box on a shelf for months or in a plastic bottle in the refrigerated section of the grocery store, homemade nut milk is fresh, pure, and free from unnecessary additives. You can trust the quality of the water you use, ensuring that your nut milk is as clean and healthy as possible. Plus, by using a nut processor like Almond Cow (https://almondcow.co/) or NutraMilk, you can easily create your own fresh batches, knowing that every sip is packed with the nutrients and flavor that only homemade can provide. It's a simple step that makes a big difference in nourishing yourself and your family with the best nature has to offer.

A Diet That Caught Me Off Guard . . . in a Good Way!

When Melissa Urban and Dallas Hartwig wrote *The Whole 30*, I read the book and decided I loved the philosophy. But when it first came out, although it was the book I wanted to write, I thought it would be too difficult for people to commit to something so challenging. But look at how it's taken off! Millions of copies have been sold and countless lives changed. The success of The Whole 30 program shows me that people are not only willing but *eager* to take on these kinds of nutrition challenges. It's reaffirmed my belief that with the right guidance, people can—and will—make the necessary changes for their health.

What's even more exciting about adopting a new diet plan within this context is that it's about more than just *your* health—it's about your future baby's health too. Now is the time to start thinking and acting as if you're already pregnant, because what you do now matters as much as when you're carrying your child.

I'm putting a lofty goal in front of you, and I fully believe you can achieve it. You might experience some fails along the way, but I've seen my patients pick themselves up, brush off the dust, and get back on track. This is about stewardship—not just of your own body but of the new life you're preparing to welcome into the world. It's about

RENEW

partnership too. You and your partner are in this together, and supporting each other throughout this journey is key. If you can commit to this process as a couple, it will strengthen your relationship and prepare you both for the journey of parenthood. Sharing a common goal sets a strong foundation for the future.

Being all in means more than just sticking to a nutrition plan. This is where the rubber meets the road. It's about committing to the creation of a new life and all the responsibilities that come with it. Once your child is here, there will be no room for wavering. You have what it takes to overcome any wobbling or uncertainty you might feel now, and it is worth summoning all your strength to do just that. You have the strength to prioritize your health in this way. The process I'm asking you to go through will help you develop the mental and emotional muscles you need. It's about building internal awareness and readiness, so when the time comes, you're fully prepared to be a parent.

Smart Splurges: Elevate Your Well-Being

Right about now, you might be feeling slightly nervous about the food you're going to be eating on this plan. Occasional indulgences, when done thoughtfully, are a key aspect of this nutrition lifestyle. I like to call these "Smart Splurges"—they're special treats that not only bring us joy but also align with our health goals.

Smart Splurges are about making choices that nourish both body and soul. Remember, it's not about perfection; it's about balance. By choosing your splurges wisely, you can enjoy life's pleasures without compromising your health. Here are a few of my favorite Smart Splurge recipes.

Almond Fudge Butter

If you're looking for a sweet treat to serve guests that might even get them hooked on your diet, these will not disappoint. Made with dairy-free chocolate chips, almond butter, and coconut oil, they taste like peanut butter cups—but without all the sugar or guilt! They're also quick and easy to make when you're craving something sweet.

What you need

Chocolate Layer

- 1½ cups dairy-free dark or semi-sweet chocolate chips (I like the Enjoy Life brand)
- ½ cup smooth almond butter
- 1 tablespoon raw honey
- ¼ cup coconut oil, melted (organic, extra virgin)

Almond Butter Layer

- 1 ½ cups almond butter
- ¼ cup coconut oil, softened (organic, extra virgin)
- 4 tablespoons raw organic honey
- 1 pinch pink or sea salt

Make!

Line a small baking dish with parchment paper. Melt the chocolate chips in a small saucepan over medium heat. Add the almond butter and honey. Stir in the coconut oil until the mixture is creamy and smooth. Pour the chocolate batter into the baking dish and place it in the freezer to set while you work on the next layer.

In a medium bowl, whisk the almond butter layer ingredients together until smooth. The consistency will still be thick enough to spread. Spread the almond butter layer over the chocolate layer. Place in the freezer to set for an hour. Cut into squares and serve! (Makes 16 squares.)

Summer Berry Tart

Perfect for warmer weather or any special occasion (like the Fourth of July!), this is a beautiful and BERRY delicious dessert to serve for family or friends, or for when you just want to treat yourself. It's made using fresh berries, coconut yogurt, and almond flour.

What you need

Dough

- 1 cup blanched almond flour
- 2 tablespoons coconut flour
- ⅔ cup tapioca flour
- ½ cup coconut oil
- 1 teaspoon (for sweet pies) or ½ teaspoon (for savory pies) maple sugar or coconut sugar
- ½ teaspoon fine-grain sea salt
- 1 large egg (pasture-raised, organic)

Filling

- Coconut yogurt (vanilla or plain)
- Toppings: Fresh organic berries (strawberries, golden raspberries, raspberries, blackberries, and blueberries)
- Mint, for garnish

Make!

In the bowl of a food processor, pulse all the dough ingredients except the egg to create thick, small pieces, then pulse in the egg until a dough forms. Gather the dough into a ball prior to rolling or pressing it into your pie dish/es. Once the dough has been pressed into the pie dish, gently pierce it with a fork all over so it does not puff up while baking.

For a fully baked crust, bake at 375° F for 15 minutes or until very lightly browned. Remove from the oven to cool slightly. Fill with yogurt and top with berries and fresh mint! (Makes 1 large or 4 mini tarts.)

Pumpkin Bars with Coconut Cream Almond Butter Drizzle

These decadent and delicious pumpkin bars are perfect when sweet temptations are in abundance. Made with naturally sweet pumpkin and honey, they will give you all the taste with none of the sugar spike!

What you need

Pumpkin Bars

- ½ cup organic pumpkin purée
- ½ cup almond butter
- ⅓ cup honey
- 2 eggs (pasture-raised, organic, cage-free)
- 1 teaspoon cinnamon
- ¼ teaspoon ground cloves
- ½ teaspoon baking soda
- 1 pinch sea salt

Coconut Cream Almond Butter Drizzle

- ¼ cup almond butter
- ¼ cup coconut cream
- 1 tablespoon maple syrup or honey
- ¼ cup almond and pecan pieces (topping)

Make!

Preheat the oven to 350° F. Mix the pumpkin bar ingredients together. Pour into a greased 8x8-inch baking dish and bake for 30 minutes. Then remove from the oven and let cool. Meanwhile, mix the drizzle ingredients together in a small bowl. Cut the pumpkin bars into 9 squares, then top with drizzle and chopped nuts. (Makes 9 bars.)

Two-Ingredient Pancakes

These yummy pancakes are made with just *two* ingredients. They're perfect for a quick breakfast or snack—or for anytime! Gluten-free and dairy-free, these pancakes are naturally sweetened with organic bananas. Add a touch of nut butter and honey for a truly special breakfast or smart splurge. Double or triple the recipe and freeze the extra to enjoy later!

RENEW

What you need

Pancake

- 1 large ripe banana
- 2 eggs

Optional Toppings

- Banana slices (organic)
- Nut butter (raw cashew butter, almond butter)
- Honey (organic)

Make!

In a medium bowl, mash the banana well with a fork, and then whisk in the eggs. Heat your skillet over medium-low heat. Spray the pan with coconut oil or lightly coat it with oil using a paper towel. Scoop ¼ cup of the mixture into the skillet. Cook for about 50 seconds on each side or until golden brown. Serve with desired toppings.

Blueberry Pineapple Smoothie

This recipe is like an ice-cream parfait, without the inflammation and blood-sugar spike. And it is so delicious and easy to make. Dairy-free, gluten-free, and sweetened with a little honey or agave nectar, this smoothie is a perfect Smart Splurge for anytime.

What you need

Pineapple Layer

- 1 cup pineapple chunks, frozen
- ½ banana, peeled and frozen
- ½ cup frozen peaches or mangos
- ½ cup coconut milk (or nut milk of choice)
- 1 tablespoon honey or agave nectar

Blueberry Layer

- ½ cup wild blueberries, frozen
- ½ banana, frozen
- 1 tablespoon honey or agave nectar
- ½ cup milk of choice
- 1 scoop Perfect Paleo unflavored protein powder (or you can use any of the Every Life Well protein powders, such as PreConceive Nutrition or Fertility Fuel, which come in various flavors)[216]
- fresh cubed mango (topping)

Make!

Blend the pineapple layer in a blender. Add it to two glasses, then wash out the blender and add the blueberry layer until smooth. Spoon the blueberry mixture on top of the pineapple layer. Top with mango. Serve cold. (Makes 2 servings.)

For more ideas on how to indulge wisely, check out my Instagram posts with #SmartSplurge, where I share more tips and inspiration.

RENEW

The Link Between the Preconception Diet and Your Baby's Epigenetics

Throughout this book, we've been talking about epigenetics—how behaviors and environment can cause changes that affect the way your genes work. But as we enter into this conversation about nutrition, I want to point out that epigenetics remind us just how deeply connected we are to our environment, and how the choices we make now can send a ripple through the generations to come.

A woman's nutritional status both prior to and during pregnancy is intricately linked to the health of her offspring, even into adulthood.[217] This concept is known as the Developmental Origins of

Health and Disease (DOHaD) or Fetal Origins of Adult Disease, and it highlights the connection between environmental influences during critical developmental times and the consequences—or benefits— these influences can have on both short and long-term health.[218]

In the 1980s, research first linked birth weight to cardiovascular risk later in life.[219] Since then, numerous studies have made connection between a mother's nutritional status and a wide range of health outcomes in her children, including diabetes, heart disease, hypertension, obesity, cognition, and even cancer. One striking example is the fetal origins of breast cancer hypothesis, which suggests that the hormonal environment during pregnancy—shaped by diet and exposure to endocrine disruptors—can modify the genetic expression in breast tissue, potentially affecting cancer risk later in life.[220]

In 2004, a study by Robert Waterland and Randy Jirtle looked at how the food a mother eats during early pregnancy can cause changes in how certain genes work in her baby. These changes don't alter the baby's DNA but can affect how certain genes are turned on or off. The researchers focused on parts of the DNA called *transposons*, which can move around within the genome, and *imprinted genes*, which are only active depending on whether they come from the mother or father.

The study found that these early changes, influenced by the mother's diet, can increase the risk of the baby developing chronic diseases like obesity, diabetes, or heart disease later in life.[221] While this particular study zeroed in on the pregnancy diet, I want to remind you that making changes to your diet usually doesn't happen overnight, and so what you do during preconception will set the stage for how you eat during pregnancy. Obesity preconception creates multiple challenges for fertility, and studies show that weight loss is a promising strategy for improving fertility outcomes.[222]

Dads, you're not off the hook here. There is plenty of research indicating that your nutritional status matters just as much as Mom's prior to conception. For instance, if you are overweight, keep in mind that one study's findings suggest that a father's obesity before conception can affect how certain genes are marked during sperm development.[223] Because these gene markers are crucial for healthy development, a father's obesity could have lasting effects on his child's health, potentially impacting them even before they are born.[224]

Even if your weight isn't an issue, it's interesting to note that levels of folate (a B vitamin that is essential for DNA synthesis and repair) in men prior to conception have been linked to epigenetic changes in their offspring. A study published in *Nature Communications* by Sarah Kimmins and colleagues found that insufficient folate in a father's diet could lead to DNA methylation changes, which could potentially cause birth defects and increase the risk of diseases in their children.[225]

Research has also shown that a father's diet can affect the quality of his sperm, including the presence of certain epigenetic markers. For instance, one study indicated that a high-fat diet in male mice could lead to altered sperm and metabolic changes in their offspring, suggesting that poor paternal diet could predispose children to metabolic disorders.[226] Furthermore, men who consume a diet rich in fiber, antioxidants, and high-quality proteins tend to have higher fertility rates.[227]

This body of research highlights just how important it is for mothers to eat well before and during pregnancy, and for fathers to be properly nourished prior to conception, because it can have long-lasting effects on their child's health. The good news? Many of these factors are modifiable. By making intentional, positive changes to your diet before conception, you can promote favorable epigenetic changes, giving your child the best possible start in life.

What to Include

Three types of food—macronutrients, micronutrients, and phytonutrients—make up a good preconception diet.

Macronutrients are the carbohydrates, fats, and proteins that your body needs regularly in order to function and create energy. But both quality and quantity make all the difference.[228]

Micronutrients are the vitamins and minerals that the body needs in small quantities. Adequate levels of micronutrients are essential for fertility and fetal development.[229]

Phytonutrients (or antioxidants) are chemicals or compounds found in certain plants that help protect them from insects, fungi, and even the sun. These chemicals and compounds have antioxidant properties. Studies show that phytonutrients carry tremendous health benefits for humans, especially in the prevention of disease in family health.[230]

What NOT to Include

What you leave out of your diet is just as important as what you include. Certain foods and additives can contribute to inflammation, disrupt hormone balance, and burden your body's detox pathways—none of which is ideal when trying to conceive. In this section, we'll go over the key offenders to avoid so you can create a cleaner, more supportive environment for fertility and overall health.

- **Bad fats:** Trans-fat is found in some fried foods, processed foods, and commercially manufactured baked goods and pastries. These fats wreak havoc on your gut microbiome, blood sugar, and cholesterol.[231]

- **Seed oils:** These are high in omega-6 linoleic acid, which is linked to inflammation.[232] When heated, seed oils produce trans-fats, and most seed oils you buy are processed. This includes corn oil, soybean oil, sunflower oil, canola oil, safflower oil, grapeseed oil, and cottonseed oil.

- **Toxins:** I've devoted an entire chapter to detoxification, and more detail is provided there. Common toxins include MSG, brominated vegetable oil (BVO), and BPA, as well as added sugars, artificial sweeteners, artificial trans-fats, and much, much more. The herbicide glyphosate is also very common in our foods.

- **Dairy:** Cow's milk, cheese, and other dairy products can be inflammatory. While some people react differently to dairy than others, I suggest avoiding dairy products altogether. (My patients' lab work always look better when they are avoiding dairy.) The link between inflammation and infertility is conclusive.[233] A recent systematic review and meta-analysis investigated the impact of dairy consumption on women with PCOS, focusing on body measurements, blood glucose, insulin, and testosterone levels.[234] The study found that dairy intake was associated with increased insulin levels and higher BMI in these women.[235]

- **Sugar:** Obesity, cardiovascular diseases, and even cognition and mood are all affected by free sugars (sugars added to food).[236] The evidence of this keeps growing.

- **Gluten:** Found in wheat, barley, and rye, gluten has been incredibly controversial in the last decade. The reason for this has been the rise of non-celiac gluten sensitivity (NCGS), where people who do not have celiac disease nevertheless experience symptoms (bloating, fatigue, digestive issues) or just subtle elevated inflammation markers in testing.[237]

- **GMO products:** Genetically modified (GMO) products continue to be controversial. Most studies on GMO foods suggest links to toxic effects, including impacts on the liver, pancreas, kidneys, or reproductive system.[238] Thankfully, GMO products must be labeled as such, so definitely keep an eye out for that label.

No Gluten or Dairy—Really?

The American diet is basically built on gluten and dairy. Gluten is a protein found in wheat, barley, and rye that helps give bread and pasta their chewy texture. Just think about the bowl of cereal millions of Americans make every morning—it's usually a cereal made from wheat and other grains, with a cup of cold cow's milk poured on top. At lunch, perhaps a sandwich made with a couple slices of cheddar. And dinner might include a wheat-based pasta with melted cheese of some variety, or dinner rolls, mac and cheese, the list goes on. Sadly, we're conditioned to think that a meal isn't a meal without gluten or dairy.

I've had many patients who struggled with the idea of cutting out these staples of their diet. It's such a huge inconvenience trying to revamp your entire way of nourishing your body; I get it! But once I explain just how much these ingredients interfere with our health, suddenly the change feels worthwhile.

One patient, Candace, was facing pretty severe hormone and thyroid disruptions. Other doctors had wanted to put her on a synthetic thyroid hormone replacement to address what they'd diagnosed as Hashimoto's thyroiditis, never once talking to her about her nutrition. I talked to her about how inflammatory gluten and dairy are, and just how powerful an effect they can have on our hormones. I encouraged her to try being strict about it for six months and then retest to see how her numbers were looking. When the six-month experiment was over, not only was she feeling so much better, she was blown away by her new test results. Her hormones had normalized, including her thyroid numbers! After that, she knew gluten and dairy were no friends of hers, and she was highly motivated to keep them out of her diet. I hope this success story will encourage you to do the same!

The Role of Nutrition in Detoxification

Nutrition doesn't just nourish the body; it also plays a critical role in detoxification. As we touched on in the last chapter, certain nutrients are critical in the final phase of cellular detoxification. Foods rich in antioxidants, fiber, and certain phytonutrients can support the body's ability to detoxify harmful substances, which is especially important during the preconception period.

A well-rounded diet rich in colorful vegetables, fruits, and high-quality proteins can help your body efficiently eliminate toxins. Cruciferous vegetables such as broccoli, kale, and brussels sprouts are particularly effective at supporting liver detoxification pathways.[239] By focusing on these foods, you're not only nourishing your body, you're also creating a cleaner, healthier environment for your future child.

Changing Your Diet: A Commitment to Future Health

Making significant changes to your diet can feel overwhelming, especially when you're doing it for reasons that go beyond your own immediate health. But remember—this is a commitment to your future, and more importantly, to the health and vitality of your future child. I hope you are feeling encouraged by how powerful your food choices really are. Every meal counts!

To set yourself up for success in this venture, based on what you know about yourself and your tolerance for change, decide now whether it's smarter to start small and build gradually or if you do better when you just jump in 100 percent. If starting small and building is your preferred path to success, begin by adding nutrient-dense foods to your diet, and as you become more comfortable, start eliminating the less healthy options. Focus on the "why" behind these changes. Each healthy choice you make is a gift to your future family—a powerful step toward ensuring that your child starts life on the best possible footing.

Your mindset is everything. Take it one day at a time, celebrate small victories, and remember that perfection isn't the goal—progress is. You're setting the foundation for a lifetime of health, and I promise the rewards will be well worth the effort.

How to Optimize Fertility and Prepare the Body for Pregnancy

The Healthy Eating Index 2015 (HEI-2015) is a tool used to assess how well a person's diet aligns with the Dietary Guidelines for Americans, which is published by the US Department of Agriculture (USDA) and the US Department of Health and Human Services (HHS). Some research shows that women who closely follow a healthy diet based on the HEI-2015 have a significantly lower risk of diminished ovarian reserve, strongly suggesting that proper nutrition may improve fertility outcomes.[240] In light of this, here's your preconception checklist for building up nutrition stores and supporting favorable epigenetics.

Eat whole foods.

Start to phase out processed, packaged food options, as well as refined sugars, industrial fats, artificial sweeteners, and chemical food additives. Instead, cook more at home with high-quality ingredients. Incorporate an abundance of colorful produce, protein with every meal, and healthful fats.

Include specific fertility foods.

These nutrient-dense options provide critical fats and micronutrients that support fertility and pregnancy:

- Dark leafy green vegetables (e.g., kale, arugula, collards, dandelion greens)[241]
- Whole eggs and egg yolks from pastured chickens[242]
- Poultry, lamb, goat, bison, pork, and beef (choose red meat that is grass-fed or regenerative)
- Low-mercury fish (sardines, anchovies, mackerel, wild salmon) in limited quantities (1–2 servings per week)[243]
- Shellfish (cooked oysters, shrimp, scallops)[244]
- Cruciferous vegetables (broccoli, cauliflower, cabbage, arugula, bok choy)
- Organic nuts and seeds (variety is key)[245]
- Colorful produce (blueberries, raspberries, red cabbage, orange sweet potatoes, beets, butternut squash, white onions, yellow peppers, green asparagus)[246]

Decrease toxin exposures.

- Eat organic to reduce pesticide and herbicide exposures.
- Eliminate alcohol and caffeine.
- Filter your drinking and cooking water and avoid plastic containers.
- Choose glass or stainless-steel food storage containers and never heat food in plastic.
- Prioritize foods and beverages that are packaged in glass.

Lower your inflammation with food.

Diets with a high anti-inflammatory potential are continuously showing promise for fertility, for both men[247] and women.[248] Food can actually function as our medicine, and one of the ways it does that is by lowering our inflammation rather than increasing it. One benefit of the fertility foods I've mentioned is that they are also anti-inflammatory. When it comes to meats, what's important is how they are prepared, their leanness, and the quality and quantity you eat. This is why grass-fed beef is so important. Quantity and quality are also good guidance for nuts and eggs.

Get adequate supplementation.

In addition to foods, spices such as turmeric, ginger, garlic, cinnamon, cayenne, black pepper, cloves, cardamom, peppermint, licorice root, and oregano are anti-inflammatory.[249] Even when eating a thoughtful and complete diet, you may still experience micronutrient gaps due to factors like soil depletion or an individual need for greater amounts of certain nutrients. In chapter 9, I'll share an in-depth look at how exactly you and your partner will be supplementing during this time.

Control your blood sugar with food.

Proteins are much better at controlling blood sugar than fiber or carbohydrates.[250] The diet I've provided here is excellent at helping you do this. In addition, studies have found that chromium, a trace element that is naturally present in many foods, is essential for controlling blood sugar levels. In fact, between 25–50 percent of the American population suffers from a chromium deficiency.[251] This may be linked to commercial farming methods, but it's also important to know that as you get older, your body finds it more difficult to absorb chromium.[252] Animal-sourced protein is a great source for chromium, including poultry and fish. Lean beef has the highest chromium count. Broccoli and green beans are also great sources, as well as egg yolks. All of these form part of the fertility-specific foods I mentioned.

Get your omega-3s.

To keep toxin exposure low, it's best to choose fish with minimal contamination, like wild-caught salmon, sardines, and other small fish, and limit servings each week. But don't skip out on omega-3s—they're essential for brain health, hormone balance, and reducing inflammation. The best sources are fatty fish and shellfish, but you can also get omega-3s from caviar, eggs, chia seeds, flaxseeds, nuts, and leafy greens. Include these nutrient-rich foods in your daily diet to support overall health and fertility.

Omega-3s offer women many benefits. They're anti-inflammatory—especially EPA and DHA—and help maintain healthy ovarian follicles, which are crucial for releasing a healthy egg during ovulation. They also assist in producing and regulating reproductive hormones such as progesterone, which is vital for preparing the uterine lining for implantation. Inflammation in the reproductive system can impair fertility, and omega-3s reduce systemic inflammation, improving the likelihood of conception. They also enhance blood flow to the uterus, creating a healthier environment for embryo implantation. In addition, DHA supports the development of a baby's brain and nervous system, so starting supplementation before pregnancy helps build maternal stores.

Omega-3s are also beneficial for men. They're critical for sperm structure, particularly in forming the sperm's cell membrane, improving motility and morphology. EPA and DHA protect sperm cells from oxidative damage, which can impair DNA integrity and fertility. Additionally, omega-3s may positively influence testosterone production, which is essential for sperm production and overall reproductive health.

There are also some shared benefits of omega-3s. Stress and anxiety can negatively impact fertility. Omega-3s are known to support mental health by reducing symptoms of stress and depression. They

RENEW

also are known to improve circulation, which benefits reproductive organs by delivering oxygen and nutrients more effectively.

The Preconception Diet

The Preconception Diet focuses on whole, unprocessed foods, with no gluten or dairy. Here is a helpful Preconception Diet quick guide to help you begin to formulate your meal planning.

Preconception Diet	Not Preconception Diet
Grass-fed meat	Gluten
Wild game	Dairy
Pasture-raised poultry	Grain
Pasture-raised eggs	Corn
Fish (*However, during preconception, I recommend reducing seafood due to mercury levels.)	Processed foods
Vegetables	Refined sugar, high fructose corn syrup
Nuts/Seeds	Syrup (rice syrup, refined maple syrup)
Fruit	Artificial sweeteners
Natural sweeteners (honey, agave, maple syrup, monk fruit)	Legumes (beans, peanuts)
Healthy oils	Artificial colors and flavors

Ten Tenets of the Preconception Diet

The foods you eat during preconception lay the foundation for your fertility, hormone balance, and overall health—before, during, and after pregnancy. The Preconception Diet is designed to provide your body with the most nutrient-dense, anti-inflammatory, and hormone-supportive foods while eliminating those that can interfere with optimal health. This approach isn't about deprivation but rather about fueling your body with the right building blocks to support conception and a healthy pregnancy. Following are the ten key principles that guide this dietary plan, focusing on whole foods, quality nutrients, and gut-friendly choices to create the best possible environment for you and your future baby.

1. **Whole Foods:** The cornerstone of the Preconception Diet is a focus on whole, nutrient-dense foods. This means eating foods in their most natural state, without the processing and additives that are common in today's diet.

2. **Lean, Clean Proteins:** The Preconeption Diet emphasizes high-quality animal proteins, such as grass-fed beef, free-range poultry, and pasture-raised eggs. These proteins are rich in essential amino acids and nutrients like iron and B vitamins, which are critical for both male and female fertility.

3. **Healthy Fats:** Contrary to outdated dietary advice, fats are not the enemy. This diet includes healthy fats from sources such as avocados, nuts, seeds, olive oil, and coconut oil. These fats are essential for hormone production, brain function, and overall health.

4. **Fruits and Vegetables:** A wide variety of colorful fruits and vegetables are encouraged on this diet plan. These foods are packed with vitamins, minerals, antioxidants, and fiber—all of which support a healthy gut, reduce inflammation, and provide the necessary building blocks for a healthy pregnancy and baby.

5. **Nuts and Seeds:** Rich in healthy fats, fiber, and protein, nuts and seeds are a staple of the Preconception Diet. They provide

essential fatty acids like omega-3s, which are important for reducing inflammation and supporting brain health in both parents and developing babies.[253]

6. **Exclusion of Gluten:** This diet is naturally gluten-free, as it excludes grains. This means you don't need to purchase "gluten-free" options. Many such options contain sugars, chemicals, artificial sweeteners, and more. There's no need to turn to processed options to be gluten-free!

7. **Exclusion of Grains and Legumes:** This diet excludes grains (such as wheat, rice, and corn) and legumes (such as beans, lentils, and peanuts). These foods contain antinutrients like lectins and phytates, which have been shown to interfere with nutrient absorption and digestion.[254] However, you can practice what is called the "modified Preconception Diet." Here, you can add a small amount of non-gluten grains such as buckwheat and rice or a small amount of chickpeas or lentils.

8. **Exclusion of Dairy:** Research showing the benefits of this type of diet does not include any animal lactation products, even ghee. You may not notice any symptoms from eating dairy, but it can contribute to inflammation, hormone imbalances, and digestive issues. Often the negative effects of dairy are insidious. The Preconception Diet encourages you to find calcium and other nutrients from nondairy sources, such as leafy greens and nuts.

9. **No Refined Sugars or Processed Foods:** These foods can spike blood-sugar levels, lead to insulin resistance, and contribute to inflammation—all of which can negatively impact fertility.

10. **Focus on Fiber:** This diet plan includes fiber-rich foods such as artichokes, avocados, broccoli, brussels sprouts, chia seeds, figs, berries, apples, and sweet potatoes.

More on the Dairy Story

I want to share a bit more on the subject of dairy in case you're struggling with the idea of going dairy-free and you'd like to know more of the reasoning behind this recommendation. First, milk naturally contains estrogens, and modern dairy farming practices, which involve milking pregnant cows, can significantly increase these hormone levels. These hormones may contribute to early puberty in children by disrupting hormonal balance, increase risks of hormone-sensitive cancers such as breast, ovarian, and prostate cancer, and affect male reproductive health, including sperm quality and testosterone levels.[255]

Insulin-like Growth Factor 1 (IGF1), which is present in milk, has been linked to elevated risks of hormone-sensitive cancers by promoting cell growth and reducing apoptosis. It's also linked to acne development through increased sebum production and skin cell turnover.[256]

Emerging research also reveals that milk is not just a nutrient source but a complex signaling system that activates mTORC1, a key regulator of growth and metabolism.[257] Lifelong exposure to cow's milk can overstimulate this pathway, contributing to health issues such as early puberty, acne, obesity, hormone-sensitive cancers, and neurodegenerative diseases like Parkinson's and Alzheimer's.[258] This overactivation is driven by milk's amino acids, growth factors, and bioactive microRNAs, which persist even after pasteurization. These findings highlight the potential risks of dairy consumption.

I hope this information helps with getting you on board for getting dairy out of your diet!

Why Is This Diet Great for Preconception?

The Preconception Diet is particularly beneficial because it provides a foundation of nutrient-dense, anti-inflammatory foods that support overall health and fertility for both men and women. Here's how it can enhance your preconception health:

- **Support Hormone Balance:** Healthy fats are essential for hormone production, which is crucial for fertility. Hormones like estrogen, progesterone, and testosterone are all derived from cholesterol, so ensuring adequate intake of good fats is key.[259]

- **Reduce Inflammation:** Chronic inflammation can interfere with fertility and increase the risk of complications during pregnancy. This diet's emphasis on whole foods, healthy fats, and the exclusion of inflammatory foods like refined sugars and processed grains helps to reduce inflammation and create a healthier internal environment for conception.[260]

- **Optimize Nutrient Intake:** The focus on nutrient-dense foods means you're providing your body with the essential vitamins and minerals needed for optimal fertility. For example, this plan is rich in zinc (from meat and shellfish), folate (from leafy greens), and omega-3 fatty acids (from fish, kelp, and nuts)—all of which are vital for reproductive health.[261]

- **Improve Gut Health:** A healthy gut is essential for overall health and fertility. The Preconception Diet's emphasis on fiber-rich vegetables, fruits, and nuts supports a diverse and balanced gut microbiome, which is linked to improved digestion, immune function, and even mood. A healthy gut can also help the body better absorb nutrients, ensuring that you and your future child get the maximum benefit from the foods you eat.[262]

- **Stabilize Blood Sugar:** Stable blood-sugar levels are crucial for hormonal balance and fertility. The Preconception Diet's focus on whole, unprocessed foods with a low glycemic index helps to prevent blood-sugar spikes and crashes, reducing the risk of insulin resistance and supporting overall hormonal health.[263]

- **Encourage Detoxification:** The nutrient-rich foods included in this diet, particularly cruciferous vegetables, support the body's natural detoxification processes. By reducing the intake of processed foods and increasing the consumption of detox-supporting foods, you help your body eliminate toxins that could interfere with fertility and fetal development.[264]

- **Enhance Sperm Quality:** For men, this diet can improve sperm quality by providing essential nutrients like zinc, selenium, and antioxidants, which are known to protect sperm from oxidative stress and support healthy sperm production.[265]

- **Enhance Egg Quality:** For women, this diet can improve egg quality by lowering inflammation, preserve DNA integrity, improve membrane fluidity and mitochondrial function, enhance oocyte maturation and fertilization potential, and regulate ovulatory cycles and healthy hormone signaling.

Tips for Implementing Dietary Changes

- **Start with the end in mind.** You can do this! Allow love to be your true motivation through all of this. You will come into conflict with so much of the culture—the advertising, the sales, the easy options available to you at the grocery store. This way of nourishing yourself might go against what you're used to, but once you get over the initial steps, it will come naturally. Set your mind to it, and you will succeed!

- **Then, add the good.** Rather than getting overwhelmed with removing foods you need to avoid, start by adding nutrient-dense options to your diet. As you incorporate more healthy foods, begin phasing out those that are less healthy.

- **Take out the bad.** "Just this one time . . ." will always catch up to you. You might need to avoid specials at the grocery store if they don't align with your goals. Some boxed or canned item might sound like a good deal, but don't allow them to get you off course.

- **Eat out the smart way.** Choose restaurants with healthy options you can enjoy. Plan for success by looking up the menu online and making your choice before you even arrive. I recommend starting by looking at your protein options and narrowing it down from there.

- **If you are overwhelmed, make incremental changes.** Each week, aim to add two Preconception Diet-friendly foods and eliminate one poor dietary choice. For example, add avocado and beets to your diet and cut out cheese. If you're addicted to sugary beverages, work on weaning off them by reducing your intake and replacing them with healthier options. (You can find many ideas for tasty, nutritious beverages on my website at https://annshippymd.com.)

- **Prioritize pure water.** Ensure your drinking water is free from contaminants by investing in a quality water purification system. I might sound like a broken record on this point but remember to avoid drinking from plastic containers. If you drink your eight glasses or more of water first, often you don't even want the unhealthy sodas!

- **Eat the fruit rather than drinking the juice.** Fruit is a fantastic source of fiber and phytonutrients. Eating the fruit is a much better choice than drinking the juice for several reasons, including that eating increases satiety[266] and regulates blood sugar better (fruit juice creates a blood-sugar spike).[267] Plus, the skin of the fruit and the pulp tend to have a higher fiber content than just the juice alone.[268]

- **Enjoy healthy snacks.** Everyone needs some satisfying, tasty snacks if they're going to stick to a nutrition plan.

Preconception Diet Recipes

Here are some recipes to get your taste buds excited and your creative juices flowing! I think you'll find these are all easy to make and don't require tons of ingredients. Choose all organic foods and beef that is grass-fed and grass-finished. For the smoothie recipes, I recommend adding in one to two servings of Preconceive Nutrition or Fertility Fuel protein powder.

Breakfasts

Banana Pancakes with Fresh Berries

What you need

- 2 ripe bananas
- 2 eggs
- ¼ cup almond flour
- ½ teaspoon cinnamon
- 1 teaspoon avocado or coconut oil for cooking
- ½ cup fresh mixed berries

Make!

Mash the bananas in a bowl. Whisk in eggs, almond flour, and cinnamon until smooth. Next, heat a skillet over medium heat, grease with avocado oil, and pour in the batter to form small pancakes. Cook until golden, flipping halfway. Serve with fresh berries.

Leek, Mushroom, and Sausage Frittata

This leek, shiitake mushroom, and sausage frittata is a flavorful and nutrient-dense dish, perfect for any meal of the day. Eggs are rich in omega-3 fatty acids, lecithin, choline, vitamins A and E, beta-carotene, protein, B vitamins, and trace elements such as copper, iron, magnesium, manganese, selenium, zinc, and iodine.

Pasture-raised eggs contain higher levels of omega-3s, vitamin E, vitamin A, and beta-carotene compared to conventionally raised eggs. Incorporating organic vegetables such as leeks and shiitake mushrooms enhances the dish's antioxidant and fiber content. This recipe is gluten-free, dairy-free, and keto-friendly.

What you need

- 2 links Italian sausage, paleo-friendly
- ½ cup shiitake mushrooms, sliced
- 1 leek, sliced (white and light green parts only)
- ¼ cup organic green onions, chopped
- 2 eggs (organic, pasture-raised)
- 1 tablespoon almond milk
- ¼ teaspoon sea salt
- ¼ teaspoon black pepper
- Pinch of red pepper flakes

Make!

Preheat the oven to 475° F. In an oven-safe, 8-inch saucepan over medium heat, cook the sausage, breaking it apart until it is crumbly and fully cooked. Add the shiitake mushrooms, leek, and green onions; cook for 4 minutes, then remove some of the mixture to reserve for the topping.

In a small bowl, whisk the eggs, almond milk, sea salt, black pepper, and red pepper flakes. Pour the egg mixture into the pan, ensuring an even layer. Top with the reserved sausage and vegetable mixture. Cook over medium heat for 1 minute. Transfer the pan to the preheated oven and bake until the frittata is puffy, about 3–4 minutes. Serve with a sprinkle of flaky sea salt.

Zucchini Fritters

Zucchini, a member of the squash family, is technically a fruit and is packed with nutrients, antioxidants, and fiber. It contains zeaxanthin, a compound that helps reduce oxidative stress. These easy and delicious fritters can be enjoyed as a side dish, snack, or lunch, and they're great for picky eaters!

What you need

- 2 medium organic green zucchinis, grated
- 1 egg, beaten
- ¼ cup coconut flour
- 1 teaspoon salt
- 1 teaspoon pepper
- 3 tablespoons avocado oil

Make!

Add the zucchini to a colander, pressing down on the shredded zucchini to drain as much liquid as possible. Transfer to a bowl and add the egg, coconut flour, salt, and pepper. Mix together until well combined. Heat a skillet over medium heat and add the avocado oil. Scoop portions of the batter into the skillet, forming fritters. Cook until each side is golden brown. Repeat with the remaining batter.

Broccoli Bacon Breakfast Skillet

This breakfast skillet is a delicious way to incorporate nutrient-rich cruciferous vegetables into your morning routine. Combining broccoli and cauliflower with classic eggs and bacon, this dish is gluten-free, dairy-free, and keto-friendly.

What you need

- 2½ cups organic cauliflower rice (frozen or freshly prepared)
- 1 head organic broccoli, cut into florets
- 3 strips organic, uncured bacon
- 2 eggs, (organic, pasture-raised)
- Pink salt and pepper, to taste
- 1 tablespoon coconut oil (optional, for frying eggs)

Make!

Preheat the oven to 375° F. Place the bacon strips on a baking sheet and bake for 10–15 minutes, or until they reach your desired crispiness. Set aside to drain on a paper towel–lined plate.

In a large skillet over medium heat, add the cauliflower rice. Cook until most of the liquid has evaporated, then add the broccoli. Continue to cook until the broccoli is softened.

In a separate stainless steel skillet, fry the eggs over low heat, using coconut oil if desired. Cut the cooked bacon into pieces and add them to the large skillet with the cauliflower rice and broccoli. Top with the fried eggs. Sprinkle with salt and pepper and serve warm.

Snacks

Avocado Deviled Eggs

What you need

- 2 hard-boiled eggs, yolks and whites separated
- ¼ avocado
- ½ teaspoon Dijon mustard
- lime juice to taste

Make!

Mix the egg yolks, avocado, Dijon mustard, and lime juice. Pipe the mixture into the egg whites.

Apple Nachos with SunButter Drizzle and Toppings

What you need

- Apples
- SunButter
- Honey
- Cashews
- Chia seeds
- Cinnamon
- Sea salt

Make!

Slice the apples thinly, arranging them in an overlapping pattern on a large plate or serving platter. (Think of this as creating a base similar to nachos.) Next, make the SunButter drizzle. In a small bowl, combine the SunButter with a teaspoon of honey. Stir vigorously until the mixture becomes smooth and slightly runny. If it's too thick, you can add a tiny bit of water or olive oil, a few drops at a time, until you reach the desired consistency. Use a spoon to drizzle the SunButter mixture evenly over the apple slices. Add crunch by roughly chopping the cashews and sprinkling them over the apples for a crunchy texture. Next, add your toppings. Lightly sprinkle chia seeds and a pinch of cinnamon over the top. For a savory twist, add a small pinch of sea salt to balance the sweetness. These apple nachos are perfect for sharing or enjoying as a special, flavorful snack that feels indulgent but remains healthy.

Frozen Blueberry and Cashew Clusters

What you need

- Frozen blueberries
- Cashews
- Honey

Make!

Mix the frozen blueberries with cashews and a drizzle of honey. Freeze the mixture on a baking sheet in small clusters for a cool, crunchy, and naturally sweet snack.

Seaweed Snacks with Avocado and Garlic Salt

What you need

- Avocado
- Garlic salt
- Seaweed snacks

Make!

Mash half an avocado and season with garlic salt. Spread a small amount of the avocado mash on each seaweed snack for a quick and nutrient-dense bite.

Cinnamon-Spiced Buckwheat Granola

What you need

- Buckwheat groats
- Coconut oil, melted
- Honey
- Cinnamon

Make!

Toss the buckwheat groats with a little melted coconut oil, honey, and cinnamon. Spread the mixture on a baking sheet and toast in the oven until golden and crunchy. Enjoy as a granola snack or sprinkle on top of smoothie bowls.

Chia Seed Pudding with Black Cherry Juice

What you need

- Chia seeds
- Black cherry juice
- Honey

Make!

Combine chia seeds with black cherry juice and a touch of honey. Stir well and refrigerate until the mixture thickens into a pudding. This makes a sweet, tart, and satisfying snack that's rich in omega-3s and antioxidants.

Other Super Quick and Easy Snack Ideas

- Sunflower seed butter on celery
- Chia seed pudding with protein powder mixed in
- Smoked salmon on avocado slices
- Almond butter-stuffed dates
- Plantain chips and guacamole

Main Dishes

Preconception Diet Pot Roast with Mushrooms and Carrots

Cold temperatures outside call for warm comfort foods inside. This pot roast recipe checks all the boxes for a winter favorite—packed with flavor, it's delicious *and* nutritious. Beef is a great source of zinc, a mineral that supports your immune system, and is especially helpful during cold and flu season. Opt for organic, grass-fed, pasture-raised (free-range) beef for better nutritional value. Pasture-raised beef contains higher levels of anti-inflammatory omega-3 fatty acids and lower levels of pro-inflammatory omega-6 fatty acids compared to conventionally fed beef. Look for labels like "100 percent grass-fed" to ensure no grain supplementation. Recommended brands are Wellness Meats and Butcher Block. To maximize nutrition, this recipe includes organic carrots, onions, mushrooms, and garlic, and uses beef bone broth for added benefits, such as improved red blood cell and hemoglobin production, reducing the risk of anemia.

What you need

- 3 tablespoons extra virgin olive oil, divided
- 2–3 cups sliced fresh porcini or baby portabella mushrooms
- 1 sweet (yellow) onion, chopped
- 3 cloves garlic, finely chopped or smashed
- 1 (3- to 4-pound) grass-fed, pasture-raised chuck roast
- 1 teaspoon pink or sea salt
- 1 teaspoon ground black pepper
- 1–1 ½ cups beef or bone broth (gluten-free)
- ½ cup red wine
- 2 tablespoons tomato paste
- 2–3 large organic carrots, sliced
- 2 cups small white or red potatoes, halved
- 1 tablespoon chopped parsley or rosemary, for garnish

Make!

Preheat the oven to 350° F. In a large Dutch oven, heat 2 tablespoons of olive oil over medium-high heat. Add mushrooms and cook, stirring occasionally, for about 5 minutes. Remove from the pot. Add the remaining 1 tablespoon of olive oil to the pot. Sauté the onions and garlic until translucent. Remove from the pot.

Sprinkle chuck roast with salt and pepper. Add to the pot and sear on all sides, about 3 minutes per side. Add broth, wine, tomato paste, cooked mushrooms, onions, carrots, and potatoes to the pot. Stir gently to combine. Cover the Dutch oven and place it in the preheated oven. Bake until fork-tender, about 1 hour per pound (approximately 3 hours for a 3-pound roast). Garnish with parsley or your preferred herb before serving.

Preconception Diet Mediterranean Chicken and Veggies

Makes 2 meals (double for more). A great way to shorten a jam-packed task list is to add meal prepping! Most of us are very busy, and making healthy meals every day can be challenging. Doubling or even tripling a recipe is also helpful when preparing nutritious meals for family and kiddos who are heading back to school. And as with all my recipes, Mediterranean Chicken and Veggies is gluten- and dairy-free. Made with organic chicken breasts, zucchini (feel free to substitute with your favorite veggies), and riced cauliflower, it's packed with protein, fiber, and healthy nutrients. Enjoy!

What you need
- 1 ½ lb. organic boneless, skinless chicken breasts
- avocado oil for coating the chicken
- ½ teaspoon garlic powder
- ½ teaspoon black pepper
- ½ teaspoon salt
- ¼ teaspoon paprika
- ¼ teaspoon dried parsley
- 1 tablespoon avocado oil
- 1 large zucchini, chopped (organic)

- 1 red bell pepper, seeds removed and chopped
- 2 garlic cloves, minced
- 2 cups cauliflower, riced (organic)
- Sea salt and black pepper, to taste

Make!

Preheat the oven to 450° F. Place the chicken in a large bowl and cover with warm water and a couple of dashes of salt. Let it brine for 15 minutes. After brining, pat the chicken dry and place it in a baking dish. Brush it with avocado oil. Combine all seasonings in a small bowl and sprinkle the seasoning mixture over the chicken until well coated. Bake for 16–20 minutes or until the chicken is cooked through. Remove from the oven and let rest for 5 minutes before slicing.

In a large skillet over medium heat, heat the 1 tablespoon avocado oil and add the zucchini and bell pepper. Sauté for about 5 minutes, then add garlic. Cook until the garlic is fragrant, then stir in the cauliflower and cook until tender, about 3–4 minutes more. Season with salt and pepper, and serve with the chicken.

Preconception Diet Turkey Meatballs with Cauliflower Tzatziki Sauce

Looking for a new appetizer to serve for a special gathering? Or just want to impress the family with a delicious and nutritious recipe that everyone is sure to enjoy? These meatballs taste as amazing as they look. And they're pretty simple to make, considering they look like something that would be served in an upscale restaurant. They're also gluten-free, dairy-free, and keto—so enjoy!

What you need

Turkey Meatballs

- 1 ½ lbs. ground turkey (pasture-raised, organic)
- 1 egg (pasture-raised, organic)
- 1 tablespoon avocado oil
- 2 garlic cloves, minced
- ¼ cup white onion, diced small

- ¼ cup almond flour
- ½ tablespoon nutritional yeast, optional
- ½ teaspoon Himalayan pink salt
- ½ teaspoon pepper
- ¼ teaspoon paprika

Cauliflower Tzatziki

- ½ cup steamed cauliflower (organic)
- 1 cup raw cashews, soaked in water for at least 8 hours in the refrigerator
- 2 garlic cloves, minced
- 1 tablespoon avocado oil
- 1 tablespoon lemon juice
- 1 tablespoon fresh dill, minced
- ¼ English cucumber, diced small
- Sea salt, to taste
- Black pepper, to taste

Make!

Preheat the oven to 375° F. In a large bowl, mix the meatball ingredients together. Using a cookie scoop or spoon, measure approximately 2-inch-diameter meatballs. Place each meatball on a parchment paper–lined baking sheet. Bake 15–20 minutes or until the meat is cooked through. Remove from oven and skim off any fat. Set aside.

In a food processor, blend the cauliflower, cashews, and about 2 tablespoons of the cashew water, scraping down the sides as you go. Add the garlic, avocado oil, and lemon juice, and blend again. Add more cashew liquid if needed. Stir in the dill and cucumber; season with salt and pepper. Place in the refrigerator to cool before serving.

Chicken and Carrot Tikka Masala

This recipe is nutritious, delicious, and full of flavor! It's packed with spices and organic veggies and made with pasture-raised chicken. Turmeric is one of the spices I especially like to include in many of my recipes for its numerous health benefits. This meal is surprisingly easy to make and a beautiful dish to serve to family or guests.

What you need

- 2 teaspoons turmeric
- 1 teaspoon garam masala
- 1 teaspoon ground coriander
- 1 teaspoon ground cumin
- ½ teaspoon pink or sea salt
- 1 ½ cups full-fat coconut milk, divided
- 1 lb. boneless, skinless chicken breast, cubed (pasture-raised, organic)
- 2 carrots, sliced (organic)
- 1 tablespoon avocado oil
- ½ onion, chopped
- 4 oz. tomato paste
- 1 cup diced tomatoes (organic)
- Almond flour tortillas and/or cauliflower rice, for serving

Make!

In a small bowl, combine the turmeric, garam masala, coriander, cumin, and salt. In a small bowl, mix half of the seasoning mixture with ½ cup coconut milk. In a large ziplock bag or storage container, add the chicken, carrots, and seasoned coconut milk; chill for 2 hours.

Heat the avocado oil in a medium pot over medium heat. Add the onion and tomato paste and cook, stirring continuously, until the onion is softened. Add the remaining spice mixture and cook for another 2 minutes.

Stir in the diced tomatoes and their juice, and bring the sauce to a simmer to thicken (this will take about 6 minutes). Add the sauce to the blender along with the remaining 1 cup of coconut milk and blend until smooth. Return the sauce to the pot, then add the chicken and marinade from the bag. Coat the chicken in the sauce and cook for about 20 minutes until the chicken and carrots are cooked through and the sauce is thick. Serve with your favorite almond flour tortillas or cauliflower rice.

Beef Kabobs with Turmeric Ranch Dipping Sauce

These beef kabobs are made with organic, grass-fed sirloin, fresh peppers, and a flavorful dipping sauce. Feel free to substitute with chicken or another meat if desired, and get creative with your vegetables—cauliflower or zucchini also work well. This recipe is gluten-free, dairy-free, paleo, and keto-friendly.

What you need

Kabobs

- 1 lb. grass-fed, organic sirloin, cut into cubes
- ¼ cup coconut aminos
- ¼ cup avocado oil
- 1 teaspoon ground pepper
- ½ teaspoon pink or sea salt
- ½ teaspoon garlic powder
- 1 lb. small organic peppers, cut into thick slices
- 1 red onion, cut into 1-inch squares
- Fresh parsley, chopped

Turmeric Ranch Dipping Sauce

- ¼ cup paleo mayonnaise
- ⅛ cup coconut milk
- ½ teaspoon dried parsley
- ¼ teaspoon onion powder
- ¼ teaspoon pink or sea salt
- ¼ teaspoon black pepper
- ¼ teaspoon turmeric

Make!

In a large bowl, toss the meat with coconut aminos, avocado oil, and kabob seasonings until well coated. Cover and marinate for 15 minutes while you prepare the vegetables.

Preheat the oven to 350° F (or prepare a grill). Thread the meat, peppers, and onions onto skewers in an alternating pattern. Place on a baking sheet or grill. If baking, cook for 15 minutes, then flip and bake for an additional 8–10 minutes until the meat is cooked through and dark brown. Remove from the oven and garnish with fresh parsley. Serve with the Turmeric Ranch dipping sauce (simply combine all ingredients and mix well).

Preconception Diet Meatballs with Carrot Purée

Looking for a nutritious twist on traditional meatballs? This recipe offers a lighter alternative by using potatoes as a binder and serving the meatballs over a vibrant carrot purée, reminiscent of a Swedish-style dish. Carrots are rich in vitamin A, beta-carotene, antioxidants, and fiber, enhancing the meal's nutritional value. This dish is gluten-free, dairy-free, and grain-free.

What you need

Meatballs

- 2 small potatoes, peeled and diced
- ½ lb. freshly ground beef (grass-fed)
- ½ lb. freshly ground pork (grass-fed)
- 1 ½ teaspoons chopped parsley
- 2 garlic cloves, minced
- 1 teaspoon pink or sea salt
- 1 teaspoon pepper
- 1 egg (pasture-raised, organic)
- Avocado oil, for cooking

Carrot Purée

- 1 lb. organic carrots, peeled and chopped
- ½ teaspoon salt
- ½ teaspoon pepper
- ¼ teaspoon garlic powder
- Parsley, for garnish

Make!

Place the potatoes in a medium pot, cover with water, and bring to a boil. Reduce to medium-low heat, cover, and cook until the potatoes are fork-tender, about 6 minutes. Drain and mash the potatoes in a medium bowl; set aside to cool until they are not hot to the touch.

In the same pot, add the carrots and cover with water. Bring to a boil, then lower the heat to a simmer, cover, and cook until the carrots are fork-tender, approximately 20 minutes. Drain the carrots, reserving some of the cooking liquid. Mash the carrots with a potato masher or blend until smooth, adding reserved liquid as needed to achieve desired consistency. Season the purée with salt, pepper, and garlic powder, and set aside.

In the bowl of the mashed potatoes, add the beef, pork, parsley, garlic, salt, pepper, and egg; combine thoroughly. Using clean hands, form the mixture into balls. Heat a skillet over medium heat and add the avocado oil. Once the oil is hot, cook the meatballs until they are browned on all sides and cooked through. Remove the meatballs from the skillet and set aside. To serve, place the meatballs over the carrot purée and garnish with parsley.

Chimichurri Steak

This is a flavorful and nutrient-rich dish that combines grass-fed skirt steak with a vibrant herb sauce. Grass-fed beef is a good source of essential minerals, including iron, zinc, phosphorus, magnesium, and potassium, which support bodily functions such as oxygen transport, immune function, bone health, and nerve function.

What you need

- 1 cup fresh parsley
- 1 tablespoon fresh oregano leaves
- 3 garlic cloves, minced
- 1 teaspoon red pepper flakes
- ¼ cup distilled vinegar (optional)
- ½ teaspoon sea salt
- ¼ teaspoon black pepper
- ½ cup avocado oil
- 1 lb. grass-fed skirt steak

Make!

In a food processor, combine the parsley, oregano, garlic, red pepper flakes, vinegar (if using), sea salt, and black pepper. Pulse until the herbs are finely chopped. Transfer the mixture to a small bowl and stir in the avocado oil until well combined.

Place the skirt steak in a resealable bag or shallow dish. Pour half of the chimichurri sauce over the steak, ensuring it is well coated. Reserve the remaining sauce for serving. Marinate the steak in the refrigerator for at least 1 hour or overnight for enhanced flavor. When ready to cook, heat a skillet over medium heat and add a small amount of avocado oil. Remove the steak from the marinade and place it in the skillet. Cook for approximately 4–5 minutes on each side, or until the steak reaches your desired level of doneness. Once cooked, remove the steak from the skillet and let it rest for a few minutes. Slice the steak into strips and serve with the reserved chimichurri sauce drizzled on top. Enjoy this gluten-free, dairy-free, and keto-friendly dish!

Bison Chili

Bison chili is a hearty and nutritious comfort food, perfect for cooler fall and winter evenings. This easy one-pot recipe incorporates organic carrots, onions, and garlic for added nutrients. Using grass-fed, pasture-raised bison provides a leaner alternative to beef, offering high protein content with lower fat and calories.

RENEW

What you need

- 1 tablespoon avocado oil
- 1 large white onion, diced
- 2–3 organic carrots, peeled and chopped
- 5 cloves garlic, minced
- 1 jalapeño, seeded and chopped
- 2 lbs. ground bison (grass-fed)
- 1 24-oz. jar organic diced tomatoes, with juice
- 1¼ cups bone broth or gluten-free beef broth

Chili Spice Mix

- 1 tablespoon smoked paprika
- 1 tablespoon chili powder
- ½ teaspoon onion powder
- ½ teaspoon garlic powder
- ½ teaspoon ground cumin
- ½ teaspoon red chili flakes
- ½ teaspoon sea salt
- ½ teaspoon black pepper
- ¼ teaspoon cayenne pepper

Toppings

- Avocado, peeled and sliced
- Organic chopped cilantro
- Jalapeño, seeded and sliced
- Red pepper flakes

Make!

In a small bowl, combine the chili spice mix seasonings and set aside. In a large stockpot or Dutch oven, heat the avocado oil over medium heat. Add the onion and carrots; cook for 3–4 minutes until the onion becomes translucent. Stir in the garlic and jalapeño, cooking for an additional minute. Add the bison, cooking until browned and breaking it into small pieces with a large spoon. Mix in the prepared chili spice mix blend, ensuring the meat is well coated. Stir in the tomatoes with their juice and the bone broth. Bring the mixture to a boil, then reduce the heat to a simmer. Cover and let it cook for 45 minutes. Serve the chili in bowls and garnish with avocado slices, cilantro, jalapeño, and red pepper flakes as desired.

Broccoli Beef

This savory and nutritious dish combines tender, marinated beef with crisp broccoli, enhanced by the flavors of garlic and ginger. It's a gluten-free, dairy-free, grain-free meal that's quick to prepare, making it perfect for any day of the week.

What you need

- 1 lb. grass-fed flank steak, cut into thin strips
- ½ cup coconut aminos, divided
- 1 lb. broccoli, cut into florets, (organic)
- 1 tablespoon coconut sugar
- ½-inch piece of ginger, peeled and grated
- 3 garlic cloves, minced
- 1 tablespoon tapioca flour
- 1 tablespoon avocado oil
- ½ teaspoon black pepper
- ½ teaspoon pink or sea salt
- ¼ cup sliced green onions
- ¼ teaspoon red pepper flakes

Make!

In a large bowl, combine the beef strips with ¼ cup coconut aminos. Marinate in the refrigerator while preparing the broccoli. Bring a large pot of water to a boil. Add the broccoli florets and cook for 1½ minutes. Drain and immediately transfer the broccoli to an ice bath to halt the cooking process.

In a jar with a lid, combine the remaining ¼ cup coconut aminos, coconut sugar, ginger, garlic, and tapioca flour. Shake well until the sugar is dissolved.

Heat a large wok or skillet over high heat. Add the avocado oil and stir-fry the marinated beef until browned on all sides. Remove the beef and set aside. Pour the prepared sauce into the wok and heat for 1 minute. Return the beef and add the blanched broccoli to the wok, tossing to ensure everything is well-coated with the sauce. Season with salt and pepper to taste. Garnish with the green onions and red pepper flakes before serving.

Ginger Garlic Baked Salmon

This Asian-inspired recipe is made with coconut aminos, a delicious gluten-free soy sauce substitute. I recommend using wild-caught sockeye salmon, which has an exceptionally firm texture and a rich, iconic salmon flavor. It is full of omega-3s and delivers more beneficial vitamin D than farm-raised salmon. This dish is gluten-free, dairy-free, and bursting with lots of flavor! Enjoy with coconut rice or carrot-cucumber salad.

What you need

- 2 wild-caught salmon fillets, about 6 oz. each
- 3 garlic cloves, minced
- 2 teaspoons grated ginger
- 3 tablespoons coconut aminos
- 1 tablespoon apple cider vinegar
- 1 teaspoon honey
- Chopped green onions (organic)
- Black sesame seeds

Make!

Pat the salmon dry, then add to a large bowl. Press garlic and ginger on the top of each filet. In a small bowl, add coconut aminos, vinegar, and honey. Pour this mixture over the salmon and cover. Refrigerate for 20 minutes. Preheat the oven to 375° F. Add the salmon to an ovenproof skillet. Pour the marinade evenly on top, spooning any minced garlic and ginger over the top. Bake for 18 minutes. Remove from the oven and top with the green onions and black sesame seeds. Makes 2 servings.

Sides

Cauliflower Rice Buddha Bowls

Buddha bowls are typically a combination of roasted vegetables with or without a protein, served over rice or quinoa in a big, round bowl. This recipe contains an abundance of beautifully seasoned roasted vegetables and is super flavorful! I opted to use riced cauliflower as the base. Cauliflower is always a great choice because it's rich in so many vitamins and minerals, is an excellent source of fiber, and contains a compound called *sulforaphane*. Sulforaphane is found in all cruciferous vegetables (including the cauliflower and brussels sprouts in this recipe) and has many health benefits attributed to it.

What you need

- 5 brussels sprouts, halved (organic)
- 1 white potato or a small sweet potato, cubed
- 1 carrot, peeled and chopped (organic)
- ½ tablespoon avocado oil
- ½ teaspoon pink or sea salt
- ¼ teaspoon pepper
- 2 cups riced cauliflower, fresh or frozen (organic)
- ½ teaspoon ground turmeric
- 1 cup sliced baby portabella mushrooms
- Fresh parsley, chopped
- Sprinkle with fresh or toasted pumpkin or sesame seeds

Garlic Sauce

- 2–3 cloves garlic, finely minced
- 1 teaspoon lemon zest
- 1 cup paleo mayonnaise
- 1 teaspoon Dijon mustard
- ¾ teaspoon pink or sea salt
- ¼ teaspoon pepper, to taste

Make!

Mix all garlic sauce ingredients in a small bowl, then cover and refrigerate until ready to use. Preheat the oven to 400° F. Line a baking sheet with foil and set aside. In a large bowl, toss the brussels sprouts, potato, and carrot with avocado oil, salt, and pepper. Spread evenly onto the baking sheet and roast for 20 minutes, shaking the pan about halfway through so the veggies cook evenly.

Heat the cauliflower according to the package directions if using frozen. Sprinkle the cauliflower with turmeric and toss until it is evenly coated. Spoon into bowls. In a small skillet, heat the avocado oil, then cook the mushrooms for about 5 minutes until softened. Construct your Buddha bowls by adding all the vegetables on top. Season with additional salt and pepper, if desired, and sprinkle with parsley. Serve with the garlic sauce. Makes 2 servings.

Broccoli and Butternut Squash Soup

This soup is especially nutrient-dense with vitamins and minerals. It's high in potassium, loaded with vitamin A, and includes half your daily dose of vitamin C. It's also a great source of fiber and sulforaphane. Enjoy!

What you need

- 1 tablespoon avocado oil
- ½ yellow onion, chopped
- 3 cloves garlic, pressed or minced
- 1 tablespoon tapioca flour
- 4 cups broccoli florets (organic)
- 1½ cups butternut squash, cubed
- 1 cup shredded carrot, divided
- 4 cups gluten-free chicken broth
- 1½ cups coconut cream, optional
- Pink sea salt and black pepper, to taste
- ½ cup chopped cooked nitrate-free bacon, about 4 slices

Make!

In a large stock pot or Dutch oven over medium heat, heat the avocado oil until hot. Stir in onion and cook for 4 minutes or until softened. Stir in garlic and cook another minute more. Add the tapioca flour and cook another minute. Add broccoli, butternut squash, and half of the carrots, then cover with chicken broth. Bring to a simmer on low heat and cook, covered, for 20 minutes.

With an immersion blender, blend the soup until no large pieces remain. Stir in the coconut cream and add the rest of the carrots. Simmer uncovered for another 5 minutes. Season to taste with salt and pepper. Top with chopped bacon, if desired.

Creamy Watercress Soup

Watercress, one of the oldest leafy vegetables consumed by humans, is often underappreciated despite its rich nutrient profile. This small leaf with a peppery taste makes a beautiful salad or soup and is packed with vitamins A, C, E, K, and B6, as well as minerals such as calcium, manganese, potassium, thiamin, riboflavin, and phosphorus. This creamy soup is a delicious and nutritious way to enjoy these nutrient-packed greens. And it's gluten-free and dairy-free.

What You Need

- 1 tablespoon avocado oil
- 1 shallot, chopped
- 1 clove garlic, minced
- 6 celery stalks, chopped (organic)
- 1 teaspoon pink salt
- Black pepper, to taste
- ½ teaspoon garlic powder
- 1 cup chopped cauliflower (organic)
- 1 cup organic coconut milk
- 1 (32-oz.) carton organic, gluten-free chicken broth or bone broth
- 2 tablespoons lemon juice
- 5 cups fresh organic watercress leaves and soft stems (remove tough stems)

Make!

Heat the avocado oil in a large saucepan. Add the shallot, garlic, and celery, along with the salt, pepper, and garlic powder, and sauté until softened. Add the cauliflower, coconut milk, and chicken stock. Cover and simmer for 20 minutes, or until the cauliflower is tender. Add the lemon juice and watercress; let it simmer for about 1 minute, until the leaves are wilted. Remove from heat, pour the contents into a food processor or blender, and blend until smooth.

Cauliflower and Chive Fritters

These fritters are a delightful alternative to hash browns, and they're suitable for breakfast, lunch, as a side dish, or as a snack. Cauliflower is rich in vitamins C, K, B6, folate, potassium, and manganese. It's also an excellent source of fiber and contains protein, niacin, magnesium, and phosphorus. Additionally, cauliflower contains sulforaphane.

What you need

- 1 head cauliflower, cut into florets (organic)
- 2 eggs, whisked (pasture-raised, organic)
- ½ cup almond flour
- 1 teaspoon pink or sea salt
- 1 teaspoon cracked pepper
- 1 tablespoon finely chopped fresh chives
- Avocado oil, for frying

Preconception Diet Ranch Dressing

- ½ cup paleo mayonnaise
- 3 tablespoons coconut milk
- 1 teaspoon apple cider vinegar
- ½ tablespoon chopped fresh dill (organic)
- ⅛ teaspoon onion powder
- ⅛ teaspoon garlic powder
- Pinch pink sea salt
- Pinch pepper

Make!

Bring a large pot of water to a boil. Add the cauliflower florets and cook at a rolling boil for about 6–7 minutes or until fork-tender. Drain well and set aside to cool slightly.

Place the cauliflower in a large bowl and mash with a potato masher until creamy but still slightly chunky. Add the eggs and almond flour, mixing thoroughly. Stir in the salt, pepper, and chives.

Heat a skillet over medium-high heat and add avocado oil. Form the batter into patties and fry on each side until golden brown. Transfer to a wire rack with a paper towel underneath to drain excess oil.

To prepare the ranch dressing, combine all dressing ingredients in a bowl and mix well. Serve the fritters warm with the dressing.

Creamy Cauliflower Soup

This soup is hearty, healthy, and delicious. Made with organic cauliflower, onion, and garlic, it's packed with nutritious vegetables and dairy-free coconut milk. Cauliflower is low in carbohydrates and rich in vitamins C, K, B6, folate, potassium, and manganese, making it an excellent source of fiber. As a member of the cruciferous family, cauliflower contains glucosinolates, sulfur-containing compounds that support detoxification. This puréed soup is the perfect comfort food as temperatures begin to fall. The flavorful toppings add a delightful crunch to this beautifully crafted dish. Serve it alone or with a salad for a complete meal.

What you need

- 3 tablespoons avocado oil
- 1 medium yellow onion, diced (organic)
- 5 garlic cloves, minced (organic)
- 1 head cauliflower, roughly chopped into pieces (organic); reserve some to sauté as a topping
- 3 cups organic, gluten-free chicken broth
- 3 sprigs fresh thyme, tied together
- 1 cup full-fat coconut milk
- Pink or sea salt, to taste
- Cracked black pepper, to taste

Toppings

- Sautéed cauliflower
- Sea salt
- Freshly cracked pepper
- Fresh thyme
- avocado oil

Make!

In a large pot over medium heat, add the avocado oil. Add the onion and cook until translucent, about 5 minutes. Add the garlic and cook for another minute. Add the cauliflower and cook for 4 minutes, stirring occasionally. Pour in the chicken broth and add the thyme sprigs. Bring to a simmer and cook until the cauliflower is tender. Remove the thyme sprigs and discard.

Blend the soup with an immersion blender until smooth. Stir in the coconut milk and season with salt and pepper to taste. Serve warm, topped with sautéed cauliflower, a sprinkle of sea salt and cracked pepper, fresh thyme, and a drizzle of avocado oil.

Cruciferous Coleslaw

This nutritious and delicious side dish combines cabbage, broccoli, and brussels sprouts, all members of the cruciferous vegetable family, which are rich in sulforaphane. Unlike traditional coleslaw recipes that often include sugar, this version offers a tangy flavor without added sugars. Enjoy it alongside your favorite pork, chicken, or beef dishes. Option: Top with broccoli sprouts for added benefits. Broccoli sprouts contain glucoraphanin, a potent antioxidant that converts into sulforaphane when activated by chewing or digestion, boosting the body's detoxification pathways and providing protection against air pollution and potential carcinogens.

What you need

- 1 cup finely shredded green cabbage (organic)
- 1½ cups finely shredded red cabbage (organic)

- 1 cup broccoli, sliced into thin strips (organic)
- 1 cup shredded brussels sprouts (a mandolin works great for this) (organic)

Coleslaw Dressing

- 4 tablespoons avocado oil
- 2 tablespoons apple cider vinegar
- 1 tablespoon mustard
- 1 tablespoon lemon juice from organic lemons
- Salt, to taste
- Black pepper, to taste

Make!

Combine all the vegetables in a large bowl. In a small jar, mix the dressing ingredients and shake well. Toss the vegetables with the dressing until evenly coated. Serve immediately.

Wild Mushroom, Caramelized Onion, and Kale Soup

This soup is a nutritious and delicious comfort food, perfect for cooler temperatures. Packed with flavor and antioxidants, a bowl of it makes a perfectly balanced and filling meal. I recommend making extra and freezing some for later!

What you need

- 2 tablespoons avocado oil
- 1 sweet onion (such as Vidalia, organic), sliced to ½-inch thickness
- 4 cloves garlic, minced
- 1 teaspoon pink or sea salt
- ½ teaspoon cracked pepper
- 2 cups shiitake mushrooms, whole
- 2 cups sliced baby portabella mushrooms (also called cremini mushrooms)
- 4 cups gluten-free chicken or vegetable broth (organic)
- 2 cups kale, roughly chopped into bite-size pieces (organic)
- ½ cup coconut milk or coconut cream

RENEW

> ***Make!***
>
> In a large pot, heat the avocado oil over medium heat. Add the onions and sauté until golden brown, about 10–15 minutes. Add the garlic, salt, pepper, and mushrooms. Continue to cook until the mushrooms are softened and golden. Pour in the broth and bring to a boil. Add the kale. Reduce the heat to low and simmer, covered, for 20 minutes. Stir in the coconut milk. Season with additional salt and pepper to taste.

Putting It All Together

All of these recipes are designed to include nutrient-dense foods that support fertility, hormone balance, and overall health for both men and women during the preconception period. You can find more recipes on my website at: https://annshippymd.com/recipes/. The following diagram shows about how much of each type of food you'll aim to eat at each meal.

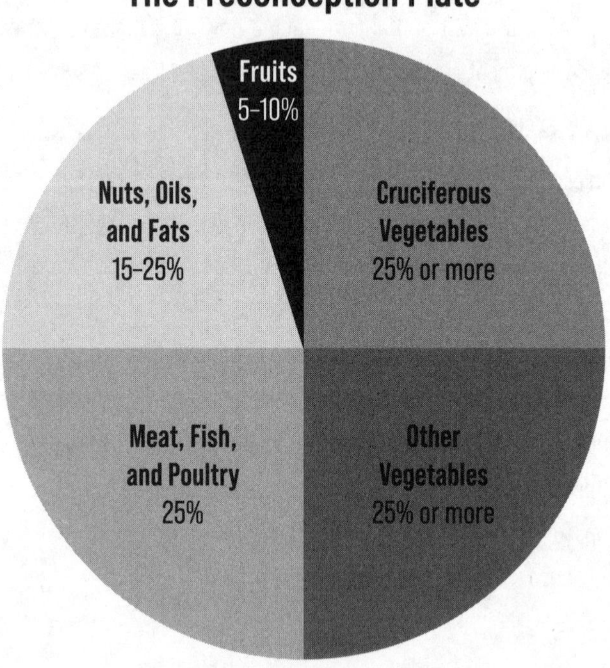

Sample Weekly Preconception Menu

Monday

Breakfast: Banana Pancakes with Fresh Berries
Lunch: Preconception Diet Pot Roast with Mushrooms and Carrots
Dinner: Chicken and Carrot Tikka Masala
Snack: Avocado Deviled Eggs

Tuesday

Breakfast: Leek, Mushroom, and Sausage Frittata
Lunch: Broccoli and Butternut Squash Soup
Dinner: Bison Chili
Snack: Frozen Blueberry and Cashew Clusters

Wednesday

Breakfast: Broccoli Bacon Breakfast Skillet
Lunch: Wild Mushroom, Caramelized Onion, and Kale Soup
Dinner: Preconception Diet Turkey Meatballs with Cauliflower
   Tzatziki Sauce
Snack: Apple Nachos with SunButter Drizzle and Toppings

Thursday

Breakfast: Zucchini Fritters
Lunch: Chimichurri Steak with Cruciferous Coleslaw
Dinner: Beef Kabobs with Turmeric Ranch Dipping Sauce
Snack: Chia Seed Pudding with Black Cherry Juice

Friday

Breakfast: Cinnamon-Spiced Buckwheat Granola with Almond Milk
Lunch: Creamy Cauliflower Soup with Cauliflower and Chive Fritters
Dinner: Ginger Garlic Baked Salmon with Cauliflower Rice Buddha Bowls
Snack: Plantain Chips and Guacamole

Saturday

Breakfast: Smoked Salmon on Avocado Slices
Lunch: Preconception Diet Meatballs with Carrot Purée
Dinner: Broccoli Beef with Steamed Cauliflower Rice
Snack: Almond Butter-Stuffed Dates

Sunday

Breakfast: Chia Seed Pudding with Protein Powder
Lunch: Creamy Watercress Soup with Toasted Pumpkin Seeds
Dinner: Preconception Diet Mediterranean Chicken and Veggies
Snack: Seaweed Snacks with Avocado and Garlic Salt

Final Thoughts

Nourishing yourself well during the preconception period is about more than just preparing for a healthy pregnancy—it's about setting the foundation for your child's future well-being. The choices you make now have the power to influence not just your child's health, but also their potential, their resilience, and their happiness. So take these steps with confidence, knowing that you're investing in something truly extraordinary—the next generation.

Q&A

Q: What if I just don't have the time in my busy life to cook this often?

A: Many of these recipes are far easier than you think! I know it seems easier to just give in and reach for the oh-so-nicely-packaged, easy-to-reach, easy-to-prepare snack or meal, but there's just no getting around it: It's not good for you. Stick to preparing your own food and you will find you *do* have the time and skills—and healthy eating will give you more energy too! It's really all about priorities and getting creative.

Q: What if I'm overwhelmed by the idea of cleaning out my kitchen?

A: It's definitely a challenge but think of it as an investment in your health and your future. Start small if you need to—clean out one shelf at a time. In the first few pages of this chapter, I offer some advice on how to do this. Even dedicating just fifteen minutes a day to revamping your kitchen will lead to significant progress over the course of a week.

Q: Isn't eating this way really expensive? I'm not sure I can afford it.

A: Following this type of diet is actually not more expensive than following any other. In fact, one of the benefits is that you don't need to shop for expensive "gluten-free" options, as the diet just eliminates these altogether and provides more natural options without the need to buy special products. It'll take some time and tweaking to figure out, but I think you will find your grocery budget won't really change much.

Q: What do I do when friends invite me over for meals? I don't want to be a pain.

A: Most of the time, your friends will want to accommodate you. They might even be intrigued by your choices and interested in learning something new. Make it easy for them and share some of your new resources and recipes!

Q: Do I need to stop eating out at restaurants?

A: You can keep eating out—you just need to be more aware of the details, such as what ingredients are in the sauces or what the garnish is. Start by choosing a protein to narrow your options and then work on it from there. Obviously, though, fast-food is a no-go!

Q: Do I need to follow this diet for life?

A: Once you enjoy the benefits of eating this way, I don't think you'll want to go back! Plus, you'll be equipped for feeding your children well. Remember, your ultimate motivation in all this is your love for your family and future generations. I promise you—the investment will be well worth it!

CHAPTER 8

Tuning In: The Art of Balanced Living

Your life and the way you live it is completely unique to you. There is no one else on this planet who is walking in your shoes. And furthermore, your life *belongs* completely to you. You and you alone are responsible for all the decisions you make. I know this can seem overwhelming, but it's also exhilarating. Your life is in your hands, and you can make the choices to bring about any changes you desire. You're truly in the driver's seat.

Think about it this way—when you and your spouse or partner have a baby, that child's life will also be your complete responsibility. At least for a while! And that child will see the choices you make in your daily living and emulate them, whether you like it or not. So let's spend some time considering how attuned to your body's needs you really are and start making shifts in the areas that call for a little improvement.

Studies increasingly show that lifestyle factors do contribute toward fertility.[269] These factors include eating, of course, but also consist of stress management, your recreation choices, and even what media you consume. A job, a life event, or even a social strain can have a negative impact on sperm quality, for instance. Two simultaneous stressful life events can worsen the impact.[270] And get this: Just the perceived stress of giving a sperm sample can see a 39 percent decrease in sperm concentration and a 48 percent decrease in motility, dropping overall semen quality.[271] The link between anxiety and sexual stress is strong, and men undergoing infertility treatment are more likely to have an anxiety disorder or depression.[272] Attending to living a balanced life is therefore absolutely imperative—for both partners.

Where to start? First, flip back to chapter 3 where you explored your current lifestyle habits, including your stress levels, exercise routine, and more. Take a look at your answers to the questions in that chapter to get a sense of your starting point. Now, let's take that foundation and build upon it with actionable advice. This chapter will guide you through essential aspects of what I like to call the art of balanced living. It really is an art form! Of course, our focus is specific to this preconception period, but I believe your life is a work of art that you continue to create and shape over time. The knowledge you'll gain here can help you through every season to come.

What Are You "Consuming"?

When we think of the word *consume*, our minds usually first go to food and beverages. But what else do we consume? We consume information—a *lot* of it. This information comes from myriad sources; in fact, I'd argue that there are more modalities for consuming information today than there ever have been in human history. As we drive down the highway, we are often listening to music or podcasts, reading billboards, and hearing advertisements. When we're in our homes, the TV is sometimes (or often) on, and we're frequently looking at our computer, phone, or tablet. At work, even more information pours in. Other than when we are asleep, there's rarely any time when we are not receiving input.

We're designed to be able to learn what we need to know about our surroundings; it's part of our survival instinct. But because we live in this moment in history, information overload has become a very real threat to our mental health.[273] And since your mental health plays a critical role in your overall health, your ability to conceive, and epigenetics, we want to spend some time and energy considering this topic. Here's a central question to help you paint a clear picture of your own information overload status: Are you consuming information, or is information consuming *you*? Keep that question in mind as you continue reading.

Mindful Consumption

Because of our unparalleled access to technology, information consumption has become habitual; we don't even think about it. But when you look at it objectively for a moment and think of our social media scrolling, the news alerts that pop up constantly on our phones, and of course, all the advertising, shows, and movies we consume on TV—it's astounding. I'm sure you could add even more to that list just thinking about your day-to-day digital life. It's no wonder our brains are "overloaded"!

Especially during this time of preconception, and into pregnancy, I encourage you to become more mindful of any negative news stories, toxic social media (often referred to as "doomscrolling"), and even relationships that drain you. Are you spending a lot of your time reading, watching, or engaging with these things? If so, think about how you can shift toward consuming content that inspires, educates, and uplifts you instead. This includes following accounts and interacting with communities that align with your values and support your journey both in life and in parenthood.

Just as we've talked about filtering the water you drink, I urge you to also filter the information and energy that enter your life. Develop a practice of checking in with yourself to assess how certain information or relationships make you feel and then make a conscious decision to reduce or eliminate anything that doesn't inspire or support you and your growth. Ask yourself, *What is my truth filter?* Start looking at all the information coming in through the lens of your future child, your partnership, future parenthood, and your life. And then ask yourself these questions: *Is it truthful? Does it resonate? Does it align with my values?*

While this is fresh in your mind, take a few minutes to write down your thoughts about how you can reduce the "noise" coming in.

Embracing Nature

Switching gears from technology completely for a moment, let's consider your relationship with someone very important—Mother Nature. Connecting with nature is one of the most grounding and restorative practices you can adopt as you prepare for conception. After all, our bodies weren't made to be indoors all the time, walking around in shoes on concrete floors, hunched in front of our computer screens under harsh LED lights, or even running on a treadmill inside the walls of a crowded gym, surrounded by the unnatural sights and sounds of TVs and music. And if we are asking our bodies to do this thing they were *actually* designed to do—reproduce—we need to be mindful of allowing our bodies to commune with nature, and even to marvel at the wonder of the creation around us.

Regardless of where you live and whether you consider yourself to be "outdoorsy," I hope you will consider the possibilities for how you can begin to create more time and space in your life for being in nature.

Natural Rhythms

On April 8, 2024, there was a solar eclipse, and I just happen to live in an area that was in the path of totality, which meant I had the privilege of watching the world around me go dark right in the middle of the day. It was a spiritual experience, one I'll never forget. As we were preparing for the big event to occur, looking through our special eclipse glasses, I noticed a phenomenon. Just before it started to get dark, all the birds began flying around and chirping loudly. I realized that they were roosting! Even though I'm sure they were thrown off by the fact that the sun had only been up for a few hours, they knew that the sky was getting dark, and it was time to go home to their nests. This was a beautiful reminder of something I take for granted—nature is dependent upon rhythms. And so are we. But somewhere between answering emails, attending Zoom meetings, running errands, and checking items off our never-ending to-do lists, we forget that. And as a result, many of us have lost touch with the rhythms of nature.

I'll go into more depth on this subject, specifically on circadian rhythms, later in this chapter, but for now, here's why all of this matters: The process of conception and birth is deeply rooted in the natural world. By tuning into these rhythms, you can prepare your body and mind for the journey ahead.

Getting Outside More

Right now, I invite you to think of three ways you can get out into nature daily. Here are some examples to get you thinking:

- **Stroll About:** Whether you live in a bustling city or out in the countryside, in the foothills or near the coast, find an outdoor space where you can comfortably and safely go for a quiet stroll. Look at your surroundings and really breathe them in. Notice the blooms on the flowers, the clouds drifting by, and the insects that cross your path.
- **Get Gardening:** There's nothing like putting your hands in the dirt and planting something beautiful. It could be

fragrant herbs in a pot on your back porch, flowers in your front yard, or vegetables in a garden—it all counts!

- **Take a Hike:** If you're up for a little more adventure, lace up your hiking boots and hit the trails! (If you're in an area with wildlife like snakes, bears, or coyotes, make sure you're taking the necessary precautions.)

- **Have a Seat:** Sometimes we just need to sit outside and breathe in the fresh air. Again, take notice of all the gifts of nature that abound. Do not tune into music or a podcast; instead, just be alone with nature.

- **Pack a Picnic:** Find a nice, sunny spot and enjoy your delicious meal under the blue sky.

- **Practice Playful Grounding:** Walking barefoot on natural surfaces is known as "grounding," and some people swear by it, especially when traveling, to help their body sync up with their new surroundings. There's no harm in taking off your shoes and walking around on the grass; it can make you feel like a kid again!

- **Gaze at the Sunset (or Sunrise):** When was the last time you were outside, watching the sun as it peeked over the horizon? Or sat and watched the sun disappear for the night? It's so awe-inspiring when you really think about it.

- **Wade in the Water:** If there's a body of water near you (and the water is safe for swimming), take a dip! Or just sit on the bank or beach and gaze at the ripples in the water, noting how they move when the breeze blows or a bird or fish disturbs the surface.

Whether you choose the same thing each day or mix it up, whether you venture out in solitude or go explore with your spouse, friend, or family member—it doesn't matter. Just know that these moments allow your body to recharge and reconnect with the natural rhythms of life.

My patient Beau is a high-powered executive with lots on his plate. He made a commitment years ago to get to the gym at least three days a week, and regardless of what's going on in his day, he's vigilant about making time for a good workout. But when his energy levels started to nosedive, I suggested we look objectively at his daily routine. It turned out, Beau was spending 95 percent of his time indoors. Up before the sun, he drove to work early in the morning, worked out in an indoor gym, and then drove home after dark most days. So we discussed whether it'd be possible for him to create time in his schedule to be intentional about getting outside. Even if he had to take a call while walking in the park, he needed to somehow spend more time in nature. It's hard for anyone to disrupt our routine, but thankfully he realized the importance of this addition, and he found a way to spend at least 20 to 30 minutes a day outdoors. He even took off his shoes and socks and made it a point to walk around in the grass barefoot. It didn't take long for his energy levels to normalize. Beau was pretty surprised at how big of an impact such a small thing could make, and you might be too!

In today's hustle and bustle, it's easy to go multiple days in a row without really getting out in nature, but as soon as you intentionally choose to do so, I think you'll find it a simple and enjoyable addition to your routine. Connecting with the natural world can help reduce stress, improve mental clarity, and enhance your overall sense of well-being, all of which can enhance your fertility—for both you and your partner. Here's why:

More Nature Equals...

- **Lower Stress Hormones:** Chronic stress leads to an increase in cortisol, which affects fertility by interfering with ovulation and sperm production. Spending time in nature has been shown to reduce cortisol levels, thereby improving reproductive hormone regulation.[274] For men, as stress is reduced, testosterone levels are increased.[275]

- **A Well-Regulated Endocrine System:** Exposure to nature can trigger the parasympathetic nervous system (the body's relaxation response), which helps regulate the endocrine system, including reproductive hormones like estrogen and progesterone. Even just twenty minutes a day can make a big difference.[276] Exposure to green spaces has also been linked to better overall reproductive health and reduced incidence of menstrual disorders.[277] Additionally, studies suggest that relaxation techniques, such as meditation in a natural environment, can help balance reproductive hormones, particularly in women undergoing fertility treatments.[278]

- **Optimized Epigenetics:** Chronic stress is known to cause harmful epigenetic modifications, such as DNA methylation, which can disrupt gene expression and negatively impact health. Lowering cortisol, however, leads to favorable epigenetic changes. Reduced stress from nature exposure can influence the expression of genes related to inflammation and immune function, potentially altering the epigenetic landscape in a positive way.[279] In fact, phytoncides, natural compounds released by trees, can influence epigenetic regulators like histone deacetylases (HDACs), which play a role in gene expression related to immune health.[280]

- **Longer Telomeres:** One intriguing bit of research indicates that people living near green spaces have been found to have longer telomeres,[281] which are protective caps on the ends of chromosomes that shorten with age. Telomere length is influenced by epigenetic factors, and the reduced stress and increased physical activity associated with spending time in nature are believed to contribute to these epigenetic changes that slow cellular aging.

Lifestyle Impacts on Male Fertility

An article in the journal *Reproductive Biology and Endocrinology* investigated how lifestyle factors, especially stress and overall quality of life, impact male fertility. It emphasized that psychological stress can negatively affect specific aspects of male reproductive health, such as semen quality, sperm count, motility, and morphology.[282] High levels of stress are linked to hormonal imbalances that disrupt sperm production.[283]

The study also found that poor lifestyle habits, including inadequate nutrition, lack of exercise, and insufficient psychological support, can exacerbate these issues. Targeted interventions such as stress-response optimization, healthy eating, regular physical activity, and mental health support, can significantly enhance reproductive outcomes.

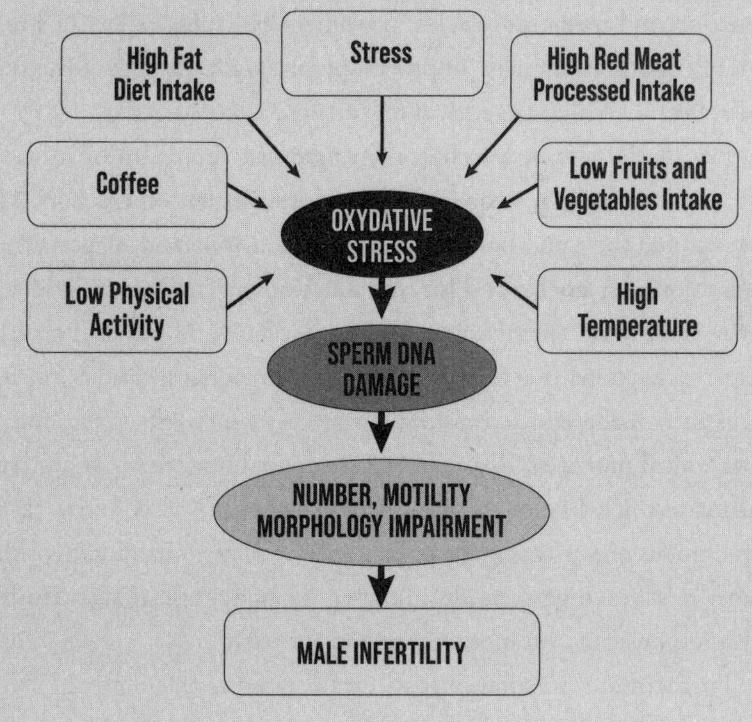

Meditation Is Medicine

Meditation and mindfulness practices can help you align your intentions with the natural flow of life. This can look different to different people, and how you choose to slow down, quiet your mind, and focus your thoughts doesn't matter as long as you're doing it on a regular basis.

Research supports the idea that meditation can positively influence fertility and hormone regulation by reducing stress, balancing the endocrine system, and promoting overall well-being. Stress is a major factor that can disrupt hormonal balance, particularly the hypothalamic-pituitary-adrenal axis, which influences reproductive hormones such as estrogen and progesterone. Studies show that when individuals engage in regular meditation or mindfulness practices, it helps to lower their cortisol levels, which in turn supports healthier ovulation and menstrual cycles in women. For men, reducing stress through meditation may improve sperm quality and testosterone levels, both of which are critical for fertility.

Dr. Joe Dispenza, a well-known figure in the realm of meditation and self-healing, is one of my favorite meditation teachers. He has explored the mind-body connection extensively and suggests that meditation can go beyond stress reduction by helping individuals rewire their brain chemistry to foster emotional and physical health. Dispenza explains that through meditative practices, the brain produces more coherent, harmonious patterns, which affect the body's biochemical processes. This can help regulate hormones that are crucial for fertility, like oxytocin and progesterone.[284] Meditative techniques focus on activating the parasympathetic nervous system, or the body's "rest and digest" mode, allowing the body to shift away from a stress response and promote reproductive health.

Furthermore, meditation can create a sense of emotional well-being and mental clarity that may benefit individuals trying to conceive. Meditation can also address emotional blockages, and this is important because unresolved trauma can manifest as physical symptoms, including fertility issues. By practicing mindfulness and meditation, individuals may be able to break free from subconscious patterns that contribute to stress and hormonal imbalances. This holistic approach suggests that aligning the mind and body through meditation not only aids in hormonal regulation but also improves the emotional state, potentially creating a more favorable environment for conception.

There are many different mediation apps available these days that can help you tailor your meditation time as you see fit, whether that means listening to a guided meditation or one that offers a soundscape. Here are a few that I recommend:

- **Headspace:** Offers guided meditations, mindfulness exercises, and sleep sounds. It's beginner-friendly and covers various aspects of well-being.
- **Calm:** Known for its guided meditations, breathing exercises, calming soundscapes, and sleep stories.
- **Insight Timer:** A free app with a large library of guided meditations and music tracks to help with relaxation and focus.
- **MyLife (formerly Stop, Breathe & Think):** Customizes meditation recommendations based on your current mood and feelings.
- **Simple Habit:** Provides quick, five-minute meditations for busy schedules alongside sleep and mindfulness tools.

I've also seen meaningful changes in stress response by combining neurofeedback with meditation using the Muse (choosemuse.com) or Sens.ai devices (sens.ai). Neurofeedback helps you to shift your brain waves to a more resilient state. The devices offer the added benefits of being able to train your brain to focus or sleep better. There are many devices available now; Muse and Sens.ai are the two that I have used personally.

You might prefer to meditate on Scripture. Or you might feel drawn to create a mantra. Just know that there's no one-size-fits-all approach to meditation, but no matter which one you choose, the health benefits will be impactful. The point is simply to create time and space in your schedule for giving your mind a break from the constancy of thoughts and point it in one direction. And know that it's working, even when you find yourself thinking about other things!

Optimizing Your Stress Response

Ah, stress . . . I believe it's one of the—if not *the*—biggest causes of chronic illness facing modern humanity. In fact, research keeps showing that female infertility patients consistently report significantly more symptoms of anxiety and depression than fertile individuals.[285] Other studies have shown that, for men, chronic stress causes severe damage to germ cells, which accounts for fertility problems in men.

Is infertility causing stress? Or is stress causing infertility? This, of course, is the age-old question, and the studies are leaning in the latter direction, especially as psychological treatments are showing promise in helping infertility challenges.[286]

According to the American Psychological Association, "Stress is a normal reaction to everyday pressures, but can become unhealthy when it upsets your day-to-day functioning. Stress involves changes affecting nearly every system of the body, influencing how people feel and behave. By causing mind–body changes, stress contributes directly to psychological and physiological disorder and disease and affects mental and physical health, reducing quality of life."[287]

That just about sums it up, doesn't it? Stress affects *everything*, and that includes your fertility and epigenetics.

You are in the driver's seat, so the question is: How do you respond to the stress that you will inevitably experience?

Create Your Unique Stress-Reduction Plan

Your first step is to identify the causes of consistent stress in your life. If you're always feeling as if you're behind the eight ball, unable to get everything done, and like so many people in your life are depending on you, then your stress might be coming from being overcommitted. If that's the case, then it's probably time to set some boundaries and take a closer look at your daily schedule to determine where you can redeem some time for yourself.

On the other hand, if you're overwhelmed by your financial situation and constantly worried about making ends meet, you might need to make some adjustments to your budget and your monthly spending or consider making some bigger changes to your lifestyle in order to balance your finances. Money is a big source of stress and anxiety for many people, but facing this issue and creating a game plan can be so empowering.

If you're stuck in an emotional rut, perhaps due to recent or past trauma, there might be some deeper work to do, maybe even with the help of a professional. There's absolutely no shame in asking for help to get out of that cycle, because as much as you might wish it would go away on its own, unresolved trauma has a way of sneaking back up on you.

Regardless of the source of your stress, identifying it is so important because then—and only then—can you create a strategy for dealing with it properly. So take some time to write down possible sources of emotional/mental stress in your life, and then start to work on strategies for reducing or eliminating those sources. Work with your partner on this; you can practice helping each other manage stress because in a family system, when one person is feeling stressed out, the rest of the family is impacted. Studies show that chronic stress exhausts a man's energy and mental resources over time in such a way that his ability to identify the support needs of his wife is greatly reduced. This puts strain on the relationship. The problem is not so much day-to-day stress. In that case, married couples still seem to be able to recognize each other's needs and provide support. But chronic stress affects both the awareness of the need for support and actual provision of the support.[288]

Plus, stress will only compound with the challenges of pregnancy and parenthood. Even though this journey is fueled by and filled with love, there are no guarantees it will be easy or stress-free—quite the contrary. But allow love to be your guide as you get a handle on how you're going to identify and strategize your stress reduction.

Stress Response Optimization Techniques

Once you have an effective strategy in place for reducing controllable sources of stress, it's important to build in some techniques to help you manage stress that is outside of your control. Because . . . life happens. A rainstorm delays your flight for a work trip. Your air conditioner goes out in the middle of summer. You get in a fender bender. Any number of uncontrollable stressors can and will pop up, but there are ways you can help yourself cope with those situations.

Earlier in the book, I introduced you to some powerful stress-reducing supplements, and I want to remind you to take those regularly, because they can really reduce the physiological impact of stress. I also want to encourage you to identify and implement daily practices that help manage and reduce mental/emotional stress. Here are some tried-and-true ideas:

- **Work Up a Sweat:** Physical activity helps release endorphins, improving mood and reducing stress.
- **Just Breathe:** Engaging in slow, deep breaths can help calm the nervous system and alleviate stress. I often recommend box breathing (slow breath in for six seconds, hold for six seconds, slow breath out for six seconds, repeat) several times a day to help your mind and body unwind.

- **Nourish to Flourish:** As discussed in the chapter on nutrition, eating a balanced diet with whole foods supports overall well-being, increases mental clarity, and helps manage stress levels.

- **Protect Your Sleep:** An adequate amount of restful sleep helps the body recover from daily stress and boosts resilience.

- **Steward Your Time Well:** Time management is key. Organizing your tasks and breaking down large projects into manageable steps can reduce feeling overwhelmed. Fasting from news and social media can be monumental.

- **Hone Your Hobbies:** Taking time for activities you enjoy provides a mental break from stressors.

- **Build "Fences":** Setting healthy boundaries, saying no to obligations that don't really fit into your life, and setting limits can help prevent overcommitment and reduce stress.

- **Laugh a Little:** Finding moments of joy and humor can lighten your mood and decrease your stress.

- **Get Social:** Talking with friends, family, or a support group can help you feel understood and less anxious about life.

- **Take Ten:** Regular breaks throughout the day can help reset your mind and reduce the buildup of stress.

If there are some ideas on that list that you haven't tried lately, work them into your routine for a while. You might be surprised by how much they help. Ultimately, you can discover what works best for you and make it a nonnegotiable part of your life.

Holistic Support

You could also consider complementary therapies such as acupuncture, massage, or aromatherapy to support stress reduction. These practices can help balance your body's energy and improve your overall sense of well-being. Many of my patients have found incorporating these types of therapies into their lifestyle has been highly beneficial.

RENEW

Prioritizing Sleep

Right up front I'm going to admit something to you—I did not prioritize sleep when I was in the preconception period. Or during my pregnancies. Yikes! I was in medical school, we were building a custom home, my husband at the time was commuting back and forth to a totally different area of Texas, and my plate was full to overflowing. In fact, during my second pregnancy, I was a second-year resident, working in the hospital wards or ICU most months and even did a month of night float. So my sleep rhythms were a mess. If I had it to do over again knowing what I know now, I'd do things differently for sure. I'm thankful I survived it, but I hope you will be able to prioritize your sleep better than I did!

Earlier in this chapter, we talked about natural rhythms, and I referred to *circadian rhythms*. According to the National Institute of General Medical Sciences, "Circadian rhythms are the physical, mental, and behavioral changes any organism experiences over a 24-hour cycle. Light and dark have the biggest influence on circadian rhythms, but food intake, stress, physical activity, social environment, and temperature also affect them. In humans, nearly every tissue and organ has its own circadian rhythm, and collectively they are tuned to the daily cycle of day and night."[289]

In a 2020 study in the *International Journal of Molecular Sciences* titled "Disruption of Circadian Rhythms: A Crucial Factor in the Etiology of Infertility," researchers considered the connection between circadian rhythms and fertility, and specifically how disruptions in these rhythms can significantly impact reproductive health. The circadian clock, regulated by specific "clock genes," controls various physiological processes like hormone secretion, which are crucial for fertility.[290]

The authors explored the mechanisms by which circadian rhythms influence fertility, highlighting the roles of hormones such as gonadotropins, estrogens, and androgens, which are all regulated by circadian rhythms. The study also examined the effects of external factors, such as stress and light exposure, on circadian rhythms and their subsequent impact on reproductive health. In male fertility, clock genes play a role in processes like spermatogenesis, while in female fertility, they regulate the estrous cycle and hormone production. Disruptions in circadian rhythms, often caused by irregular sleep patterns, were highlighted as a contributing factor to infertility. Such disruptions can alter hormone secretion, particularly those related to reproductive health, leading to issues with the hypothalamic-pituitary-gonadal axis.[291]

Furthermore, the study reviewed genetic models in mice that show how mutations in clock genes can lead to fertility issues, such as irregular estrous cycles, reduced sperm quality, and impaired steroidogenesis. In humans, the study linked shift work and disrupted circadian rhythms to prolonged time to pregnancy and menstrual irregularities.[292] (By the way, in case you were wondering, steroidogenesis is the process your body uses to make steroid hormones, which are essential for many functions such as energy, metabolism, stress response, and reproduction. Imagine a hormone factory inside your cells, specifically in your adrenal glands, ovaries (in women), and testes (in men). The process starts with cholesterol. Your body takes cholesterol and converts it into pregnenolone, which is like the "master ingredient" for all steroid hormones. From there, it gets transformed into different hormones depending on what your body needs.)

As you can see, our hormones are highly influenced by our circadian rhythms. What's the most powerful way to maintain healthy circadian rhythms? *Having a regular sleep pattern.*

Improving Sleep Hygiene

Your mission is simple: Focus on establishing a consistent sleep routine that supports restorative rest for at least seven hours per night in a dark room. I know that can be difficult in practice, but I've found that when I task my patients with creating a set bedtime and waking time each day, they do well. It's all about putting some intention behind it. You might need to evaluate your pre-sleep routine to make sure it doesn't include screens at least one hour prior to going to bed and ensure your sleep environment is conducive to rest (e.g., a cool, dark, quiet room). You can also use blue-light-blocking glasses in the evenings. Again, just putting a little thought into your sleep routine can go a long way toward establishing a healthy rhythm for sleep.

Supporting Sleep with Supplements

Safe supplements including magnesium glycinate, glycine, and theanine can promote relaxation and improve sleep quality. If you have trouble sleeping, consider adding these as part of your nightly routine.

Limiting Stimulants

If the number of Starbucks in every neighborhood is any evidence, our society is pretty much fueled by coffee. If you can't imagine making it through the day without a few cups of joe (or—*gasp*—energy drinks), then we need to have a little talk. Caffeine is a stimulant, and it can disrupt sleep patterns as well as affect your adrenal health. For some people, even having small amounts of caffeine in the morning can affect the quality of their sleep at night. Gradually cutting back will also help ease the transition when you need to eliminate caffeine entirely during pregnancy. Consider drinking caffeine-free organic herbal teas instead; there are so many delicious ones on the market!

Nicotine is another obvious stimulant best to be avoided. The connection between sudden infant death syndrome (SIDS) and maternal smoking is well documented.[293] However, preterm birth, low birth weight, and poor intrauterine growth are also linked to smoking, as well as further complications such as respiratory and other infections, neurodevelopmental issues, and mental health challenges.[294] Vaping also exposes you to many toxins.[295]

Smoking has been shown to harm male fertility by reducing sperm motility, concentration, and morphology while causing genetic and epigenetic damage to sperm. Nicotine and its metabolite, cotinine, can cross the blood–testis barrier, leading to DNA fragmentation, genome instability, mutations, and chromosomal abnormalities. These effects compromise sperm quality and increase the risk of fertility issues.[296]

What might be less obvious, however, are the medical products you use that contain stimulants. Pseudoephedrine is a nasal decongestant and a common drug used in sinus medication, and something to avoid during preconception. Also, by no means is taking appetite suppressants or energy pills a safe idea!

Exercise

Physical activity plays a vital role in fertility and overall health, benefiting both men and women. Recent research from the Broad Institute of MIT and Harvard underscores the extensive cellular and molecular changes triggered by physical activity across multiple organs.[297] This includes implications for the reproductive system, where exercise can influence hormonal balance and inflammatory responses. Even the most basic exercise has been shown to improve fertility outcomes.[298] Studies point to cyclic exercise (walking, cycling) as a common approach, as well as a combination of cyclic exercise and training in the circuit or "boot camps."[299] However, yoga also produces positive results—including enhanced blood flow, reduced inflammation, relaxation response, and modulation of the hypothalamic-pituitary-adrenal axis (which regulates metabolism, immune responses, and the autonomic nervous system). Yoga also has a positive effect on oxidative stress, oxidative DNA damage, epigenetic changes, hormonal balance, ovarian function, and menstrual irregularities, and can help tremendously with stress reduction.[300]

Choosing the Right Exercise

Exercise plays a big role in supporting fertility for both men and women. Gentle, low-impact activities such as yoga, walking, swimming, and Pilates can help lower stress, improve blood flow, and keep hormones balanced. These types of movement can also reduce pain, ease anxiety and depression, and even improve birth outcomes by lowering the chances of needing assisted delivery.

For men, regular movement doesn't just boost overall health—it can also improve sperm quality. Studies show that yoga, in particular, can create positive changes in nearly four hundred genes linked to sperm health, helping set the stage for a healthier baby. Whether it's yoga, stretching, or a relaxing evening walk, prioritizing movement can make a big difference in your fertility journey.

Consistency over Intensity

Aim for regular, moderate exercise rather than sporadic, intense workouts. Daily movement, whether it's a morning walk, stretching, or a short exercise session, is more beneficial in the long run. If I don't work out first thing in the morning, I know I probably won't get to it, so I protect my early morning schedule for working out at the gym or on a Pilates Reformer.

Exercise with a Partner

Exercising with your spouse or partner builds a shared routine and strengthens your relationship. Consider activities you can enjoy together, such as hiking, dancing, yoga, or even simple stretching exercises at home.

Pelvic-Floor Health for Women

Ideally, every woman would see a pelvic-floor physical therapist before and after their pregnancy to help make sure her pelvic floor is functioning well. If you have access to one, I encourage you to make an appointment.

At a minimum, incorporate pelvic-floor exercises into your daily routine because they go a long way toward helping your body prepare for pregnancy and childbirth. Integrating these exercises into daily activities, like while waiting at traffic lights, can make them a seamless part of your routine. Pelvic-floor exercises are essential for addressing and preventing issues such as urinary incontinence and pelvic pain, and they can speed up your postpartum recovery. These exercises help strengthen the muscles supporting the pelvic organs, enhancing both functionality and quality of life. Here are two examples of pelvic floor exercises you can start doing today:

Kegel Exercises

Sit or lie down in a comfortable position. Identify your pelvic floor muscles by pretending like you're trying to stop the flow of urine midstream or by imagining you are trying to prevent passing gas. Once you've located these muscles, tighten them gently, hold the contraction for about five seconds, and then relax for five seconds. Aim to repeat this process ten to fifteen times in a row. Gradually increase the duration of the contractions and the number of repetitions as your strength improves.

Kegel exercises strengthen the muscles of the pelvic floor, improving bladder control and reducing symptoms of urinary incontinence. They also help support the pelvic organs and can be beneficial in preparation for childbirth and postpartum recovery.

Bridge Exercise

Lie on your back with your knees bent and feet flat on the floor, hip-width apart. Place your arms by your sides with your palms facing down. Engage your core and pelvic floor muscles as you lift your hips off the ground, forming a straight line from your shoulders to your knees. Hold this position for five to ten seconds, then slowly lower your hips back to the ground. Repeat the exercise ten to fifteen times.

This bridge exercise targets the glutes, lower back, and pelvic floor muscles. It helps strengthen the muscles supporting the pelvic region, improves overall stability, and can aid in relieving pelvic pain and discomfort. This exercise also promotes better posture and core strength.

Pelvic Floor Insight from an Expert

Stephanie Hahn, PT, DPT, a pioneering expert in women's pelvic health, has dedicated her career to empowering women facing these challenges. She established the first women's health program focused on pelvic-floor disorders in Austin, Texas, and coauthored *A Woman's Guide to Pelvic Health*, which provides practical advice for restoring pelvic-floor health through targeted exercises.

Hahn's work emphasizes the importance of integrating pelvic-floor exercises into daily routines. Her approach not only addresses the physical aspects of pelvic health but also helps overcome the embarrassment and stigma often associated with these issues. Beyond structured therapy, Hahn encourages women to adopt simple, consistent physical activities to support their well-being. She let me interview her for the purposes of sharing some specific information with you in this book:

The pelvic floor is a group of muscles at the base of the pelvic basin surrounding the anal, vaginal, and urethral openings. These muscles serve three essential roles: (1) *Support*: They hold up the pelvic organs, maintaining proper placement and support during movement and rest; (2) *Control*: They help with sphincter function, preventing leakage of urine or feces when sneezing, laughing, or coughing; and (3) *Sexual Health*: The tone and flexibility of these muscles impact sexual arousal and satisfaction, an essential factor in reproductive health.

The pelvic floor acts as a "diaphragm" at the base of the pelvis, coordinating with the respiratory diaphragm. This coordination means that the pelvic floor will gently rise and fall with each breath, maintaining both elasticity and strength. However, various life factors can disrupt this balance, resulting in either excessive or insufficient muscle tone.

There are a number of reasons for pelvic-floor issues in women of childbearing age. One of these reasons is ***too much tension (hypertonicity)***. Overly tight pelvic-floor muscles are common among high-stress individuals and can stem from factors such as trauma, excessive sitting, or even chronic stress that leads to "clenching." When the pelvic floor muscles are too tight, this can lead to pain during rest or sexual intercourse, or even bladder issues like urgency and frequency. Some women may unknowingly clench their pelvic-floor muscles, just as many of us unconsciously clench our jaws. This hypertonic state can interfere with healthy, pain-free sexual function and make vaginal delivery more challenging.

Another reason is ***not enough tension (hypotonicity)***. Chronic constipation, obesity, and hypermobility can lead to weakened pelvic-floor muscles. In these cases, the muscles are underactive and lack the tone required for adequate pelvic support, which is particularly problematic during pregnancy. Women with connective tissue disorders like Ehlers-Danlos syndrome often experience this lack of tension. With added weight and the hormonal changes of pregnancy, the condition can worsen, potentially leading to issues such as urinary incontinence.

Prepregnancy Assessment and Support

Before conception, it is beneficial to consult a pelvic-floor specialist (typically a physical therapist) who can assess muscle tone, alignment, and posture. Tailored therapy can address any muscular imbalances before the additional stress of pregnancy, promoting a smoother pregnancy and delivery process.

Key Exercises for Pelvic-Floor Health

A well-functioning pelvic floor is essential for overall stability, core strength, and preparation for pregnancy. Engaging in mindful exercises that promote both awareness and relaxation can help optimize pelvic health and support the body's changing needs. The following movements focus on breathing coordination, gentle pelvic-floor engagement, and foundational strength from the ground up, ensuring a balanced and supportive core system.

- **Diaphragmatic Breathing:** Lie on your back with your knees bent. Place one hand on your lower abdomen and inhale deeply, letting your abdomen rise and your pelvic floor relax and lower slightly. Exhale, feeling a gentle lift in the pelvic floor and a subtle contraction of the abdomen. This gentle, rhythmic breathing engages and relaxes the pelvic floor in harmony with the diaphragm.

- **Pelvic-Floor Awareness Exercise:** While lying down, place your hand over your perineum (the area between the anus and the genitals) to feel the gentle expansion on inhalation and contraction on exhalation. Practice without forcing movement to develop awareness of the natural rhythm of your pelvic floor, avoiding active kegels at this stage to focus solely on relaxation.

- **Short-Foot Exercise for Arch Support:** Pregnancy often increases foot size and arch flattening due to the hormone *relaxin*. This "short foot" exercise can help strengthen the arch. Stand and press your big toe down without gripping, creating an arch by shortening the space between your toes and heel. Repeat for five repetitions on each foot. This exercise improves posture from the ground up, supporting the entire pelvic region.

Core Strengthening and Postural Alignment

Strengthening the core is foundational, but not all core exercises are created equal. Hahn advises working on the transverse abdominis, obliques, and rectus abdominis in balance:

- **Transverse Abdominis Activation:** While lying on your back, gently pull your belly button toward your spine on an exhale. This activates the deepest abdominal layer, creating a corset-like support around your pelvis.
- **Oblique Strengthening:** Twisting motions that engage the side body (like seated twists) strengthen the muscles essential for both stability and the active pushing phase during delivery.
- **Postural Alignment:** Stand with your weight centered on the arch to heel (rather than the toes). Avoid letting your pelvis or midsection "sway" forward. Visualize aligning your ear, shoulder, hip, knee, and ankle in a straight line. Maintaining this posture helps with breathing and pelvic support.

Upper Body and Postural Support for Both Partners

As you begin to transition to life with a baby, upper body strength and posture become increasingly important, especially for dads, who often take on more carrying and lifting responsibilities postpartum. Shoulder blade and upper back strengthening combined with chest stretching can prevent common issues such as back and shoulder pain.

Again, a big thank-you to Stephanie Hahn for sharing such detailed advice. It's important for both partners to work together to get stronger and to optimize your posture. Whether through Pilates, stretching, or integrating exercises into daily life, the goal is to create a sustainable routine that enhances both physical and emotional health. Engaging in regular, moderate exercise, including pelvic-floor work, can significantly benefit overall health and fertility, highlighting the importance of a holistic approach to physical well-being.

RENEW

Final Thoughts

Living well in the preconception period is about more than just physical health—it's about creating an environment of love, positivity, and readiness. By being mindful of what information you consume, managing stress, prioritizing sleep, and incorporating regular exercise, you prepare not only your body but also your mind and spirit for the incredible journey of parenthood.

Q&A

Q: How can I involve my partner in these lifestyle changes to ensure we're both prepared for conception?

A: Involving your partner in lifestyle changes can strengthen your relationship and help align your goals for parenthood. Earlier in the book, I encouraged you to discuss your mutual desire for a healthy preconception period, so now is the time to continue that conversation and discuss shared activities like exercising, cooking nutritious meals, or practicing mindfulness. Collaboration ensures both of you are on the same page and committed to creating a balanced lifestyle that prepares you for parentship.

Q: I live in a city with limited access to nature. How can I connect with the natural world?

A: Urban living can still provide opportunities to connect with nature. Visit local parks or botanical gardens regularly and bring nature into your home with houseplants or small garden spaces. You can also plan weekend getaways to natural settings. Even small daily habits, such as pausing to appreciate the weather or watching a sunset from your balcony, can help you feel more in tune with the natural world.

Q: Are there specific meditation techniques that are particularly beneficial during the preconception period?

A: Mindfulness meditation and loving-kindness meditation are particularly beneficial during preconception. Mindfulness meditation helps you become more aware of your thoughts and reduces stress, which is important for overall well-being and hormonal balance. Loving-kindness meditation, which focuses on cultivating compassion and positivity, can help promote emotional well-being. You can also find fertility-specific guided meditations on YouTube.

Q: How does information overload impact fertility, and what steps can I take to mitigate its effects?

A: Information overload can increase stress, which negatively impacts hormonal balance and fertility. It can also make it harder to focus on important tasks or decisions. To mitigate its effects, set limits on screen time and be intentional about what information you consume. Prioritize uplifting, educational, or inspiring content. You can also schedule regular digital detoxes or set specific times of day for media consumption to reduce overstimulation.

Q: How can I manage stress if I have a high-pressure job that I can't change right now?

A: I understand that managing stress in a high-pressure job can be extra challenging. It requires building stress-reduction techniques into your daily routine. Break tasks into manageable steps, set realistic priorities, and take short breaks throughout the day to reset. Practice mindfulness techniques, like deep breathing or short meditations, during stressful moments. Outside of work, ensure you're engaging in activities that help you recharge, such as some of the topics we covered in this chapter—physical exercise, hobbies, or time in nature. It may also help to discuss workload adjustments or stress-management support with your employer if possible.

Q: How can I practice mindfulness in daily activities beyond formal meditation sessions?

A: You can practice mindfulness in everyday tasks by paying attention to the present moment. For example, when eating, savor the flavors and textures of your food. During a walk, observe your surroundings and engage with the sights, sounds, and smells. When doing household chores, like washing dishes or folding laundry, stay focused on the task at hand and your breath. This helps cultivate a sense of calm and presence throughout your day.

Q: What are some strategies for setting healthy boundaries to prevent overcommitment and reduce stress?

A: Start by recognizing your limits and identifying tasks or commitments that don't align with your values or goals. Politely say no to additional obligations and protect time for self-care and rest. Establish clear boundaries with work, friends, and family to avoid burnout. It may also help to schedule personal downtime or quiet moments throughout the week. Setting boundaries not only reduces stress but also helps you maintain a healthy balance in your life.

Q: How can I find supportive communities or groups that align with my journey toward balanced living and parenthood?

A: Look for local or online groups focused on wellness, fertility, or mindfulness. Many communities offer wellness classes, yoga sessions, or workshops that promote balanced living. Online forums, social media groups, and virtual wellness communities are also excellent resources for finding support, sharing experiences, and exchanging advice. Engaging with these groups can offer encouragement and practical tips for maintaining a balanced lifestyle as you prepare for parenthood.

RENEW

Believe

Introspect

Renew

Thrive

Hope

Section IV Introduction

The *Thrive* section is all about building resilience, vitality, and well-being for both partners before conception, ensuring you're both prepared to create the healthiest foundation for your future child. Thriving isn't just an individual goal; it's a shared investment in the health of the next generation. In this section, you'll gain the knowledge and tools to flourish together, supporting each other's health as you build a strong base for your future family.

Chapter 9: Smart Supplements: Powering Up for Parenthood provides guidance on key nutrients and supplements that benefit both men's and women's fertility and overall vitality. This chapter offers research-backed recommendations for supporting reproductive health, enhancing energy, and optimizing wellness in preparation for conception. With strategic supplementation, you're giving yourselves and your future child an important advantage in health and resilience.

Chapter 10: Gut Genesis: Your "Garden" of Generational Health highlights the essential role of gut health, which impacts immune function, hormone balance, and genetic expression in both partners. You'll learn how fostering a balanced gut microbiome (as well as other microbiomes in your body) benefits the whole body and supports reproductive health. Together, you'll build a stable, supportive foundation that can positively influence your child's health.

Chapter 11: Harmonizing Your Hormones emphasizes the importance of balanced hormones for each partner, exploring how nutrition, lifestyle, and stress management play a role in achieving harmony. By prioritizing hormonal health as a team, you'll both enhance fertility and create a balanced environment that supports conception.

Chapter 12: Taming Inflammation explores how chronic, low-grade inflammation—whether driven by histamine intolerance, oxalate buildup, or autoimmune triggers—can quietly sabotage your fertility and future child's health. This chapter helps you uncover these often-overlooked culprits, understand their impact on your hormones and epigenetics, and take practical steps to cool the fire within. By calming inflammation now, you're creating a more welcoming environment for conception and laying a healthier foundation for generations to come.

Chapter 13: Fertility GPS: Navigating Your Reproductive Journey helps you map out a shared path toward conception. This chapter covers tracking cycles, understanding fertility signals, and recognizing each partner's contributions. With these insights, you'll approach conception with a sense of teamwork, clarity, and confidence, both understanding your rhythms and maximizing your fertility potential.

Together, these chapters in *Thrive* will empower you to reach your fullest health potential as a team, creating a nurturing and robust environment for your future child to flourish.

CHAPTER 9

Smart Supplements: Powering Up for Parenthood

I'm going to give it to you straight: Prenatal vitamins are *not* enough. And they're *really* not enough if you wait until a positive pregnancy test before you start taking them. I believe all of us—in every season of life—need to be on supplements because our food supply simply can't give us all the nutrients we need to have optimal health. As we touched on in the nutrition chapter, our food simply isn't what it once was, so we really need supplements in order to get all the nutrients our bodies need. It's especially important to be supplementing during a time when you're asking your body to put its best foot forward and create an egg or sperm with optimized epigenetics! By supplementing, you can improve the quality of the "ingredients" necessary for creating a healthy baby.

Researchers have learned so much about how certain supplements can impact our epigenetics, and that information can have a far-reaching impact on your family tree. You have the ability to influence not only your own gene expression, but that of your children's and their children's. I get excited about how effective proper supplementation can be, mostly because I've seen it work wonders in my practice over the years.

At just twenty-seven years old, Ellen's journey to motherhood had already been an uphill battle. Her irregular menstrual cycles had always been a source of frustration and confusion, but when she and her husband decided they were ready to start a family, those irregularities took on a new meaning. After trying to conceive for over a year without success, Ellen sought help from not one but two fertility specialists. Both offered the same solution: in vitro fertilization (IVF).

The process was emotionally and physically taxing. Ellen's first IVF cycle yielded seven follicles, but only three eggs fertilized, and of those, just one embryo made it to day five. The hope she had clung to was shattered when she learned that the embryo had an abnormal chromosome. The specialists told her that her eggs were small and appeared older than her age suggested. Those words felt like a cruel verdict.

Feeling heartbroken and hopeless, Ellen couldn't bring herself to go through another round of IVF. She decided to look for alternative options and eventually found her way to my practice. During our first meeting, Ellen's sadness was palpable, but so was her determination to uncover the root causes of her struggles. Together, we embarked upon a comprehensive journey to understand what was happening inside her body.

Her lab work painted a complex picture. We discovered that Ellen had a sensitivity to gluten, as well as underlying issues including parasites, yeast overgrowth, and methylation challenges due to the MTHFR gene mutation. Her bloodwork revealed Factor V Leiden, a genetic predisposition that increased her risk of blood clotting. Additionally, her nutrition was far from optimal, lacking the essential building blocks needed to support a healthy pregnancy.

Over the next eight months, Ellen committed fully to the plan we created. She overhauled her diet, eliminating gluten and dairy and focusing on nutrient-dense, anti-inflammatory foods. We addressed the infections and imbalances in her gut, restoring harmony to her microbiome. We also implemented a supplement routine tailored to her needs.

Ellen's transformation was remarkable. As her body healed, so did her spirit. Her cycles became more regular, her energy improved, and she began to feel hopeful again. Then, one morning, Ellen called me, her voice trembling with emotion. "I'm pregnant," she said, tears of joy spilling over. Against all odds, she had conceived naturally.

By optimizing her body's systems through proper nutrition and supplementation, Ellen was able to rewrite her story and embrace the role she had longed for: becoming a mother.

Assimilating Supplements

Because supplements have such a profound effect on your body chemistry, I want to remind you that if you're currently on any medications or under a physician's care for any condition, make sure you discuss this with your doctor before proceeding. You know your body better than anyone else, so if you feel like you need a little extra time to assimilate new supplements, then give yourself that time before adding in new ones.

Quality Counts

When it comes to selecting specific supplement brands, remember that they're not all created equal. It's critical that you choose products with high-quality ingredients that have been tested and designed to be as bioactive as possible. But don't worry; I've done the work for you by curating this specific list based on the highest of quality standards.

A whole world of supplements exists these days, but for our purposes, I'm zeroing in on the ones I see as nonnegotiable for preconception. Because I know you'll be more apt to follow through on taking them daily if you understand why they're so important, I'm going to spend a little time explaining each of them.

Also, you can use this QR code to go to a page on my Every Baby Well website that gives you a current list of all the preconception supplements I recommend, as well as links to purchase.

Supplements by Purpose

To help you get a better sense of which supplements are working to accomplish which goals, I've created a simple supplement pyramid. At the bottom of the pyramid, you'll find foundational supplements, and

Preconception Supplement Pyramid

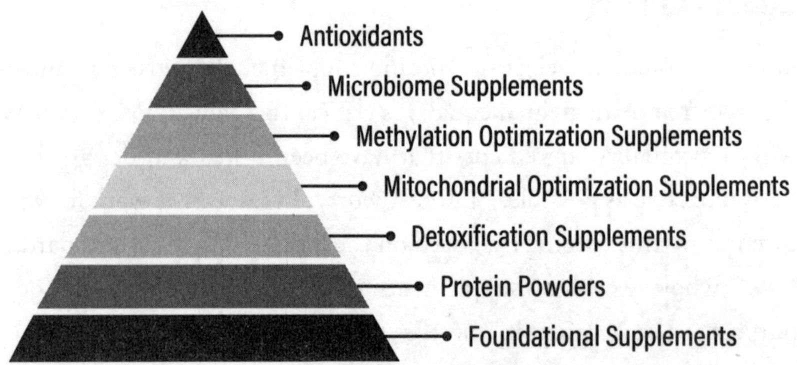

then you'll work your way up the pyramid. Each level builds on the next. You don't want to pick and choose supplements or do just one thing in isolation. Instead, the idea is to address each of these layers so you can build your structure for fertility and epigenetic optimization. As you read through the various supplement descriptions, you'll find that many of them fit into more than one category, but I chose to place them into the one that fits best.

Foundational Supplements

Women's Wellness + Fertility Force

Recommendation: Women's Wellness + Fertility Force—Comprehensive Nutritional Support for Preconception Health (by Every Baby Well)

This supplement is a targeted formula designed to support preconception health, hormone balance, and reproductive wellness by delivering a powerful combination of essential vitamins, omega-3 fatty acids, and phytonutrients in convenient daily packets. Here are the ways in which this supplement supports fertility and preconception health for women:

- Provides foundational nutrition: A comprehensive blend of bioavailable vitamins and minerals ensures essential nutrients for egg quality, hormone regulation, and reproductive function.
- Supports detoxification and liver health: Milk thistle, artichoke, dandelion root, and turmeric aid liver function, promoting the elimination of toxins and excess hormones that can impact fertility.
- Enhances antioxidant protection: Resveratrol, turmeric, and garlic reduce oxidative stress, protecting egg and cellular integrity while supporting a healthy inflammatory response.
- Boosts essential fatty acids for reproductive health: EPA, DHA, and DPA omega-3s from high-quality fish oil improve

hormonal balance, egg quality, and uterine health, while also supporting fetal brain development.

- Strengthens gut health and microbiome: Nutrients like turmeric and garlic promote a healthy gut, which plays a critical role in nutrient absorption, hormone metabolism, and immune function—key factors in fertility and pregnancy wellness.

Suggested Use:

Take one packet daily.

Men's Wellness + Fertility Force by Every Life Well (men only)

Recommendation: Men's Wellness + Fertility Force is a comprehensive formula that provides the foundation for improving sperm count, motility, and optimizing overall reproductive health by addressing certain key factors.

It supports cellular energy production with acetyl L-cartinine and alpha lipoic acid, enhances immune function with N-acetyl cysteine and resveratrol, and provides powerful antioxidants like green tea extract (ECGC) to protect sperm DNA.

This formula also aids in detoxification, helping to remove environmental toxins that can impair sperm quality.

Preconception Omegas

Recommendation: Preconception Omegas—Essential DHA by Every Baby Well

This supplement is a high-concentration DHA fish oil formula designed to support fertility, pregnancy, and early childhood development. DHA is a vital omega-3 fatty acid that plays a crucial role in hormonal balance, egg and sperm quality, brain health, and fetal development. Since the body cannot produce DHA on its own, supplementation is essential for optimal preconception health and a strong foundation for pregnancy.

Each soft gel provides 580 mg of DHA in its natural triglyceride form, ensuring absorption and bioavailability. This formula is sourced off the Chilean coast, where the cold, fresh waters provide one of the cleanest, most sustainable sources of fish. Purified and vacuum-distilled, it undergoes independent testing to ensure heavy metals, pesticides, and contaminants are removed to undetectable levels. Here's how it's helpful with preconception:

- Supports fertility: DHA is essential for egg and sperm membrane integrity, promoting optimal reproductive function.
- Enhances fetal brain development: Rapid brain growth occurs in the third trimester and early postnatal months, making DHA critical during pregnancy.
- Promotes a healthy pregnancy: DHA supports cardiovascular health, proper blood flow to the placenta, and a balanced inflammatory response.
- Improves postpartum mood balance: Research shows low DHA levels are linked to a higher risk of postpartum mood challenges, while DHA supplementation can provide protective benefits.
- Supports newborn cognitive development: Studies suggest maternal DHA intake during late pregnancy and breastfeeding enhances cognitive function, improves sleep patterns, and may even boost IQ in early childhood.

Choline and Phosphatidylcholine

According to numerous studies, "supplementing the maternal diet with additional choline has been shown to improve offspring cognition, neurodevelopment, and placental functioning, and to protect against neural and metabolic insults."[301] Choline is an essential nutrient that impacts mood, muscles, and other brain and nervous system functions, and it helps modulate gene expression, cell membrane signaling, lipid transport and metabolism, as well as early brain development.[302] Bottom line: Choline is a vital part of your mission to create a healthy baby, and our bodies simply cannot produce enough of it on their own, so supplementation is critical.

Phosphatidylcholine (PC) is a phospholipid that contains choline as part of its structure. PC is another "desert island" supplement; I always have it with me. The reason is simple: Nothing in the body can work properly without adequate amounts of phosphatidylcholine. It is perhaps the most important molecule among tens of thousands of molecules that comprise a cell, accounting for nearly 50 percent of the cell membrane. In fact, there isn't one function of the body that doesn't rely on phosphatidylcholine. The cell membrane is where virtually all the important metabolic reactions occur, making PC critical for healthy cell membrane composition and function. But lowered phospholipid availability may sometimes limit these essential functions.

PC is so important for our cell and mitochondrial membranes to be healthy, but studies show that 60 to 70 percent of people are choline deficient. We do get some choline from foods like spinach, egg yolks, beets, and meat, but it's not enough. And while the body can biosynthesize (which is the process of creating complex molecules from simpler substances through chemical reactions in the body's cells) phospholipids from other substances, the process requires many enzymes and a great deal of energy. On top of that, some of us don't absorb PC very well due to genetics.

Not only does phosphatidylcholine support healthy cell membrane composition and function, it also supports healthy choline levels and increases brain acetylcholine formation. Acetylcholine is a neurotransmitter important for memory as well as other bodily functions.

When cells membranes are healthy, cells are healthy, which lead to healthy tissues, healthy organs, and, ultimately, healthy bodies and minds. Since our goal is to support your body at a cellular level while you're preparing to conceive a baby, optimizing your levels of phosphatidylcholine is a top priority.

Daily PC supplementation may also help maintain healthy liver function, healthy cholesterol levels already within the normal range, and gastric mucosal protection. PC is widely used to support healthy aging.

As you can see, both choline and phosphatidylcholine play crucial roles in preconception health, but they serve different functions and provide distinct benefits. Both are important for optimal fertility and fetal development, but they are not interchangeable. Now, let's take a detailed look at the benefits of each.

Choline: A General Overview

Choline is an essential nutrient that is critical for various physiological processes, including cell membrane integrity, methylation, and neurotransmitter synthesis. It is especially important for preconception and pregnancy because it influences fetal brain development, placental function, and reduces the risk of neural tube defects (NTDs).

Key Benefits of Choline for Preconception

- **Supports Methylation:** Choline acts as a methyl donor, contributing to the methylation cycle. This is important for DNA synthesis and repair, which is critical for reproductive health, egg quality, and early fetal development.
- **Neural Tube Development:** Adequate choline intake in the mother reduces the risk of neural tube defects, similar to folate. It supports healthy brain and spinal cord formation in the fetus.
- **Enhances Cognitive Development:** Choline is necessary for the production of acetylcholine, a neurotransmitter crucial

for brain function and memory. During pregnancy, it helps support fetal brain development and cognitive function.

- **Promotes Liver Function:** Choline aids in fat metabolism and liver health, reducing the risk of liver disorders that can interfere with fertility and hormone regulation.
- **Improves Sperm Health:** In males, choline is beneficial for sperm motility and integrity, improving overall fertility.

Phosphatidylcholine: General Overview

Phosphatidylcholine (PC) is a phospholipid that contains choline as part of its structure. It is the primary component of cell membranes and lipoproteins, playing a key role in maintaining cellular integrity and signaling. PC also serves as a reservoir for choline in the body, which can be broken down when additional choline is needed.

Key Benefits of Phosphatidylcholine for Preconception

- **Cell Membrane Health:** PC is a structural component of cell membranes, which are critical for cell division, growth, and communication. This is essential for reproductive cells like oocytes (eggs) and sperm cells, as well as for the rapid cell division that occurs after conception.
- **Placental Health:** PC supports the structural integrity of the placenta, ensuring proper nutrient and oxygen delivery to the developing fetus. A healthy placenta is crucial for pregnancy viability and fetal growth.
- **Fat Metabolism and Lipid Transport:** PC is involved in fat metabolism and the formation of lipoproteins (such as HDL and LDL), which transport fats and fat-soluble vitamins throughout the body. This ensures adequate delivery of essential nutrients to reproductive organs and the developing fetus.

- **Liver and Gallbladder Support:** PC helps support bile production and liver function, improving fat digestion and detoxification. This is particularly important for hormonal balance and detoxification of toxins that may affect fertility.
- **Choline Reservoir:** PC can be broken down into free choline when your body's demand for choline increases, such as during preconception and pregnancy. This helps ensure a steady supply of choline for methylation and fetal development.

Differences Between Choline and Phosphatidylcholine for Preconception

Choline is typically consumed as a free nutrient, while PC provides choline in a phospholipid form. PC can be broken down into free choline as needed, but it also provides structural benefits for cell membranes, whereas free choline primarily supports methylation and acetylcholine production.

Choline primarily supports *methylation, neurotransmitter production*, and *brain development* in the fetus. It is also crucial for overall reproductive health and early fetal neural development. **PC** primarily supports *cell membrane integrity, placental health*, and *fat metabolism*. It plays a structural role in the body and provides a secondary source of choline when needed.

Why You Need Both Choline and Phosphatidylcholine for Preconception

Both *choline* and *phosphatidylcholine* are vital for preconception health, but they work in complementary ways. Choline is essential for methylation, neurotransmitter production, and brain development, while phosphatidylcholine supports cell membrane integrity, fat metabolism, and placental function. Ensuring you get enough of both can improve egg and sperm quality, promote optimal methylation, and create the best possible environment for conception.

- **Optimal Methylation and DNA Synthesis:** Choline is a major methyl donor in the body, supporting proper DNA synthesis and repair, which is crucial for reproductive health and embryo development. PC, while it contains choline, also plays a role in maintaining the health and function of reproductive cells and tissues.

- **Brain and Cognitive Development:** Choline is essential for acetylcholine production, which supports brain development in the fetus. While PC contains choline, it is less directly involved in neurotransmitter production, but it is crucial for cell membrane fluidity, which is important for brain function.

- **Placental Health and Nutrient Transport:** PC contributes to the formation of a healthy placenta, ensuring that nutrients and oxygen are properly delivered to the fetus. This is important for sustaining a healthy pregnancy and promoting fetal growth.

- **Liver Health and Detoxification:** Both choline and PC support liver function, which is essential for hormone balance and detoxification. This helps optimize fertility and reduces the risk of complications during pregnancy.

Recommended Supplementation and Food Sources for Preconception

The recommended daily intake of choline is 500–1,000 mg per day, and for phosphatidylcholine the recommended intake is 1,200–2,400 mg per day. Some experts suggest aiming for higher intake due to choline's role in fetal brain development.

Eggs (especially yolks), liver, beef, chicken, soybeans, and cruciferous vegetables (e.g., broccoli and cauliflower) are rich in choline. PC-rich foods include egg yolks, soy lecithin, sunflower lecithin, and organ meats.

Vitamin D

Recommendation: Every Life Well D3 5000 IU (once daily)

On your bloodwork, we want to see your vitamin D25 levels between 50–80 ng/ml. On average, I find that patients need to supplement with 5,000 IU to be in that range. But physicians will recommend dosing ranges anywhere between 1,000 IU and 10,000 IU.

According to a study published in *BMC Pregnancy and Childbirth*, "In reproductive medicine, there is major interest in vitamin D because its deficiency has been associated with various infertility issues, such as polycystic ovarian syndrome, endometriosis, myoma-induced infertility, male infertility, premature ovarian failure, anti-Müllerian hormone production, steroidogenesis and ovarian folliculogenesis, endometrial receptivity and implantation, and poor prognosis in in vitro fertilization (IVF) (via its crucial role in hypothalamic-hypophyseal system regulation)."[303] As if that wasn't compelling enough, vitamin D also benefits the heart, colon, prostate, and lungs.

Though we call it a "vitamin," vitamin D is technically an essential secosteroid hormone,[304] and despite its importance in many different bodily functions, research indicates that most people are deficient in vitamin D.[305] Especially in the cooler months when you're not out in the sun as much, be sure to take plenty of vitamin D.

Calcium

Calcium is the most abundant mineral in our bodies. Our bones are mostly made of calcium, and the same is true of our teeth. Calcium even plays a role in how our blood vessels contract and dilate, as well as how our muscles function and our blood clots.[306] It's a basic building block of the human body, so it only makes sense that you want to be taking enough calcium during the preconception period.

High-Calcium Foods That *Aren't* Dairy?

I know we all grew up believing that milk and other dairy products are the only way to work calcium into your diet, but I've got exciting news for you! There are plenty of high-calcium foods that do not include dairy and are actually better sources of calcium, in my opinion. These foods are excellent options for people who are lactose intolerant, follow a vegan or paleo diet, or prefer nondairy sources of calcium.

Leafy Green Vegetables

- Collard Greens: 1 cup cooked = 268 mg calcium
- Turnip Greens: 1 cup cooked = 197 mg calcium
- Bok Choy (Chinese Cabbage): 1 cup cooked = 160 mg calcium
- Kale: 1 cup cooked = 177 mg calcium
- Spinach: 1 cup cooked = 245 mg calcium (spinach contains oxalates, which can reduce calcium absorption, so it may not be as bioavailable, meaning the extent to which it is absorbed and used by the body as other greens)
- Mustard Greens: 1 cup cooked = 165 mg calcium
- Broccoli Rabe: 1 cup cooked = 100 mg calcium
- Swiss Chard: 1 cup cooked = 100 mg calcium

Cruciferous Vegetables

- Broccoli: 1 cup cooked = 62 mg calcium
- Brussels Sprouts: 1 cup cooked = 56 mg calcium
- Cauliflower: 1 cup cooked = 24 mg calcium

Legumes and Beans

(These are not part of the Preconception Diet, but small amounts are fine for most people. They shouldn't be a huge source of calcium for you.)

- White Beans (Navy Beans): 1 cup cooked = 161 mg calcium
- Black-Eyed Peas: 1 cup cooked = 211 mg calcium
- Chickpeas (Garbanzo Beans): 1 cup cooked = 80 mg calcium
- Soybeans (Edamame): 1 cup cooked = 100 mg calcium
- Tempeh: 1 cup = 184 mg calcium
- Lentils: 1 cup cooked = 38 mg calcium

Nuts and Seeds

- Almonds: 1 ounce (about 23 almonds) = 75 mg calcium
- Sesame Seeds: 1 tablespoon = 88 mg calcium
- Tahini (Sesame Seed Paste): 2 tablespoons = 130 mg calcium
- Chia Seeds: 1 ounce (about 2 tablespoons) = 179 mg calcium
- Flaxseeds: 1 tablespoon = 26 mg calcium
- Brazil Nuts: 1 ounce = 45 mg calcium
- Hazelnuts: 1 ounce = 56 mg calcium
- Sunflower Seeds: 1 ounce = 20 mg calcium

Fortified Plant-Based Milks

- Almond Milk (Fortified): 1 cup = 300–450 mg calcium
- Soy Milk (Fortified): 1 cup = 300–400 mg calcium
- Rice Milk (Fortified): 1 cup = 288–300 mg calcium
- Coconut Milk (Fortified): 1 cup = 300 mg calcium

Fortified Plant-Based Foods

- Fortified Orange Juice: 1 cup = 300 mg calcium
- Fortified Tofu: can provide 200–300 mg calcium per serving (depending on brand)

Sea Vegetables

- Wakame (Seaweed): 1 cup = 150 mg calcium
- Kelp: 1 cup = 136 mg calcium
- Nori (Dried Seaweed): 10 sheets = 70 mg calcium
- Hijiki: 1 cup = 629 mg calcium

Fish and Seafood

- Canned Sardines (with bones): 3 ounces = 325 mg calcium
- Canned Salmon (with bones): 3 ounces = 181 mg calcium
- Shrimp: 3 ounces = 125 mg calcium
- Mackerel (with bones): 3 ounces = 240 mg calcium
- Anchovies (with bones): 1 ounce = 100 mg calcium

Grains and Pseudo-Grains

(These are not part of the Preconception Diet, but they are OK for most people in small amounts.)

- Amaranth: 1 cup cooked = 116 mg calcium
- Quinoa: 1 cup cooked = 31 mg calcium
- Teff: 1 cup cooked = 123 mg calcium
- Brown Rice: 1 cup cooked = 20 mg calcium
- White Rice: 1 cup cooked = 16 mg calcium
- Buckwheat: 1 cup cooked = 18 mg calcium

Fruits

- Figs (Dried): ½ cup = 120 mg calcium
- Oranges: 1 medium orange = 60 mg calcium
- Blackberries: 1 cup = 42 mg calcium
- Rhubarb: 1 cup cooked = 348 mg calcium
- Kiwi: 1 medium = 23 mg calcium
- Mulberries: 1 cup = 55 mg calcium

Vegetables (Non-Leafy)

- Sweet Potatoes: 1 medium = 40 mg calcium
- Butternut Squash: 1 cup cooked = 84 mg calcium
- Okra: 1 cup cooked = 123 mg calcium
- Artichokes: 1 medium = 56 mg calcium
- Carrots: 1 cup cooked = 48 mg calcium

Other Plant-Based Foods

- Blackstrap Molasses: 1 tablespoon = 172 mg calcium

These foods can help you meet your calcium needs without relying on dairy products. Incorporating a variety of them into your diet ensures a broad intake of calcium along with adding other important nutrients like magnesium, vitamin K2, and vitamin D, which help with calcium absorption and bone health.

Iron Glycinate

Recommendation: Iron Glycinate (women only, but men should have their levels checked and supplement if those levels are low)

With iron, you need to proceed with caution and only take supplements if your bloodwork shows that you are low in iron. You can easily get iron overload, and at that point, it starts depositing in your organs, damaging your adrenal glands, liver, heart, brain, and more. I don't want to scare you, but it's important to pay attention to this. On the other hand, iron deficiency can contribute to infertility in both women and men, though the mechanisms and effects can vary. Be sure to check your levels regularly when taking iron, as too much iron can damage your organs.

How Low Iron Affects Fertility in Women

Iron is essential for ovulation and egg quality, making it a key nutrient for female fertility. Low iron levels can reduce the chances of conception. Iron also plays a role in maintaining egg health. When iron is deficient, eggs may be lower in quality, making fertilization and a healthy pregnancy more difficult. Here's more detail:

- **Ovulatory Function:** Iron is crucial for the proper functioning of the ovaries and the production of healthy eggs. Studies have shown that women with iron deficiency are more likely to experience anovulation (lack of ovulation), which directly reduces the chances of conception.

- **Egg Health and Quality:** Iron supports cellular functions, including energy production and DNA synthesis, which are vital for maintaining egg quality. Poor iron status may compromise these processes, leading to lower-quality eggs and decreased fertility.[307]

- **Uterine Health:** Iron is essential for maintaining healthy uterine tissue and supporting a suitable environment for embryo implantation. Low iron can interfere with the uterus's ability to support a pregnancy, increasing the risk of miscarriage or early pregnancy complications.

- **Hormonal Imbalance:** Iron deficiency anemia can disrupt hormone levels, particularly those related to the menstrual cycle and ovulation. Proper hormone regulation is critical for fertility, and disruptions may reduce the chances of conception.

How Low Iron Affects Fertility in Men

Iron is just as important for male fertility, as it helps support sperm production, motility, and overall quality. Sperm cells require iron to develop properly and function efficiently. Too little iron may result in lower sperm count and poor motility, making it harder for sperm to reach and fertilize an egg. Maintaining healthy iron levels can help optimize sperm health and improve the chances of conception.

- **Sperm Health:** In men, iron is involved in the production of healthy sperm. Iron deficiency has been linked to reduced sperm count, motility, and overall sperm health. Oxidative stress caused by low iron levels can also damage sperm DNA, contributing to infertility.[308]

- **Testosterone Levels:** Iron deficiency may indirectly affect testosterone production, which plays a key role in maintaining male fertility. Hormonal imbalances caused by low iron levels can impair spermatogenesis.

Research supports the idea that women with iron deficiency are at higher risk for infertility, and supplementation may improve ovulation rates and overall fertility outcomes. Similarly, iron is important for sperm production and male fertility. Addressing iron deficiency can be a critical part of preconception care for both men and women.

You've probably heard that iron supplements are often recommended to pregnant women. Here's why: Hemoglobin is a protein in your red blood cells, and it's responsible for carrying oxygen to your tissues. Your body uses iron to make hemoglobin. During pregnancy, your blood volume increases dramatically, and your body uses iron to make that blood, which in turn supplies oxygen to your growing baby. Thus, it's important that you have adequate iron stores before becoming pregnant. Without enough iron, you could develop iron deficiency anemia, which will affect both you and your baby.[309]

In iron glycinate, ferrous iron is reacted with glycine to form bisglycinate chelate, a nonelectrically charged compound that is totally nutritionally functional. The absence of electrical charge, uncommon for an iron supplement, makes it less likely that iron glycinate can interfere with absorption of other minerals such as calcium, vitamin E, or vitamin C. Iron can be hard on the digestive tract, but iron glycinate is the form I've found to be the most tolerable.

Magnesium Glycinate

Recommendation: Every Life Well Magnesium Glycinate 125

Magnesium deficiency is typically subclinical, meaning it lacks obvious symptoms and standard blood tests do not accurately measure intracellular magnesium levels, but this "invisible deficiency" affects a large portion of the American population, with around 50 percent of people consuming less than the recommended amount.[310] And that's a real problem because magnesium is crucial for over six hundred enzymatic processes in the body, including maintaining ionic balance, protein synthesis, and mitochondrial function.[311] A deficiency during pregnancy can interfere with fetal growth, increase the risk of preterm labor and preeclampsia, and potentially lead to long-term consequences such as metabolic syndrome in the child.[312] Pregnant women are at a higher risk of magnesium deficiency.[313] And as we've touched on, we aren't getting enough magnesium from diet alone, mostly because soil quality has become increasingly depleted over the years. So supplementation is critical.

There are ten different types of magnesium that you could take as supplements, but I recommend magnesium glycinate and dimagnesium malate, both of which are in Every Life Well Magnesium Glycinate. They are well absorbed and less likely to cause gastrointestinal upset as some forms of magnesium. Glycine is a calming amino acid that supports brain health, digestion, and joint function and promotes sleep. Malic acid (from malate) supports energy metabolism and antioxidant systems in the body.

We've already talked about how magnesium supports your conception journey, but magnesium also:

- is required for detoxification (we need sufficient levels of magnesium to help clear toxins out of our bodies)
- supports cardiovascular health
- supports healthy muscle function
- supports healthy nerve conduction
- supports bone health
- supports energy production
- helps the heart maintain a steady rhythm
- helps the pancreas function
- is needed for any muscle activity (if you frequently get muscle cramps, it could be because you are low in magnesium)
- is required for blood vessels to dilate and contract (sometimes high blood pressure is a symptom of not having adequate amounts magnesium)
- is helpful to keep your bowels moving (taking magnesium can be a gentle, non-laxative, non-habit-forming way to help you have daily bowel movements)
- is necessary for our neurotransmitters (which means a happier mood and better mental focus)

Protein Powders

Protein is a foundational nutrient for fertility, playing a key role in everything from hormone production to embryo development. High-quality protein powders can be an easy and effective way to support your body's detox pathways, balance key nutrients, and create the best possible environment for conception. In this section, we'll explore why protein is so important and how choosing the right protein powder can help fuel your fertility journey.

Preconceive Nutrition or Fertility Fuel

Recommendation: Preconceive Nutrition or Fertility Fuel Protein Powder

These delicious protein powders are designed to support comprehensive detoxification and create a healthy environment for improved fertility and overall health. Their formulas contain bone-broth protein, vitamins, minerals, and phytonutrients that support and balance Phase I and Phase II detoxification pathways and antioxidant status. (There are vegan versions available as well, which use pea protein instead of bone-broth protein.) These powerhouse protein powders also include a variety of herbs that promote healthy liver function and GI elimination. Proteins and their amino acids are vital for fertility, playing an essential role from conception to the development of a healthy fetus. They support the reproductive system every step of the way, from successful fertilization to the fetus's growth.

From fertilization onward, amino acids are crucial, creating a nutrient-rich environment in the reproductive tract for the embryo's development. Key amino acids such as arginine, leucine, and glutamine are particularly important for promoting the growth of the embryo and fostering the critical interaction between the mother's uterus and the embryo. This interaction leads to proper placental growth and ensures the baby develops well, ultimately supporting a positive outcome for the pregnancy.

The bone-broth protein in Preconceive Nutrition has an excellent amino acid profile and is formulated without dairy, gluten, or lactose, ensuring a smooth texture and pleasant taste. By enhancing detoxification processes and providing essential nutrients, a good protein powder creates an optimal internal environment that supports fertility and overall wellness.

Folic Acid or Folate?

Folic acid is still the most widely available form of vitamin B9, but it differs from folate. Folic acid is synthetic and inexpensive, but it is not chemically the same as the natural folates found in food. It is also not active. The body needs to transform folic acid into methyl folate to be used by cells.

If you have MTHFR mutations or other challenges in activating folic acid, the folic acid may remain unmetabolized and accumulate in your blood. Folic acid use may induce pseudomethylenetetrahydrofolate syndrome, where blood levels of folic acid look normal or high, but there is a functional deficiency of active folate available to cells. This can lead to high levels of folic acid in the blood, but not enough of the active form that your body actually needs. As a result, important processes—like breaking down homocysteine—may not work properly. When homocysteine levels are too high, it can increase the risk of blood clotting issues, cardiovascular problems, and complications during pregnancy.

Unmetabolized folic acid is found in the cord blood of newborns where the mother supplements with folic acid and in formula-fed infants, since formula might contain folic acid instead of folate. In addition, the use of folic acid can mask a vitamin B12 deficiency. Vitamin B12 is another critical methylation nutrient needed for fertility, pregnancy, and fetal development.

Using supplemental folate has a significant advantage over folic acid. It can replete folate levels without the risk of folic acid buildup or masking vitamin B12 deficiency. It also minimizes the risks associated with low folate levels.

- You may be getting supplemental dosages of folic acid and not even know it, although if you're following the diet I recommend, it's unlikely. Folic acid is found in many processed, refined, and fortified foods, including:
  - Bread, pasta, and baked goods made with white "enriched" flour
  - Fortified protein powders, cereals, and bars
  - Energy drinks and supplements
  - Infant formula and processed foods marketed to kids

THRIVE

Be sure to read labels to avoid this potentially harmful ingredient. While avoiding folic acid is one piece of the puzzle to support optimal methylation, the other is to increase folate levels in your body. Adults need 400 mcg of DFE (dietary folate equivalents) per day from their diet. (For reference, 1 mcg of folate equals 1 DFE.) Pregnant women need at least 600 mcg DFE per day and lactating women need at least 500 mcg. You'll find most prenatal vitamins contain around 800 mcg DFE, and it's safe to take even more, depending on individual needs and tolerance.

Detoxification Supplements

Refer to chapter 6 for supplements that aid in detoxification. And if you have specific gut problems, you can refer to chapter 11 to find more information about specific gut-related detoxification supplements.

Zeo Binder

Recommendation: Every Life Well Zeo Binder, QuickSilver Scientific Ultrabinder, and GI Detox by Biociden Botanicals

See page 188 for more information on Zeo Binder.

Liver Detox Supplements

Recommendation: Clean Beginnings—Essential Liver Detox for Preconception Health

Clean Beginnings is a targeted liver support formula designed to help both men and women eliminate toxins, balance hormones, and optimize reproductive health before conception in the following ways:

- **Supports Phase I and II liver detoxification:** Ensures harmful toxins are processed and eliminated effectively.

- **Promotes hormone balance:** Helps the liver metabolize excess hormones, such as estrogen, which can impact fertility in both men and women.
- **Enhances egg and sperm quality:** Reduces oxidative stress and toxin burden, key factors in DNA integrity and reproductive health.
- **Supports bile production and digestion:** Aids in the elimination of fat-soluble toxins, ensuring a clean, well-functioning system for conception.
- **Strengthens immune balance:** Reduces the immune burden from toxins, supporting a healthy inflammatory response crucial for fertility.

PectaSol Powder or Capsules

Recommendation: PectaSol

PectaSol Powder is a modified citrus pectin naturally derived from the pith of citrus fruit peels, including lemons, limes, and oranges. It has been shown to halt the protein galectin-3 (Gal-3), which, if elevated, impacts cellular health and kidney and liver function, as well as immunity.[314] Levels of Gal-3 seem to elevate with age.

Glutathione

Recommendation: Liposomal Glutathione

See page 187 for an overview on glutathione.

Many glutathione supplements available on the market can break down in the digestive system without being absorbed, which is why I chose to package the glutathione in phosphatidylcholine liposome for optimal absorption, bioavailability, and cell support. Every Life Well Liposomal Glutathione provides 500 mg of pure glutathione and activated B vitamin cofactors delivered in phosphatidylcholine liposomes for optimal absorption and bioavailability support.

See the appendix for a more extensive list of the toxins that glutathione is particularly effective at detoxifying.

Glutathione also plays a critical role in maintaining overall health by protecting cells from oxidative damage, supporting the immune system, and promoting cellular repair. Its antioxidant properties are vital in helping prevent the cellular damage that leads to aging, as well as diseases such as cancer and cardiovascular issues.[315] Glutathione enhances immune function by playing a role in activating T-cells and natural killer (NK) cells, which are essential in defending the body against infections and malignancies.[316] This immune-boosting ability is particularly valuable for anyone with a weakened immune system or those prone to chronic infections.

One of glutathione's most important roles is in mitochondrial function and ATP production, the energy currency of the cell. By supporting mitochondria, it helps boost energy levels and enhances cellular repair mechanisms, making it a valuable asset in managing conditions related to chronic fatigue or cell damage.[317] Glutathione's anti-inflammatory properties are also crucial, as it helps reduce pro-inflammatory cytokines, providing relief for individuals with chronic inflammatory conditions such as autoimmune diseases and metabolic syndromes.

In terms of skin health, liposomal glutathione's antioxidant capabilities are known to lighten skin, reduce hyperpigmentation, and offer protection against UV damage, promoting a healthier complexion.[318] It also shows promise in preventing neurodegenerative diseases such as Alzheimer's, Parkinson's, and multiple sclerosis by reducing oxidative stress in the brain.[319] Moreover, since it's been shown to decrease lipid peroxidation—a process contributing to plaque buildup in the arteries—glutathione can help protect against cardiovascular diseases, improving heart health.[320]

Additionally, liposomal glutathione offers benefits for athletic performance by reducing muscle fatigue and enhancing recovery after exercise. It supports liver health by aiding detoxification and protecting against damage from toxins, alcohol, and fatty liver disease. In respiratory health, particularly for individuals with chronic obstructive pulmonary disease (COPD) and asthma, glutathione helps reduce airway inflammation and improve lung function. Furthermore, it enhances glucose metabolism and insulin sensitivity, making it beneficial for individuals with metabolic syndrome and type 2 diabetes. By supporting gut health and reducing oxidative stress, liposomal glutathione may also help manage "leaky gut" syndrome and inflammatory bowel disease (IBD).

Lastly, liposomal glutathione has been linked to improvements in cognitive function and mood, particularly for individuals experiencing depression or cognitive decline, as well as offering protection in autoimmune diseases by reducing tissue damage and immune dysregulation. I know it sounds too good to be true, but all the evidence points to glutathione being a "super supplement," and one you'll always want to have on hand.

Mitochondrial Optimization Supplements

MitoQ Mitoquinol

Recommendation: MitoQ Mitoquinol Pure (daily)

MitoQ Mitoquinol is a special form of CoQ10, an antioxidant that targets mitochondria. It is designed to help minimize the impact of oxidative stress, as well as help your cells' vitality. I recommend this product to many of my patients, but right now let's zero in on how it can help you in terms of fertility and epigenetics.

One study showed the antioxidant in MitoQ has been found to help improve fertility and egg quality in both animals and humans. It helps protect human eggs (as well as the eggs of young and old mice) from developing problems with their chromosomes and supports egg development in lab settings. This effect was most noticeable in older eggs, which usually have more chromosomal issues.[321] MitoQ reduces harmful molecules (reactive oxygen species) that can interfere with the high energy needed for egg growth. It also increased fertilization and development in mouse eggs.[322]

MitoQ may also help maintain eggs in people with obesity or type 2 diabetes. These conditions can lead to higher fat levels in the fluid around the eggs, which can be harmful. In an animal study that simulated obesity-related problems, MitoQ improved the quality of developing embryos by reducing oxidative stress.[323] It was also shown to reverse issues related to PCOS, including problems with ovarian cysts and thickened uterine lining, which can affect fertility.[324]

MitoQ has been studied for its potential use in pregnancies with low oxygen levels (hypoxia) in sheep and rats. It helped improve heart function in offspring compared to controls.[325] In cases where low oxygen caused growth problems in the womb, MitoQ prevented heart issues in the later stages of pregnancy.[326]

Lastly, in lab-created ovarian tissue models, MitoQ helped follicle growth and development, protected supporting cells from oxidative stress, and improved the ability of lab-grown eggs to mature.[327]

CoQ10

Recommendation: Every Life Well CoQ10 Plus Softgels (200–300 mg; take one softgel per day with a meal)

Every Life Well CoQ10 Plus Softgels contain CoQ10 as ubiquinol (the active, antioxidant form of CoQ10), the more readily absorbed and more biologically active form that serves as an antioxidant. Coenzyme Q10 (CoQ10) is a nutrient that performs important functions throughout the body. It is particularly critical for the health of hardworking organs like the heart, liver, pancreas, and kidneys. The most important roles CoQ10 plays are in energy generation and antioxidant function.

The body uses two forms of CoQ10. The first form, *ubiquinone*, also known as the oxidized form, is better known and is used primarily for energy production in the electron transport energy cycle inside the cell. The second form, *ubiquinol*, plays a primary role in decreasing oxidative damage caused by lipid peroxidation within mitochondria. According to research, plasma ubiquinol is decreased in patients with hyperlipidemia (high levels of fats in the blood, such as triglycerides). CoQ10 Plus features a unique combination of ubiquinol and geranylgeraniol (GG), two physiologically essential molecules with complementary and synergistic actions. This composition enables better absorption—approximately 100 percent higher than the individual compound and 18 to 19 percent higher than other leading brands of solubilized ubiquinol.

CoQ10 occurs naturally in certain foods (especially animal foods such as red meat, poultry, and seafood), but the vast majority is produced inside the body. GG is also produced endogenously, which means inside the body. This internal synthesis may not always be sufficient, particularly in individuals taking pharmaceutical drugs that affect the pathway by which CoQ10 is produced.

Synthesis of CoQ10 and GG declines naturally during aging, and the use of certain pharmaceutical drugs (particularly for treating high cholesterol and osteoporosis) inhibits its synthesis, potentially resulting in a need for supplementation.

CoQ10 Benefits for Women

- **Improves Egg Quality:** CoQ10 is a potent antioxidant that protects eggs from oxidative damage caused by free radicals, which can lead to reduced fertility. As women age, their natural levels of CoQ10 decline, and eggs become more vulnerable to oxidative stress. Supplementing with CoQ10 may help mitigate this effect.

- **Supports Mitochondrial Function in Oocytes:** Eggs rely on mitochondria for energy during ovulation, fertilization, and early embryonic development. CoQ10 enhances mitochondrial energy production, supporting healthier eggs and improving their developmental potential.

- **Helps with Age-Related Fertility Decline:** Studies suggest that CoQ10 supplementation may improve ovarian reserve and fertility outcomes in older women by enhancing the energy supply to aging eggs.

CoQ10 Benefits for Men

- **Improves Sperm Quality:** CoQ10 increases sperm motility and count, which are critical factors for successful conception. Its antioxidant properties help reduce oxidative stress, a significant cause of sperm DNA damage and reduced fertility.

- **Protects Sperm DNA:** By neutralizing free radicals, CoQ10 helps preserve the integrity of sperm DNA, which is essential for creating healthy embryos.

Beta Carotene/Vitamin A

Vitamin A is crucial for pregnancy but taking too much can be harmful. In developed countries, excessive vitamin A intake, particularly during the first sixty days after conception, can lead to birth defects, especially in the central nervous and cardiovascular systems.[328] High doses of vitamin A supplements or foods rich in preformed vitamin A, like liver, are not recommended during pregnancy because of the potential teratogenic (causing birth defects) effects.[329] Therefore, while it's essential to ensure adequate vitamin A levels during pregnancy, there is a fine balance to avoid overconsumption.

Beta carotene, a safer form of vitamin A, is preferable, as the body converts it to vitamin A only as needed, reducing the risk of toxicity.

Vitamin A is crucial for the development of the fetus, especially for lung development and overall growth.[330] It is estimated that beta carotene from diet provides around 10 to 15 percent of the daily recommended vitamin A intake, and it's vital because if the mother's vitamin A supply is inadequate, the fetus and, later, the breastfed infant will also be deficient.

Maintaining sufficient beta carotene intake is crucial to supporting healthy fetal development and preventing developmental disorders.[331] For these reasons, I highly recommend that women take beta carotene during preconception, to ensure their bodies have plenty of vitamin A stores leading into pregnancy.

As for men, vitamin A plays a crucial part in their fertility because it's required for the production of sperm, a process known as spermatogenesis.[332] Spermatogenesis involves the continual production of sperm throughout a male's life, starting at puberty. Vitamin A plays a key role in pushing early-stage sperm cells, known as spermatogonia, into the pathway where they begin to differentiate and eventually undergo meiosis—a process where the number of chromosomes is halved, leading to the formation of mature sperm.[333] Without sufficient vitamin A, spermatogenesis halts, and only undifferentiated spermatogonia are present in the testes. Studies in mice have shown that supplementing vitamin A in animals that are deficient actually restarts spermatogenesis.[334]

Astaxanthin

Recommendation: Every Life Well Astaxanthin

Astaxanthin (pronounced "as-ta-ZAN-thin") is a powerful carotenoid derived from the microalgae *Haematococcus pluvialis*, known as one of the richest sources of this nutrient. Its characteristic reddish pigment gives crustaceans such as krill, lobster, shrimp, and salmon their vibrant pink color. Astaxanthin has been studied extensively for its numerous health benefits, including its protective effects against cardiovascular diseases, cancer, diabetes, neurodegenerative disorders, and immune system dysfunctions. It is also known for its anti-inflammatory, anti-aging, antiviral, neuroprotective, and nephroprotective (protecting the kidneys from damage or disease) properties. One of its unique features is its ability to interact with cell membranes, supporting their structural integrity and providing antioxidant protection against lipid oxidation, which can cause cellular damage.

In addition to these benefits, astaxanthin has shown promise in enhancing fertility. For men, its potent antioxidant properties protect sperm from oxidative stress, which is a key factor in reducing sperm quality and motility.[335]

The Benefits of Astaxanthin

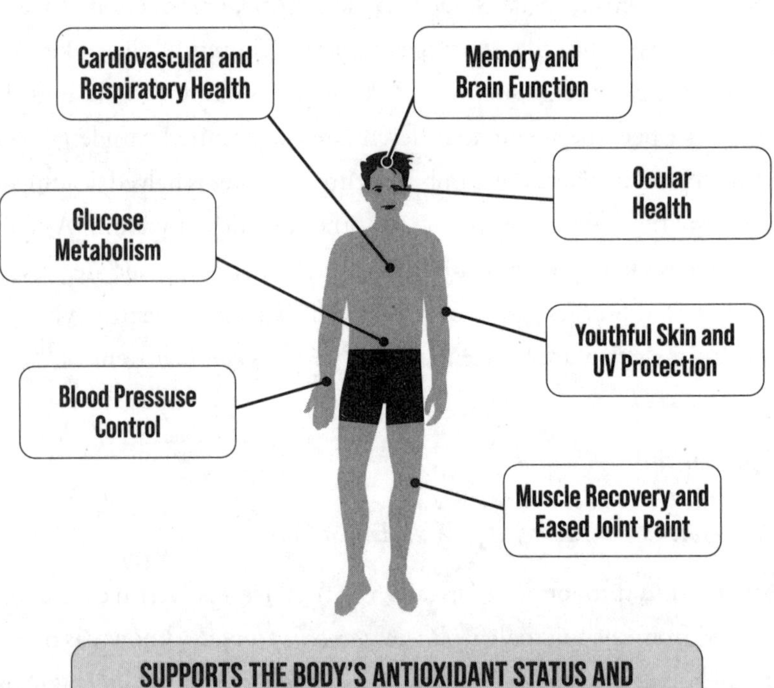

For women, astaxanthin's anti-inflammatory and antioxidant effects can enhance ovarian function and improve egg quality.[336] Oxidative stress is known to negatively impact egg quality and ovarian health, so the antioxidant support provided by astaxanthin can be particularly beneficial during the preconception period. By supporting cell membrane integrity, astaxanthin ensures the proper functioning of reproductive cells and tissues, contributing to an optimal environment for conception.

Given its role in reducing inflammation and oxidative damage, astaxanthin supports overall reproductive health and helps the body prepare for conception. By protecting cellular structures and maintaining the health of reproductive cells, it can play a significant role in improving the chances of a healthy pregnancy. Therefore, incorporating astaxanthin into your preconception regimen has a powerful potential to enhance your fertility and support successful conception.

Myo-inositol or Inositol

Myo-inositol (often just called inositol) is a natural compound that helps your cells communicate, balance hormones, and support metabolism. While "inositol" refers to a group of related compounds, the most useful form for the body is myo-inositol.

Inositol is especially important for mitochondria—the tiny energy factories inside your cells. It helps your body use insulin more effectively, ensuring your cells get a steady supply of energy. It also protects mitochondria from damage caused by oxidative stress, which can harm DNA and slow energy production. Plus, inositol helps regulate calcium levels in cells, which is crucial for keeping mitochondria running smoothly. Research even suggests that it may help your body create new mitochondria and improve how fats are used for energy— both of which are essential for overall health and fertility.

These compounds have shown considerable benefits specifically in preconception, fertility, and general human health, for both men and women. They help with the proper development of eggs and embryos by acting as a messenger for hormones like gonadotropins and insulin. Research shows that taking myo-inositol supplements can increase the chances of getting pregnant and lower the risk of pregnancy complications for both mothers and babies.[337] Specifically, it has been shown to help women with infertility, especially those with PCOS, by triggering ovulation and helping to restore a regular menstrual cycle.[338]

Myo-inositol is particularly well-researched in the context of female fertility due to its impact on ovarian function and hormonal balance. Here's how it supports women's reproductive health.

Polycystic Ovary Syndrome (PCOS) Management

Myo-inositol is commonly used to help regulate hormonal imbalances associated with PCOS. It can help lower elevated androgen (male hormone) levels and improve insulin sensitivity, which is critical for managing PCOS and restoring normal ovulation.

Women with PCOS often have insulin resistance, which exacerbates hormonal imbalances. Myo-inositol works by improving the body's response to insulin, thereby reducing insulin resistance. This helps normalize LH and FSH ratios, promoting regular ovulation and improving the chances of conception.

Myo-inositol has also been shown to promote regular ovulation in women with PCOS, enhancing fertility. In fact, it is often considered a natural alternative or adjunct to medications like clomiphene for inducing ovulation.

Egg Quality

Myo-inositol improves the quality of oocytes (eggs) by supporting proper cellular signaling and energy production. This is crucial for healthy eggs, especially in women undergoing IVF treatments. Improved egg quality directly influences the success of embryo development post-conception, contributing to healthier pregnancy outcomes.

Hormonal Balance in Non-PCOS Women

Even for women without PCOS, myo-inositol supports healthy ovarian function by improving cellular responses to hormones like FSH and estrogen. This balance is key to achieving and maintaining fertility in all women.

Myo-inositol and Inositol for Men's Fertility and Preconception

Inositol, especially myo-inositol, also plays a role in male fertility by influencing sperm quality and hormonal balance.

Improvement in Sperm Health

Myo-inositol enhances sperm motility, which is crucial for successful fertilization. It works by supporting mitochondrial function in sperm cells, thereby increasing energy production and improving movement.

Inositol can also improve sperm count and morphology. Research has shown that myo-inositol supplementation can lead to better sperm parameters, which are critical for fertility in men.

Hormonal Balance in Men

Myo-inositol helps regulate testosterone levels in men, which is important for maintaining reproductive health. It can reduce excess estrogen and support healthy testosterone production, contributing to improved libido and sperm production.

Oxidative Stress Reduction

Myo-inositol has antioxidant properties that protect sperm from oxidative stress, a common issue that can negatively affect sperm health. This is important for preserving the integrity of sperm DNA and reducing the risk of infertility or miscarriage due to damaged sperm.

Other Benefits of Myo-inositol and Inositol for General Health

Insulin Sensitivity and Metabolic Health

Both men and women can benefit from myo-inositol's ability to improve insulin sensitivity. This is especially helpful for individuals with insulin resistance, metabolic syndrome, or type 2 diabetes. Better insulin regulation supports overall hormonal balance and metabolic health, which indirectly benefits fertility.

Mental Health and Mood Disorders

Inositol, particularly myo-inositol, has been studied for its effects on mental health. It helps modulate neurotransmitter signaling, especially serotonin, which can reduce symptoms of anxiety and depression. This is significant because stress and mood disorders can negatively affect reproductive health and conception efforts.

Studies suggest that inositol may be effective in reducing the frequency and severity of panic attacks, potentially making it a natural alternative to certain medications for anxiety disorders.

Thyroid Health

Myo-inositol has been shown to improve thyroid function, particularly in individuals with subclinical hypothyroidism or Hashimoto's thyroiditis. By enhancing the thyroid's ability to process hormones efficiently, inositol can support hormonal balance, which is important for reproductive health and overall well-being.

Lipid Metabolism and Cardiovascular Health

Myo-inositol can help lower triglycerides and improve HDL (good) cholesterol levels. Since high cholesterol is linked to reduced fertility and overall health issues, myo-inositol's lipid-lowering effect is an added benefit for preconception health.

By improving metabolic health and reducing inflammation, myo-inositol also contributes to cardiovascular protection, reducing the risk of heart disease.

Weight Management

Myo-inositol can help with weight loss, particularly in women with PCOS or individuals struggling with obesity. By improving insulin sensitivity, it aids in fat metabolism, reducing abdominal fat and promoting healthy body weight, which is crucial for fertility.

Dosage and Supplementation

For Women with PCOS: A common dosage is 2,000 mg twice daily (4,000 mg per day), often combined with 200 mcg of D-chiro-inositol in a 40:1 ratio. This combination has been shown to improve ovulation, insulin sensitivity, and fertility outcomes in women with polycystic ovary syndrome (PCOS).

For Women Without PCOS: Women looking to support hormone balance, egg quality, and general fertility may benefit from 1,000–2,000 mg per day of myo-inositol. This lower dose can still promote healthy ovarian function and metabolic support.

For Men: A dosage of 2,000–3,000 mg per day is commonly used to improve sperm quality, motility, and hormonal balance by reducing oxidative stress and supporting mitochondrial function.

For General Health: 1,000–2,000 mg per day may be enough for benefits related to mental health, metabolic regulation, and insulin sensitivity, even for those without fertility concerns.

Other Interesting Aspects of Myo-inositol and Inositol

- **Cell Signaling:** Myo-inositol is a critical component of phosphatidylinositol, a type of fat in cell membranes that helps regulate various cellular functions, including signal transduction (the process your cells use to receive, process, and respond to signals from their environment), cell division, and growth. This is vital for maintaining the health of reproductive tissues like the ovaries, testes, and endometrium.

- **Antioxidant Effects:** In addition to its role in fertility, myo-inositol acts as an antioxidant, helping reduce oxidative damage in various tissues, including the brain, reproductive organs, and cardiovascular system.

Hopefully, by now you have a good grasp on how both myo-inositol and inositol play important roles in improving fertility, particularly for women with PCOS and men with sperm quality issues. In women, myo-inositol helps regulate hormones, promote ovulation, and improve egg quality, while in men it enhances sperm motility and count and overall reproductive health. Beyond fertility, inositol supports metabolic health, mental well-being, thyroid function, and cardiovascular health, making it a valuable nutrient for preconception and general health.

L-Carnitine

Recommendation: Every Life Well L-Carnitine (Suggested use: 1 capsule three times per day)

L-carnitine is an amino acid essential for the transport of fatty acids into the cell mitochondria.[339] Research has shown that L-carnitine stimulates the use of fat for fuel and boosts metabolism, which plays a key role in weight management.[340] L-carnitine has also been found to help support cardiovascular health and to increase aerobic capacity during exercise.[341]

The heart and skeletal muscles, as well as many other tissues, depend on fatty acid oxidation as a source of energy. L-carnitine is an essential nutrient required for the transportation of long-chain fatty acids into the mitochondrial matrix. Within the mitochondria of each cell, a metabolic process called beta-oxidation occurs, resulting in the production of energy.[342]

L-carnitine also aids in the transport of short-chain and medium-chain fatty acids out of the mitochondria and helps liberate coenzyme A, an important component of cellular energy.

This particular L-carnitine formulation provides 500 mg of L-carnitine per capsule, delivered using quick-release, fast-absorbing Licaps® technology. These cutting-edge advancements in capsule filling, sealing, and nutrient delivery ensure therapeutic potency and efficacy.

Oral NAD+

Recommendation: NAD+ by Every Life Well

NAD+ Shield is a dietary supplement designed to support the body's natural cellular repair processes, enhance antioxidative status, and promote healthy aging. It contains clinically relevant amounts of Niagen® (nicotinamide riboside chloride), resveratrol (as Veri-te™), and pterostilbene. Nicotinamide riboside, a form of vitamin B3, serves as a precursor to nicotinamide adenine dinucleotide (NAD+), a coenzyme involved in over five hundred bodily reactions, including gene expression, stress response, and DNA repair. Resveratrol and pterostilbene are plant-derived compounds known for their antioxidant properties and support of healthy cellular function.

Research indicates that NAD+ levels decline with age, contributing to oxidative stress and mitochondrial dysfunction in the ovaries.[343] NAD+ is essential for energy production and cellular repair. Reduced levels of NAD+ impair the cells' ability to combat oxidative damage and maintain mitochondrial health, which are critical for ovarian function and fertility.[344] Increasing NAD+ levels activate proteins like sirtuins and PARPs (Poly ADP-Ribose Polymerases), which play crucial roles in egg maturation and early embryo development.[345]

I recommend boosting NAD+ levels to help mitigate these age-related effects and support healthier ovarian aging.

Microbiome Supplements

Probiotics

Recommendation: Every Life Well Daily Probiotics (men and women) and Preconception Probiotics by Every Baby Well (women only)

A healthy gut microbiome plays a huge role in your overall health, fertility, and epigenetics. Probiotics have become super popular, and the market is flooded with all types and varieties, so it can be a little overwhelming to figure out which ones to use.

Probiotics are live bacteria that are good for your body, especially your digestive system. We usually think of "bacteria" as germs that cause diseases, but your body is full of bacteria, both good and bad. Probiotics are often called "good" or "helpful" bacteria because they help keep your gut healthy.

Supplementation with probiotics has many health benefits, which include:

- Supporting metabolic activity and the production of short-chain fatty acids and vitamins
- Nutrient absorption
- Helping good bacteria thrive in your gut by attaching to the protective lining of your intestines. This supports digestion, nutrient absorption, and immune function while keeping harmful bacteria in check.
- Helping to establish populations of good bacteria after disruption in balance
- Supporting immune function
- Promoting intestinal epithelial cell survival
- Supporting healthy bowel function

- Breaking down oxalates, natural compounds found in foods like spinach, nuts, and chocolate. This helps prevent oxalate buildup, which can contribute to kidney stones and interfere with mineral absorption.

You might have experienced side effects when taking probiotics. When first using them, some people experience gas, bloating, or diarrhea. This is because changes in the gut microbiota can result in bacteria producing more gas than usual. However, this usually clears up within a few days or weeks of taking the probiotics.

Every Life Well Daily Probiotics provide four researched strains of beneficial bacteria, totaling 30 billion CFU† per capsule. Careful organism selection is also a critical aspect of supporting digestive survival. The four strains included in daily probiotics formula include:

- *Bifidobacterium lactis HN019®*: Discovered in 1899, *B. lactis* plays a key role in the human microflora throughout a person's life. Researchers have identified strain HN019® as having excellent probiotic potential based upon its ability to survive the transit through the human gastrointestinal tract, adhere to epithelial cells, and proliferate. *B. lactis* HN019® has been extensively studied, and its safety and effectiveness are well accepted.
- *Lactobacillus acidophilus (Lactobacillus acidophilus La-14)*: This common inhabitant of the human mouth, intestinal tract, and vagina is also found in some traditional fermented milks (e.g., kefir) and is widely used in probiotic foods and supplements.
- *Lactobacillus plantarum Lp-115*: This bacterium was isolated from plant material and is abundantly present in lactic acid-fermented foods, such as olives and sauerkraut.
- *Bifidobacterium longum (Bifidobacterium longum Bl-05)*: *Bifidobacterium longum* is a beneficial probiotic bacterium

that plays a key role in gut health, digestion, and immune function. It is naturally found in the human gastrointestinal tract and is one of the first beneficial bacteria to colonize the gut in infancy. This strain helps break down complex carbohydrates and dietary fiber, producing short-chain fatty acids (SCFAs) like butyrate, which support gut lining integrity and reduce inflammation.

Bifidobacterium longum is also known for its ability to help balance the gut microbiome by outcompeting harmful bacteria and producing antimicrobial compounds. It has been studied for its potential to reduce symptoms of irritable bowel syndrome (IBS), support mental health through the gut-brain axis, and enhance immune function by modulating inflammation and promoting a healthy immune response.

Preconception Probiotics is a targeted formula designed to support a stable vaginal ecosystem and optimal urogenital health, both of which are crucial in the preconception phase. These probiotic supplements provide two specific species of *Lactobacilli*: *L. reuteri* and *L. rhamnosus*. These two species are backed by human clinical studies to establish a healthy, stable vaginal ecosystem.[346] Every area of the human body has a unique ecology and therefore a unique microbiome.

- The gut microbiome is spoken about frequently, but less commonly discussed are the specific microbiomes contained in other areas such as the skin, lungs, mouth, and even the vagina. The vaginal microbiome is abundant in *Lactobacillus* species, as they contribute heavily to the production of lactic acid.[347] The lactic acid maintains a pH of 4, which if elevated is a risk for vaginal microbiome challenges.
- Urogenital concerns are experienced frequently by women, and the most common interventions do little to address the

state of vaginal ecology, and therefore, repeated challenges are often experienced. *Lactobacillus rhamnosus* GR-1 and *Lactobacillus reuteri* RC-14 have been studied and proven to support healthy vaginal ecology and promote microbial balance.[348]

By taking this probiotic blend daily, you can help your body maintain a healthy vaginal microflora, support urogenital tract health, and help establish a healthy vaginal pH and remove unwanted organisms, all of which help you prepare for conceiving and carrying a baby.

Antioxidant Supplements

Lycopene

Lycopene is a powerful antioxidant that protects your cells from damage caused by free radicals. It is instrumental in mitochondrial testicular function and modulates lipid peroxidation.[349] Lycopene is found in foods such as tomatoes, watermelon, and pink grapefruit, but it's difficult to obtain enough through diet alone. This is where a lycopene supplement will be helpful.

Naringenin

Naringenin is a natural substance found in oranges, grapefruits, and even tomato skins. It's part of a family called *flavonoids*, which are known for their health benefits. Naringenin is excellent at protecting your liver (acting as an antioxidant and reducing inflammation), lowering cholesterol and blood pressure, and reducing inflammation throughout your body.[350] It's been shown that when naringenin is packaged into tiny particles (called *nanoparticles*), it becomes even more effective at protecting the liver and fighting cell damage[351]— hence, the benefits of taking a naringenin supplement.

Polyphenols

Polyphenols are a diverse group of plant compounds found in many fruits and vegetables, tea, coffee, and other plant-based foods. They are known to possess antioxidant properties and possess anti-inflammatory effects, as well as contribute to cardiovascular health.[352] Some polyphenols (such as resveratrol and quercetin) can enhance sperm production and increase fertility.[353]

Nitric Oxide

Nitric oxide plays many vital roles in your body. It's a gas that is produced naturally by your cells and acts as a signaling molecule, meaning it helps different parts of your body communicate with each other. Key functions include blood vessel dilation, cardiac function regulation, and healthy blood pressure support. Nitric oxide also helps with erectile function.[354] While it's found in leafy greens and beets (which contain nitrates that your body can convert into nitric oxide), a supplement is hugely helpful.

Nitric oxide plays a crucial role during the preconception period by supporting key biological processes. It promotes protein synthesis, cell migration, and wound healing while reducing proteolysis (cellular breakdown). In terms of fertility, nitric oxide enhances spermatogenesis and improves sperm quality, supports embryo survival and growth, and may aid in detoxification and reducing the risk of preeclampsia.[355] Additionally, it is linked to better milk protein production, highlighting its broad benefits for reproductive health and overall cellular function.

Nitric oxide plays a key role in male reproductive health by helping the body produce important hormones, support blood flow for erectile function, and improve sperm quality. It also helps sperm mature properly (sperm capacitation) and release enzymes needed to fertilize an egg (the acrosome reaction). Additionally, nitric oxide supports Sertoli cells, which are special cells in the testes that help protect and nourish developing sperm while maintaining the blood-testis barrier—a natural defense system that keeps harmful substances from affecting sperm production.[356] In women, nitric oxide triggers the inflammatory response needed for ovulation, regulates hormone production in luteal and granulosa cells, and acts as a signaling molecule to mediate reproductive cycles and support implantation.[357] Its role underscores its importance in optimizing fertility for both partners.

A supplement I suggest is Neo40 or Berkeley Life, which increases nitric oxide production and delivers all the benefits as I described. These are quick-dissolve tablets (which you take once a day) with no artificial sweeteners. They're also non-GMO and gluten-free.[358]

Intravenous Supplementation Therapy

IV therapy is the intravenous delivery of specific nutrients and compounds that are naturally found in the body but become depleted because of age, illness, stress, or injury. IV supplementation therapy is an effective and fast way to help restore and replenish nutrient deficiencies that can occur with absorption problems, aging, and illness.

Higher doses of therapeutic nutrients are delivered directly into the bloodstream and avoid the GI system. This is especially advantageous for anyone with GI issues like "leaky gut," poor digestion, or compromised absorption. Bypassing the digestive tract and going straight to the bloodstream means nothing gets lost along the way. Your blood, cells, and tissues are getting the full effects of the nutrients where they are needed most.

By flooding the cells with vitamins, minerals, antioxidants, and molecules, you're replenishing your body with vital nutrients at a cellular level. And since diseases and aging often originate in the cells, restoring optimal levels of these nutrients can have a profound impact on your health. Following are the preconception-specific IVs that I recommend you do.

Pharmaceutical Grade Phosphatidylcholine IVs (PK Protocol)

The PK Protocol, an intravenous therapy involving phospholipid exchange, has been shown to repair damaged cell membranes, support detoxification, and eliminate accumulated toxins, including heavy metals. By aiding in the removal of these metals and other harmful substances, the PK Protocol enhances cellular health and function.[359] This detoxification process is especially powerful for individuals preparing for conception, as it helps create a cleaner, healthier foundation in the body, which is essential for reproductive health and fetal development. (During these IVs, also ask for folic acid in the form of leucovorin and glutathione.)

NAD+ IVs

I touched on oral NAD+ earlier in this chapter; it's also available as an IV. To get an idea of what NAD+ does for you, think of it as the premium car wash for your cells. It powers the "cleaning crew" that keeps your cell and mitochondrial membranes pristine, allowing everything to operate smoothly and efficiently. NAD+ is also like a DNA detailer, helping repair any "scratches" in your genetic code and removing some of the "grime" left by toxins in the form of epigenetic marks. There's even promising evidence that NAD+ might fine-tune certain enzymes, like those that process fructose, though more research is needed. Overall, NAD+ provides a full-service refresh for your cellular health, enhancing mitochondrial function and maintaining peak cellular performance.

NAD+ is the active cofactor form of vitamin B3 (niacin), a carrier molecule used by every cell in the body for energy metabolism. We are born with a set amount of NAD+, but levels decline as we age. When NAD+ is depleted, it causes "mitochondrial dysfunction"—a condition that is linked to aging as well as virtually all chronic diseases. NAD+ impacts DNA repair, epigenetic modifications, inflammation, circadian rhythm, and stress resistance. It's natural, restorative, and protective.

As for its effects on your preconception journey, a study titled "NAD+ Repletion Rescues Female Fertility during Reproductive Aging" found that restoring NAD+ levels in aged female mice improved oocyte quality and fertility. This suggests that NAD+ supplementation could be a potential strategy to support fertility in women of advanced reproductive age.[360]

Another study titled "Impact of NAD+ metabolism on ovarian aging" explores how declining NAD+ levels contribute to ovarian aging, affecting oocyte quality and overall ovarian function. It suggests that supplementing with NAD+ precursors may enhance oocyte quality and mitigate ovarian aging, offering a potential strategy to improving fertility in women of advanced maternal age.[361]

Final Thoughts

Like everything on this journey toward conceiving a child, smart supplementation is a true commitment. In case you need a little reminder, your motivation is your deep love for your future child, as well as your responsibility to go to any length necessary to set that child up for a healthy, vibrant life. Whether or not your child faces a lifetime of chronic health problems or disease is not merely the luck of the draw—it's dependent upon *your choices right now.*

Short of moving to an isolated area, regenerating the soil, and growing our own food, it's pretty much impossible for us to single-handedly change the fact that our food does not offer us the same nutrient density that it once did. But the supplements we've talked about in this chapter can fill in the gaps, plus some. They can truly optimize your health and epigenetics and change the future for your child.

As you move forward, remember that this is your opportunity to take control of your health in a way that has profound and lasting effects. You're not just supplementing—you're empowering your body to perform at its best, paving the way for a healthy, thriving family. So take this knowledge and use it to make informed, conscious decisions that will support you every step of the way on this remarkable journey to parenthood.

Q&A

Q: Why isn't taking prenatal vitamins enough?

A: Prenatal vitamins alone are better than no supplementation at all, but studies continue to show that they don't provide the appropriate doses of key micronutrients such as folate, iron, vitamin D, calcium, and DHA. Furthermore, the combinations of vitamins found in prenatals can also sometimes work against adequate absorption. A full supplementation program is needed to make up the nutritional imbalance, since our food simply lacks what we need on an ongoing basis, especially in light of what you're asking your body to do—conceive new life.

Q: Why is our food not good enough?

A: Industrial farming and chemicals such as pesticides and fertilizers, as well as added sugars, processed foods, and cooking methods, all contribute to nutrient loss in our food today. Studies repeatedly show that the nutritional values in our food have dropped significantly since 1950.

Q: I'm on a budget. What are the most important supplements to take?

A: Although it's ideal to test and see which supplements are most important, it is important for everyone to do four to six months or more of detox supplements, preconception vitamins, and some mitochondrial support.

Q: Can I accidentally "oversupplement"?

A: Yes, especially with certain vitamins or minerals such as vitamin D, vitamin A, and iron, you can overdo it. And some supplements can cause side effects if you don't use them properly.

Q: Some people say the body doesn't actually absorb supplements. Is this true?

A: The effectiveness of supplements largely depends on their bioavailability, which refers to how well a nutrient is absorbed and utilized by the body. It's true that some forms of vitamins and minerals are not easily absorbed, making them less effective. For instance, cheaper forms like magnesium oxide have lower bio-availability compared to forms like magnesium glycinate or magnesium citrate, which are absorbed more efficiently. Similarly, fat-soluble vitamins (A, D, E, and K) require fat to be absorbed properly.

Both the quality and form of a supplement play a significant role in its absorption. Supplements that are difficult for the body to process, or those missing key cofactors for absorption, may pass through the digestive system without being fully utilized. It's also important to consider factors like gut health and enzyme levels, as these can impact the body's ability to absorb nutrients.

To ensure better absorption, it's essential to choose high-quality, well-formulated supplements tailored to individual needs. By focusing on the right forms and ratios of nutrients, and addressing any underlying factors that may affect absorption, you can maximize the effectiveness of your supplements.

CHAPTER 10

Gut Genesis: Your "Garden" of Generational Health

I'm so passionate about the health of your gut microbiome that I couldn't help but try my hand at a little poetry.

In the garden of your being, life's roots are deeply sown,
The balance of this sacred soil is where true health is grown.
What thrives within your body, you pass to child and kin,
A legacy of balance, where future health begins.

What do you think? Does that paint a poetic picture of the significance of balancing your gut? I hope so. (If not, maybe it's worth a little chuckle.) But seriously, I hope you'll be willing to adopt a new perspective on what's going on inside your gut because it's truly the genesis of your health—and the health of your future family. Imagine with me for a moment that your gut is the ultimate garden, a vibrant ecosystem where the seeds you plant and the care you provide determine the vitality of the entire system. Just like a garden, the gut thrives when it is tended to with the right balance of nutrients, diversity, and love.

Optimizing Your Microbial Garden

Think of your gut lining as the nutrient-rich soil that provides the foundation for the health of the entire garden. Just like healthy soil nourishes plants, the gut lining supports a flourishing microbiome—the community of microorganisms in our gut. (In fact, your microbiome has approximately 100 trillion bacterial cells!) This collection of trillions of microorganisms includes bacteria, viruses, fungi, and other microbes, which live in and on our bodies. These tiny life forms are essential for so many of our bodily functions, including digestion, immune system regulation, and even mental health.[362]

The microbes (bacteria, fungi, viruses) are the plants of your "gut garden." Just as any garden may have a variety of plants—flowers, fruits, vegetables, herbs—your microbiome has a variety of microbes. Some of these are beneficial (like flowers and fruit-bearing plants), while others are neutral, and still some others are like weeds—harmful to the garden. The goal is to cultivate the beneficial bacteria while keeping the harmful ones in check. Probiotics and prebiotics, found in fermented and fiber-rich foods, help feed the beneficial bacteria, just like how compost nourishes plants.

The foods we eat, the stress we manage, the quality of our sleep, and the environment we expose ourselves to act as the water and nutrients for this gut ecosystem. When we nourish our gut with a diverse, nutrient-dense diet rich in fiber, whole/unprocessed foods, and fermented products, we cultivate a flourishing microbiome that supports every aspect of our health. Probiotic-rich foods like yogurt, kefir, sauerkraut, and kimchi add healthy bacteria to the microbiome. Prebiotics—fibers that feed beneficial bacteria—also contribute to the "compost" and are found in foods like garlic, onions, and asparagus.

A healthy, well-tended garden helps us break down food into essential nutrients, supports immune function, and protects the body from harmful pathogens. Eating a balanced diet with plenty of fiber, healthy fats, and antioxidants is like giving your garden the right mix of nutrients to thrive.

But just as neglecting or poisoning a garden with chemicals will lead to poor growth, neglecting our gut through a poor diet, chronic stress, exposure to glyphosate and other toxins, and overuse of antibiotics lead to an imbalanced microbiome. This imbalance, or dysbiosis, allows invasive weeds of inflammation, poor digestion, and disease to take root.

Pathogenic bacteria and harmful microbes are the weeds in our garden analogy. If your garden is neglected or overrun with unhealthy foods, sugar, or processed foods, the weeds can take over, much like how dysbiosis happens. These "weeds" can choke out the beneficial plants and disrupt the balance, leading to disease and poor health. Pull the weeds! Limit processed foods, sugar, and alcohol, which fuel harmful bacteria, much like how weeds thrive on neglect.

You are the gardener of your gut, and it's your responsibility to make lifestyle choices that support the necessary balance. Stress management, exercise, and good sleep are like sunlight, fresh air, and water. By carefully tending to your garden, feeding the beneficial bacteria, and keeping the harmful ones at bay, you create a rich, diverse environment where the whole system can flourish—improving not only your digestion but your overall health, immunity, and even mental well-being.

The impact of our gastrointestinal tract health goes far beyond the digestive system—what we sow in the gut, we feel throughout our entire body. When our microbiome is in balance, it helps us think clearly, feel emotionally stable, and defend against infections. Conversely, an unhealthy microbiome can send signals of distress to the brain, contributing to feelings of anxiety, depression, or mental fog. This connection, often referred to as the gut-brain axis, shows that the health of our gut soil directly influences the health of our mind. The gut produces many of the neurotransmitters that regulate mood, including serotonin, which is often called the "feel-good" chemical. When the soil is rich and thriving, we feel the benefits in our mental and emotional well-being.

Beyond our minds, the garden of the gut is also the foundation of our immune system. Just as a garden with healthy soil grows strong plants, a healthy gut cultivates a strong immune system, helping to identify and fend off harmful invaders. Approximately 70 percent of the immune system resides in the gut, where it learns to recognize the difference between harmful pathogens and harmless substances. A well-tended microbiome ensures that this immune system knows when to fight and when to stand down. If the garden becomes filled with toxins, inflammatory foods, or stress, the immune system may become confused, leading to allergies, autoimmune diseases, or chronic inflammation.

Keep in mind—you don't always "feel" bad right away when these processes are going on inside your body. You might actually feel just fine at the beginning stages of chronic inflammation or auto-immunity starting to take root inside your body. This is why testing, which we talked about earlier, is so essential. It helps you find out what's actually going on inside your gut and body.

In functional medicine and precision medicine, we view the gut as the soil from which all health grows. By nurturing your gut garden with care—through mindful eating, stress response optimization, and attention to lifestyle—you can harvest the rewards of good health in every area of your life. What you plant in your gut truly determines what you will reap in terms of energy, vitality, mental clarity, and resilience against disease. Just as a healthy garden blooms and bursts with life, a healthy gut creates the foundation for a life of balance, strength, and well-being.

The study of the gut microbiome and the gut-brain axis has fascinated medical professionals for generations. Research published in 2022, titled "The History of the Intestinal Microbiota and the

Gut-Brain Axis," highlights how physicians as far back as ancient Greece and China observed the links between digestion, mood, and overall health.[363] From early fecal transplants in ancient Chinese medicine to the eighteenth-century discoveries of bacterial communities in the digestive system by Antonie van Leeuwenhoek, curiosity about the gut's influence on the body and mind has persisted across centuries.[364]

Physicians in the nineteenth century, for example, often looked to the gastrointestinal system as the source of emotional and mental disturbances, a theory that remains relevant today in light of modern findings about the gut-brain connection. Modern research, such as that done by the Human Microbiome Project, has only deepened our understanding of this delicate ecosystem, revealing that the diversity and balance of gut bacteria can influence everything from metabolism and immune response to mood and cognitive function.[365]

In fact, the gut is often referred to as the "second brain" because of the complex network of neurons and the significant role it plays in regulating various bodily functions.

The gut contains the *enteric nervous system (ENS)*, an incredible network of about 100 million neurons embedded in the walls of the digestive tract. This network can operate independently of the brain and spinal cord and is capable of complex reflexes and behaviors.

- The gut and the brain are in constant communication via the *vagus nerve* and through *biochemical signaling*. This bi-directional communication is known as the gut-brain axis. Through this axis, the gut can influence brain function and vice versa.

- The gut produces a significant amount of the body's neurotransmitters. For example, it produces about 90 percent of the body's serotonin, a neurotransmitter that plays a key role in regulating mood, sleep, and appetite. It also produces other neuroactive compounds like dopamine and GABA, a neurotransmitter that regulates nervous system activity. GABA helps calm the brain and plays a role in reducing anxiety, promoting relaxation, and improving sleep. The emerging field of psychobiotics focuses on how certain gut bacteria can produce serotonin, directly impacting mental health and mood regulation.[366]

- Because of the gut-brain connection, changes in the gut microbiome can influence mood, stress levels, and even behavior. This is why conditions like irritable bowel syndrome (IBS) are often associated with anxiety and depression.

- The gut is home to over 70 percent of the body's immune system. It helps regulate inflammation and immune responses, which can also impact mental health and overall well-being.

- The ENS can regulate many digestive processes autonomously, without input from the brain, including the coordination of muscle contractions for peristalsis (the wavelike muscle contractions that move food through the digestive tract), the release of digestive enzymes, and the regulation of blood flow to the gut.

There are many factors that play a role in the gut-brain axis.[367]

As you can see, the health of our gut garden impacts nearly *every* aspect of our lives, and every aspect of our lives impacts the health of our gut garden. But where it gets really exciting in terms of conceiving a child is in the area of research that supports the idea that preconception gut health plays a significant role in shaping the health of future generations through epigenetic mechanisms.

Studies suggest that the maternal microbiome during preconception and pregnancy not only influences the developing fetus but can also lead to long-lasting epigenetic changes that affect the baby's health.[368] For example, the composition of the maternal gut microbiota has been shown to influence the expression of genes related to

Regulators of Gut-Brain Axis

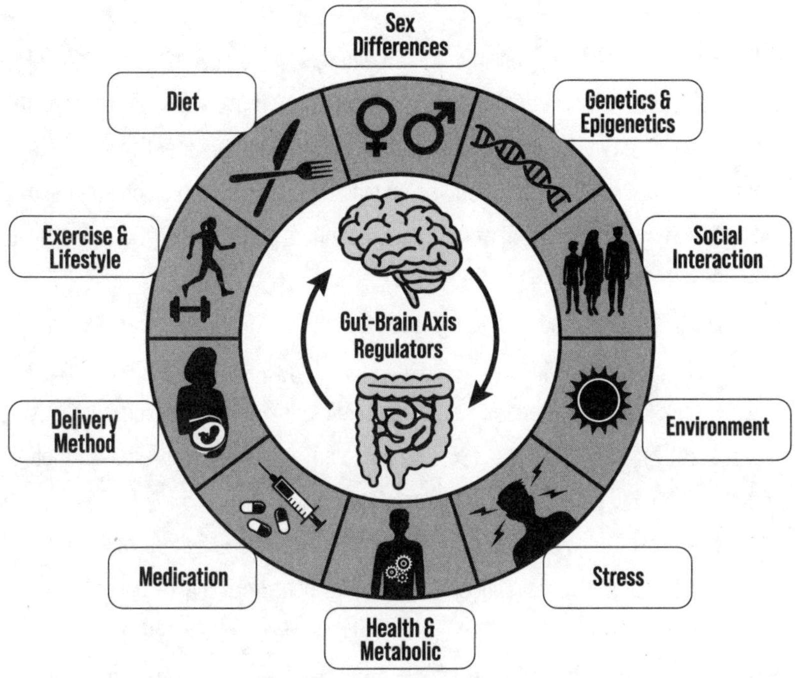

the immune system, metabolism, and even the development of the enteric nervous system in the fetus.[369]

This epigenetic influence is crucial because the gut microbiota produces metabolites that can affect gene expression in both the mother and the developing fetus. Factors such as diet, stress, and even antibiotic use before conception can disrupt the balance of beneficial gut bacteria, potentially impacting the child's health through altered gene expression. This means that nurturing a healthy gut before conception not only supports the mother's health but also provides a strong foundation for the next generation, influencing the risk of metabolic diseases, immune responses, and even cognitive development.

Let's delve a little deeper into how the state of your gut can make a significant difference in your preconception journey and why you will not have the "green light" to conceive a child unless your microbiome is balanced and thriving.

Gutsy Research

Microbiome research is a fascinating and emerging area of study that is one of the fastest growing areas of medical research today. That's why a lot of money is being invested in it. The global market for microbiome therapeutics was estimated at $919.4 million in 2023, and some market reports even project it to reach $21.5 billion by 2030, growing at a compound annual growth rate of 56.9 percent from 2023 to 2030.[370]

This is driven by the increasing recognition of the microbiome's role in conditions like metabolic disorders, immune system regulation, and gut health. As of this writing, key players in this field include Microbiotica, a UK-based company that recently raised £50 million ($67 million) to advance microbiome-based therapeutics for conditions such as ulcerative colitis and cancer.[371]

All of this funding is part of a larger trend in Europe, where both public and private entities are significantly investing in microbiome research.[372] The National Institutes of Health (NIH) and global agencies are also heavily invested in exploring how the microbiome influences human health through initiatives like the Human Microbiome Project.[373] In addition to private companies, universities like University College London and Cambridge in the UK and Johns Hopkins University in the US are conducting cutting-edge microbiome research, with some projects aimed at understanding how the microbiome influences immunity and mental health.[374]

This all underscores the need for further exploration in areas like gut-brain interactions and microbiome-based therapies and highlights why it would be wise to pay close attention to this aspect of your health when it comes to epigenetics.

The Microbiome and Hormone Regulation

A balanced gut microbiome allows the female body to clear estrogen metabolites and maintain hormonal equilibrium. When the microbiome is imbalanced, it can lead to hormone dysregulation, particularly affecting estrogens, which play an important role in reproductive health. This interaction between the gut and hormones, which is part of what is called the "gut-liver axis," is so intricate that the microbiome is often referred to as an endocrine organ.

The gut-liver axis is mediated by the estrobolome, a collection of gut bacteria capable of metabolizing estrogens.[375] When this system is disrupted (gut dysbiosis), it can result in altered estrogen levels, potentially leading to conditions like PCOS or uterus lining issues (e.g., endometriosis), both of which can severely impact fertility, as well as pregnancy complications.[376]

For instance, an increase in bacteria that produce an enzyme called β-glucuronidase can elevate circulating estrogen levels, which can contribute to endometriosis and certain cancers.[377] On the flip side, if there's too little of this enzyme, the body may struggle to maintain healthy estrogen levels, potentially leading to conditions where estrogen is too low, such as metabolic syndrome.

This delicate balance shows just how closely linked the gut is to the regulation of hormones, and why maintaining a healthy gut is so important for your preconception journey. A diet rich in fiber supports gut health and estrogen metabolism. This includes eating fermented foods such as kefir, sauerkraut, and yogurt.

The Gut Microbiome and Hormonal Balance in Men

While much of the conversation around gut health and hormones tends to focus on women, men are equally impacted by the state of their microbiome when it comes to regulating key hormones, particularly testosterone. The gut microbiome interacts with the endocrine system to influence the levels of various hormones, including testosterone and cortisol, which play essential roles in male health and fertility. Studies have found that men with gut dysbiosis or high levels of pro-inflammatory bacteria have poorer sperm motility and morphology, leading to reduced fertility.[378] The estrobolome also affects men. Estrogen is not exclusive to women—men need small amounts for proper physiological functioning, including bone health, cardiovascular health, and sexual function. Like with women, the estrobolome helps in circulating estrogen in men.

A well-balanced gut can help promote healthy testosterone and estrogen levels, while an imbalance in the microbiome may disrupt hormone regulation, potentially leading to issues like low testosterone (or "low T," as you might have heard it called).

Testosterone is crucial for maintaining male reproductive health, muscle mass, and energy levels. When the gut is in balance, it supports proper absorption of nutrients, reduces inflammation, and helps the body produce the hormones it needs. However, when the gut microbiome is compromised—due to poor diet, stress, toxins like glyphosate, and antibiotic use—it can increase inflammation and affect the body's ability to produce or regulate testosterone. This can lead to symptoms like fatigue, reduced libido, and even emotional disturbances.

Moreover, chronic gut issues like dysbiosis can elevate cortisol, a stress hormone, which further suppresses testosterone production. High cortisol levels often signal the body to prioritize short-term survival over long-term health, which may include reducing testosterone production. This interplay between the gut and hormone levels is one reason why men who experience stress or have poor gut health may also report symptoms of low testosterone, such as decreased muscle mass or mood changes.

Given the big role the gut plays in hormone regulation, it makes sense that it would also directly impact matters related to male fertility. A review article in *Frontiers in Microbiology* from May 2024 showed some fascinating insight on this connection:

- Gut microbiota can influence sperm motility and overall quality. A proper balance of estrogen and testosterone is needed for healthy sperm development. A disruption in the estrobolome can reduce sperm quality. Certain gut bacteria can produce metabolites that aid in the production of nutrients and hormones, which are vital for healthy sperm development. For instance, some beneficial bacteria can produce short-chain fatty acids (SCFAs) and polyunsaturated fatty acids (PUFAs), which are known to improve sperm membrane stability and energy supply, crucial for sperm motility.[379] Probiotics have also been shown to repair spermatogenic impairment, improving sperm concentration and motility. (How about that for a little-known positive side effect of probiotics?)

- The gut microbiota can impact the structure of the testes by affecting the blood-testis barrier (BTB) and testicular inflammation.[380] An imbalance in gut bacteria can lead to an increase in endotoxins, such as lipopolysaccharides (LPS), which can cause inflammation in the testes and damage the BTB.[381] This barrier is crucial for protecting developing sperm cells from harmful substances. Damage to this barrier can lead to conditions like orchitis (testicular inflammation) and disrupt normal spermatogenesis.

Another key influence of the microbiome on fertility is its role in regulating inflammation and immune function. Chronic inflammation, often a by-product of dysbiosis, can interfere with sperm production and quality. The gut microbiome assists in modulating the immune response, and an imbalance can trigger excessive immune activity, harming sperm cells and reducing fertility. Furthermore, an unhealthy microbiome is associated with metabolic conditions like obesity and insulin resistance, both of which are linked to reduced fertility. An imbalance in the gut bacteria that process estrogen (the estrobolome) can also affect men, leading to either too much estrogen being reabsorbed or not enough being properly broken down, which may impact hormone balance. This would then reduce testosterone levels. Dysbiosis has also been linked to weight gain and a disrupted metabolism. Estrogen also has a protective effect on the cardiovascular system for both men and women, and an imbalance can increase risk in this area. Dysbiosis in the estrobolome has been associated with increased risk of hormone-related cancers in men, such as prostate cancer.

The male microbiome also has a profound effect on the health of your future children, particularly through epigenetic changes. Epigenetic modifications can be influenced by diet, lifestyle, and microbiome health, affecting sperm DNA and potentially impacting the child's development and long-term health. For instance, paternal obesity, often associated with dysbiosis, can influence epigenetic markers in sperm, increasing the risk of metabolic disorders like diabetes and obesity in offspring. Additionally, a man's microbiome may affect his child's immune health. An imbalanced microbiome contributing to low-grade systemic inflammation can impact sperm quality and may influence the child's immune programming, raising the likelihood of autoimmune diseases, allergies, and other inflammatory conditions. While the mother's microbiome is the primary source for an infant's microbiome at birth, recent studies suggest that paternal factors can indirectly shape the child's microbiome. Through shared diets and environments, a father's microbiome can influence the home microbiome, potentially impacting the child's gut health and long-term wellness.

Optimizing a man's microbiome can enhance fertility and positively influence the health of future children. A diet rich in fiber, probiotics, and prebiotics supports beneficial bacterial growth in the gut, with foods like dairy-free yogurt, kefir, sauerkraut, and fiber-rich fruits and vegetables providing essential nutrients for a balanced microbiome. Minimizing processed foods, sugar, and alcohol can help reduce harmful microbial growth. Probiotic supplements containing strains such as *Lactobacillus* and *Bifidobacterium* can improve gut health, manage inflammation, and may even boost sperm quality.

Physical activity and stress management techniques, such as meditation and yoga, promote a healthy microbiome by reducing inflammation and supporting immune function, both of which are crucial for fertility. Additionally, being cautious with antibiotic use is vital, as antibiotics can disrupt the gut balance by killing beneficial bacteria.

Building a Healthy Gut

Fortunately, by this stage in this preconception program, you've already taken significant steps toward building a healthy gut microbiome. You've focused on detoxing, reducing the influx of toxins, and feeding the good bacteria by managing stress, avoiding unnecessary antibiotics, and supplementing with probiotics. You've adopted healthy stressless strategies, and you've optimized your overall lifestyle. You've also focused on improving gut health probiotics, eating a high-fiber diet, and reducing sugar and processed foods that fuel harmful bacteria. All of these contribute to a healthy gut microbiome, so keep up the great work!

The stool testing you completed can provide valuable insights into your gut health, allowing for targeted treatments. For example, if issues like small intestinal bacterial overgrowth (SIBO) are present, natural solutions are the first line of defense. However, when necessary, antifungals or antibiotics may be required to restore balance. This is why that data collection from the stool tests up front, and again after you've adopted these strategies for six to eighteen months, is so essential—so you can understand how to best address your unique microbiome needs.

Top Twelve Toxins That Can Harm Your Microbiome

Hold your breath, because we're diving into the toxic terrain of the top offenders that tamper with your gut's ecosystem. These notorious toxins—from heavy metals and pesky pesticides to plasticizers and processed preservers—can do a number on your microbiome, creating a hostile takeover in your gut. They're the gut disruptors, the bacterial bouncers, and the microbial mischief-makers that shift the scales away from health and harmony.

Each of these substances—all of which we've already discussed to some degree—disrupts your body's delicate microbial balance, either by wiping out the good guys, boosting the bad, or sending your hormones into a tailspin. Ready to meet this cast of characters? Whether they creep into your system through food, water, or everyday products, these twelve toxins make a clear case for cleaner living—think organic, avoid the artificial, and embrace the natural. Get to know them well so you can keep them out of your gut and let your microbiome thrive!

Toxin #1: Antibiotics

Antibiotics have a significant impact on the microbiome. Over 80 percent of antibiotics used in the US are administered to livestock, meaning that people can consume residual antibiotics through food, which can further alter gut health.[382] Antibiotics kill both harmful and beneficial bacteria, which disrupts your microbiome balance. Frequent use can lead to long-term dysbiosis and reduced bacterial diversity. Sources of antibiotics include prescription medications and conventionally raised livestock.

Toxin #2: Glyphosate

Glyphosate, the very common herbicide you are now familiar with, is present in more products than even previously thought. In 2022, the Detox Project, which works at creating transparency in the food market, found high levels of the herbicide even in products labeled as "non-GMO." Organic foods, thankfully, are less likely to be contaminated with glyphosate.[383] Glyphosate disrupts gut bacteria by reducing beneficial strains like *Lactobacillus* and *Bifidobacterium*, while supporting pathogenic bacteria, leading to an unhealthy microbial balance. This toxin is found mainly in nonorganic crops such as corn and soy.

Toxin #3: Artificial Sweeteners (e.g., Aspartame, Sucralose)

Artificial sweeteners are often marketed as a "healthier" choice, but increasingly there is evidence showing that issues like cardiovascular disease, metabolic syndrome, and nonalcoholic fatty liver disease may be associated with their use. Artificial sweeteners are also associated with potential weight gain, altered glucose homeostasis, decreased satiety signaling, increased food intake, and an altered gut microbiome.[384] Sweeteners such as aspartame and sucralose alter gut microbiota, promoting dysbiosis and impairing glucose metabolism, which may contribute to metabolic diseases. They're commonly found in diet sodas, sugar-free foods, and low-calorie sweeteners.

Toxin #4: Heavy Metals (Lead, Mercury, Arsenic, Cadmium, Aluminum)

Despite efforts to reduce exposure, low-level lead poisoning remains pervasive in the US, especially in underserved communities.[385] In fact, over four hundred thousand deaths per year in the US are caused by lead exposure.[386] Mercury exposure, primarily from certain types of fish, also continues to be a concern, although efforts are being made to reduce it. More than 80 percent of fish consumption advisories in the US and Canada are due, at least in part, to mercury contamination.[387] Heavy metals can disrupt gut health through various mechanisms. They increase harmful bacterial growth while reducing beneficial strains, leading to inflammation and oxidative stress in the gut. Heavy metal sources include contaminated water, seafood, rice, industrial pollutants, and aluminum cookware. They're also found in some vaccines.[388]

Toxin #5: Bisphenol A (BPA)

BPA is a hormone-disrupting chemical found in plastics, food packaging, and water bottles, making exposure almost unavoidable. It can negatively impact gut health by disrupting the balance of gut bacteria, which may increase the risk of metabolic issues such as insulin resistance and obesity. Studies have shown just how widespread BPA exposure is. In 2003–2004, the CDC tested urine samples from thousands of people and found BPA in 93 percent of them.[389] A follow-up study in 2012 found similar results, confirming that most people in the US are regularly exposed to this endocrine disruptor.[390]

Toxin #6: Pesticides

The Environmental Working Group has determined that over 75 percent of nonorganic produce contains pesticide residues, and 95 percent of nonorganic produce listed in their "dirty dozen" contains pesticide residues,[391] which can reduce microbial diversity in the gut. Pesticides, particularly organophosphates, reduce beneficial bacterial diversity and promote inflammation. Sources include nonorganic fruits, vegetables, and grains. (The "dirty dozen," or most-contaminated fruits and vegetables, are strawberries, greens including spinach, kale/collard greens/mustard greens, grapes, peaches, pears, nectarines, apples, bell peppers, hot peppers, cherries, blueberries, and green beans.)

Toxin #7: Processed Foods

Diets high in processed foods have been linked to an increased risk of gut inflammation and dysbiosis. In fact, researchers have found that people who eat five or more servings per day of processed foods are at an 82 percent higher risk of IBD—and eating one to four servings per day can increase your risk even as high 67 percent.[392] It's the components in these foods that can negatively alter gut bacteria. Processed foods that are high in refined sugars, unhealthy fats, and preservatives promote harmful bacterial growth and reduce beneficial species. The biggest offenders include packaged snacks, fast-foods, and processed meats.

Toxin #8: Alcohol

Drinking alcohol—especially in excess—can damage tissues and organs, leading to serious health issues. It's been linked to liver disease (ALD), weakened immune function, pancreatitis, heart disease, and even disruptions to your body's natural sleep-wake cycle (circadian rhythm). Over time, these effects can increase the risk of both short-term and long-term health problems. What is interesting about the findings, however, is that it is not necessarily the alcohol on its own that produces health concerns, but the alcohol-induced *changes* in intestinal microbiota.[393] Chronic alcohol intake leads to dysbiosis by reducing beneficial bacteria and increasing gut permeability, contributing to "leaky gut" syndrome. Sources include all alcoholic beverages.

Toxin #9: Phthalates

Phthalates are chemicals that are used to make solvents, plastics, and many personal care products. An EPA study has shown that these were detected in 58 percent of individuals in the study. It gets worse when you look at frequency. Some types of phthalates were found to have a frequency in 98 percent of the women in the study (16–49 years), and up to 99 percent in children aged 6–17.[394] Phthalates affect digestion and metabolism by disrupting gut bacteria and endocrine functions. They can be found in plastic packaging, cosmetics, and personal care products.

Toxin #10: Triclosan

According to an article in the medical journal *Gut Microbes*, "This compound is frequently detected in the human body: the National Health and Nutrition Examination Survey showed that TCS was detected in ~ 75% of the urine samples of individuals tested in the United States. Also, TCS causes ubiquitous contamination in the environment and is listed among the top ten pollutants found in the rivers of the United States."[395] Triclosan, an antimicrobial agent, reduces bacterial diversity, leading to microbial imbalances and potentially promoting antibiotic-resistant bacteria. It's found in antibacterial soaps, toothpaste, and cleaning products.

Toxin #11: Preservatives (e.g., Sodium Benzoate, Potassium Sorbate)

Increasingly, studies are showing that long-term exposure to preservatives and food additives induce changes in the gut microbiota.[396] Preservatives inhibit the growth of beneficial bacteria and may promote harmful strains, disrupting the gut microbiome balance. Packaged snacks, sodas, and processed foods commonly contain preservatives.

Toxin #12: Microplastics

Research has found that 93 percent of bottled water contains microplastics, which may affect gut health when ingested.[397] Microplastics cause gut inflammation and may alter the composition of gut microbiota, leading to potential long-term health effects. Besides bottled water, microplastics can also be found in seafood and synthetic fabrics.

(Un)Lucky Number 13 on the Toxin List

As we've explored in previous chapters, per- and polyfluoroalkyl substances (PFAS) are a group of man-made chemicals that are resistant to oil, water, and heat. We've talked about various ways they wreak havoc on your health, but did you know that they're especially disruptive to your gut microbiome? Indeed, studies have shown that PFAS exposure is associated with changes in the composition and function of gut bacteria, potentially leading to dysbiosis and associated health effects. Here's a closer look at how PFAS can impact the microbiome.

- **Altered Microbial Diversity:** PFAS exposure has been linked to a decrease in microbial diversity. Lower diversity is often associated with an imbalanced gut and increased susceptibility to various health issues, including inflammation, metabolic disorders, and kidney damage.[398]
- **Increase in Pathogenic Bacteria:** Some studies suggest that PFAS may encourage the growth of potentially harmful bacteria while reducing the presence of beneficial bacteria. This shift can disrupt gut homeostasis and weaken the gut barrier, increasing the risk of infections and inflammation.[399]
- **Promotion of Gut Inflammation:** PFAS compounds can trigger immune responses and inflammation.[400] The presence of inflammatory markers in the gut can alter the microbiome, which may lead to inflammatory bowel conditions, as well as an overall disrupted gut environment.[401]
- **Influence on Short-Chain Fatty Acid Production:** Beneficial bacteria in the gut produce short-chain fatty acids (SCFAs), like butyrate, which are essential for gut health and immune regulation.[402] PFAS exposure has been shown to alter SCFA production, leading to reduced levels of these beneficial compounds, potentially affecting gut lining integrity and overall health.[403]

THRIVE

- **Potential for Metabolic Disruptions:** The microbiome plays a role in metabolic regulation, and PFAS exposure has been linked to metabolic syndrome and obesity.[404] This connection may be due in part to PFAS-induced microbiome changes, which can affect how the body processes and stores nutrients and fat.

- **Hormone Disruption Through Microbiome Alteration:** PFAS are known endocrine disruptors, and the gut microbiome is involved in hormone metabolism.[405] Changes in the microbiome due to PFAS exposure may further disrupt hormone balance, compounding the endocrine effects of PFAS themselves.

Mitigating PFAS Impact on the Microbiome

While addressing PFAS exposure can be challenging, there are several strategies that may help support the microbiome, all of which we've discussed in various areas of this book. They include:

- **Consuming prebiotics and probiotics** to support beneficial bacteria growth and improve microbial diversity.

- **Including fiber-rich foods** in your diet to encourage SCFA production and support gut health.

- **Getting detoxification support** through a diet rich in antioxidants (e.g., fruits and vegetables) and hydration to support liver and kidney function, which help clear toxins.

Shaping Your Microbiome Through Diet

As you might expect, your diet plays a pivotal role in shaping the composition and abundance of your microbiome. And the good news is, it doesn't take long for changes to take effect. Research shows that an acute change in diet can alter the microbial composition within twenty-four hours, but those changes are reversible within forty-eight hours of discontinuation.[406] This is why a *consistently* healthy, nutrient-rich diet is the best way to maintain a balanced gut microbiome.

Refer to chapter 7 for more information on how to eat a diverse, nutrient-dense diet that will give your gut microbiota just what they need. Remember: Sugar, gluten, and dairy do not do your microbiome any favors—quite the opposite, in fact. But consuming a variety of healthy foods, including cruciferous vegetables, grass-fed beef, pasture-raised poultry, organic fruits and vegetables, and good fats such as avocados, coconut oil, olive oil, and nuts, supports a diverse gut bacteria population.

The 5 "Rs" for a Healthy Gut

Not to be a broken record, but comprehensive stool testing is the only way to get a good picture of what is going on in the digestive tract as far as microbiome health, the presence of any pathogens, inflammation, and digestive function. This testing allows you to personalize what's called the "5R Protocol" for a healthy gut microbiome. 5R stands for:

- Remove
- Replace
- Reinoculate
- Repair
- Rebalance

Whether you're experiencing uncomfortable gut-related issues (such as heartburn, loose stools, constipation, bloating, and gas) or not, this protocol can help you shape a healthy, balanced microbiome. As we dive into each R, note that while some of this information is repeated from earlier chapters, sometimes we need to hear things more than once for them to really sink in!

Number One: Remove

Remove refers to removing anything that is irritating or damaging to the digestive system along with treating any infections.

- Remove inflammatory foods and foods you are sensitive to. This may require taking a food sensitivity test or completing an elimination diet. Following the Preconception Diet is a good place to start. From there, you can personalize your approach.
- Remove food additives, toxins, and artificial sweeteners.
- Remove medications such as NSAIDs (nonsteroidal anti-nonflammatory drugs, a group of medications that help reduce pain, inflammation, and fever. Examples include ibuprofin and aspirin) that are contributing to issues. Be sure to talk with your doctor about prescription medication before making any changes.
- Treat gut infections per testing.

Number Two: Replace

With the Remove phase, we take out what is not needed and with the Replace phase, we add in what is missing for healthy digestive function. This includes:

- Hydrochloric acid and pectin (for protein digestion), such as Digestive Support by Every Life Well
- Digestive enzymes (for protein, carbohydrate, and fat digestion)
- Bile salts
- Digestive bitters to stimulate the body's own production of acids and enzymes

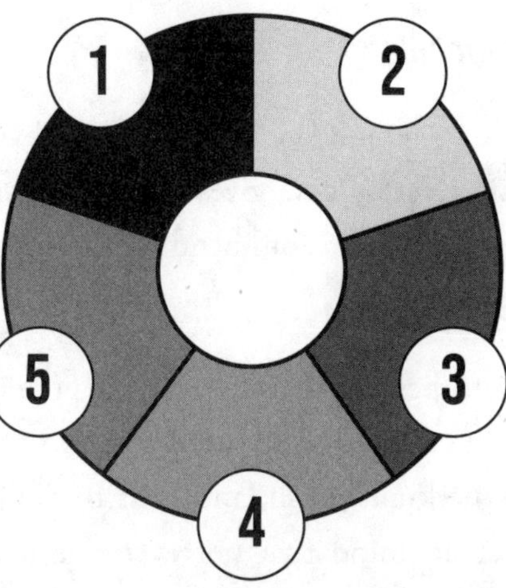

Number Three: Repair

Repair and heal the lining of the digestive system and correct any "leaky gut" symptoms. Specific nutrients and herbs that can help support the Repair stage include:

- Vitamins, including vitamins A, C, and D
- Zinc (as zinc carnosine)
- Omega-3 fats
- The amino acid l-glutamine as a supplement and from collagen protein or bone broth
- Soothing, mucilaginous herbs such as aloe, marshmallow, and DGL (GI Defend by Every Life Well)

Combination products, such as GI Defend, include several of these nutrients and herbs in a single formula.

Number Four: Reinoculate

Reinoculate means to repopulate the beneficial bacteria that make up the microbiome. Testing data gives clues about specific levels and imbalances and is useful for recommending specific probiotic supplements and dietary strategies.

- Reinoculate beneficial bacteria with probiotic supplements and fermented foods. Add small amounts of fermented foods such as sauerkraut, miso, and kefir to daily meals, as tolerated. Keep in mind that not everyone tolerates fermented foods well, so if your symptoms worsen at all, stop eating them and know that you can still heal without them.
- Increase prebiotics in order to feed the probiotics, help them proliferate, and establish robust colonies. Prebiotic foods include berries, artichokes, onions, garlic, asparagus, chicory, burdock root, bananas, green banana flour, potato starch, and leafy green veggies. (You'll know if you overdo it, as you will experience bloating and gas. More isn't necessarily better in this case!)
- Including a prebiotic fiber supplement may be helpful as well. Every Life Well's Exceed Greens + Reds is a great all-in-one option, with prebiotics, probiotics, digestive enzymes, and fiber.

Number Five: Rebalance

Rebalance means to look deeper into the issues that contributed to the imbalances in the first place. Often, these are lifestyle factors. Keep the GI tract healthy and happy by prioritizing sleep, stress management, and exercise. The digestive system works best when the nervous system is in a parasympathetic or "rest and digest" state. When we are constantly stressed and in "fight or flight," digestion is compromised. Eating while relaxed improves digestion and absorption considerably. Even taking a few deep breaths before a meal helps.

The goal of the 5R Protocol is to heal the gut in order to restore the natural balance to the digestive system. I love this approach, and I think you will too!

Aluminum and the Microbiome

Emerging research suggests that aluminum exposure may influence the gut microbiome, potentially leading to dysbiosis. When heavy metals like aluminum accumulate in the gut, they can support the growth of pathogenic bacteria and decrease populations of beneficial bacteria. This shift in microbial balance can increase inflammation, impair immune function, and contribute to gastrointestinal concerns.

Aluminum in the gut has been associated with elevated oxidative stress and inflammation, both of which weaken the integrity of the gut barrier. This compromised barrier may allow harmful bacteria and toxins to pass into the bloodstream, contributing to conditions like "leaky gut." Furthermore, oxidative stress from aluminum exposure can alter microbial populations in ways that affect digestion and immune resilience, as beneficial microbe decline, while others, less supportive of health, may flourish.

Studies also highlight how aluminum exposure can reduce populations of key bacteria like *Lactobacillus* and *Bifidobacterium*, which are essential for producing vitamins, supporting digestion, and maintaining immune health. A decrease in these beneficial strains may compromise the microbiome's ability to support overall health.

You can reduce your aluminum exposure through dietary and environmental choices to help support a healthy microbiome.

THRIVE

- Minimize processed foods, which often contain aluminum-based additives, and avoid the use of aluminum cookware and aluminum foil.

- Choose a water filter that removes heavy metals, including aluminum, to reduce exposure from drinking water.

- Pharmaceutical companies use aluminum adjuvants in vaccines to enhance the immune response, causing the body to produce a stronger and longer-lasting immunity with a smaller dose of the active ingredient. However, concerns about aluminum exposure during preconception stem from its potential to accumulate in the body and disrupt neurological and immune functions. Avoiding vaccines during this sensitive period may help minimize unnecessary exposure to metals, supporting a healthier environment for conception and fetal development.

While aluminum is not often discussed as a microbiome disruptor, its prevalence in the environment and potential to impact gut health make it a topic worth consideration. Further research will help clarify aluminum's specific effects on the microbiome, but until then, I encourage you to avoid it as much as possible.

One Body, Multiple Microbiomes

Believe it or not, microbial cells outnumber human cells by approximately 1.3 to 1 (estimated to about 30 trillion human cells to approximately 39 trillion microbial cells).[407] In fact, these microbes are so much a part of our makeup that they can even get "jet-lagged,"[408] which explains why we might experience gastrointestinal symptoms when we travel.

Most of these microbes are found in the gut, but they also exist on the skin, in the mouth, and in other mucosal surfaces. The gut microbiome alone consists of trillions of microorganisms. These bacteria are particularly dense in the colon, where they help break down complex carbohydrates and produce important vitamins (such as vitamin K and certain B vitamins).[409]

In terms of genetic material, the microbiome's genetic contribution vastly outweighs that of the human genome. While humans have around 20,000–25,000 genes, the collective microbiome encodes approximately 2–20 million microbial genes—over 100 times more genetic material than human DNA![410] This has led some scientists to even argue (fascinatingly) that humans are not solely shaped by their human genome, but are instead a "superorganism" whose functions and health are deeply influenced by their microbial genetic diversity.[411] The microbiome therefore also influences epigenetic changes. Gut bacteria, for example, can produce metabolites that trigger or suppress gene expression in both microbial and human cells, impacting everything from inflammation to metabolic processes.[412]

Throughout this chapter, we have been focusing primarily on the gut microbiome, and a little on the vaginal and urogenital microbiome. But I want to take a moment and share that your body actually hosts several distinct microbiomes, each residing in different organs or tissues. These microbiomes are composed of trillions of microorganisms, including bacteria, viruses, fungi, and other microbes, and they play essential roles in maintaining health.

Gut Microbiome

This is the most obvious one, and the one we've been paying closest attention to in our discussion so far. The gut microbiome, particularly in the intestines, is the largest and most studied at this time. It houses a vast diversity of bacteria, mainly in the colon, and has far-reaching effects on every aspect of your physical and mental health.

The gut microbiome plays a crucial role in regulating metabolism, immune function, hormone production, and inflammation—factors that directly affect fertility. The gut microbiota can influence insulin sensitivity, weight management, and the production of hormones like estrogen, which plays a vital role in ovulation and pregnancy maintenance.

Gut dysbiosis has been linked to insulin resistance, PCOS, and endometriosis, all of which can impair fertility. Studies show that restoring gut microbiota balance can improve outcomes in women with reproductive challenges. An estimated 10 to 15 percent of women of reproductive age are affected by conditions like PCOS and endometriosis, both of which are tied to gut dysbiosis.[413]

Oral Microbiome

Your mouth contains a complex and diverse microbiome, with bacteria residing on the teeth, gums, tongue, and other surfaces. The oral microbiome is responsible for breaking down food particles, maintaining oral health, and preventing infections. Imbalances in this microbiome are linked to dental issues like cavities and gum disease and may even contribute to cardiovascular disease.

But there's more. Intimate kissing—the kind where saliva is exchanged—is a courtship staple unique to us humans and very common in most world cultures. During an intimate smooch, you're probably not thinking about what's happening inside your mouth or your beloved's. As "unsexy" as it sounds, our mouths do contain a thriving microbiome. Microbes are key role players in gene expression, diet, age, and yes—even sexual behavior.

In a study in the journal *Microbiome*,[414] Dutch researchers observed how bacteria are exchanged between partners during an intimate kiss. The results were very surprising—so surprising that I wrote a blog post about it![415] Remember, when you're kissing, you're not only giving your heart away but millions of bacteria . . . so you'd better make them good ones!

Vaginal Microbiome

The healthy vaginal microbiome is dominated by *Lactobacillus* species of bacteria, which help maintain a low pH (about 3.5–4.5) and protect against harmful bacteria and infections.[416] A healthy vaginal microbiome is crucial for maintaining fertility, as an imbalanced vaginal flora can lead to infections like bacterial vaginosis (BV) or vaginal yeast infections (often caused by *Candida albicans*). These infections can also create a hostile environment for sperm, making conception more difficult and increasing the risk of complications during pregnancy.

A healthy vaginal microbiome is therefore critical for preventing these infections and sexually transmitted diseases. Around 29 percent of reproductive-age women will experience BV at some point, which has been linked to a higher risk of preterm birth, miscarriage, and infertility.[417] As we discussed in chapter 10, our Every Life Well Woman's Balance Probiotic is a great solution for maintaining a healthy vaginal microbiome.

Skin Microbiome

The skin microbiome consists of microorganisms that reside on the skin's surface. Different areas of the skin, such as oily, dry, or moist regions, host distinct microbial communities. These microbes play a role in protecting the skin from pathogens, supporting wound healing, and regulating immune responses. Imbalances in the skin microbiome can lead to conditions like acne, eczema, and psoriasis.

Respiratory Microbiome

The respiratory tract, including the nasal passages, sinuses, and lungs, contains its own microbiome. These microorganisms play a role in defending against pathogens that can enter the respiratory system,

THRIVE

helping to regulate immune responses. Alterations in this microbiome are linked to conditions like asthma, COPD, and respiratory infections.

Urogenital Microbiome

Apart from the vaginal microbiome in females, the urogenital tract (bladder and urethra) in both males and females also harbors its own microbiome. These microorganisms are involved in maintaining the health of the urinary system, and imbalances can lead to urinary tract infections (UTIs) and other urological disorders. Recent research even suggests that the bacterial communities in the male urogenital tract, particularly in the urethra, seminal fluid, and testes, can influence sperm health and reproductive outcomes.[418]

An imbalance in this microbiome has been associated with conditions like prostatitis, urethritis, and low sperm quality, all of which can negatively impact fertility. Healthy microbiota in the male urogenital tract can help protect against infections and inflammation, both of which can impair sperm production and function. In fact, certain beneficial bacteria may help regulate local immune responses, ensuring that inflammation does not damage sperm or the tissues involved in their production.[419]

Conversely, the presence of pathogenic bacteria or an overgrowth of harmful species can lead to oxidative stress,[420] which negatively affects sperm motility and DNA integrity, reducing the likelihood of conception. Additionally, men with a more diverse and balanced seminal microbiome tend to have better sperm quality compared to those with an overabundance of harmful bacteria. These harmful bacteria can produce toxins and inflammatory signals that reduce sperm viability and may even interfere with the sperm's ability to fertilize an egg.

The vaginal and urogenital microbiome plays a vital role in women's reproductive health and fertility and significantly impacts the microbiome of a vaginally born child. This microbial community, primarily in the vagina, consists of diverse microorganisms, with beneficial bacteria like *Lactobacillus* species leading the way in maintaining the health of the reproductive tract. These bacteria support a balanced microbial environment, crucial for both preventing infections and promoting fertility.

A key component of the vaginal microbiome's role in fertility is maintaining a low pH. *Lactobacillus* species help sustain an acidic vaginal pH, typically around 4.5, which creates an environment that prevents harmful bacteria and pathogens from thriving. This low pH is also essential for fertility, as it creates a supportive environment for sperm survival and motility. Disruptions to this balance can increase pH levels, allowing potentially harmful bacteria like *Gardnerella vaginalis*, associated with BV, to flourish.

Additionally, a well-balanced microbiome plays a role in preventing infections, such as UTIs and sexually transmitted infections (STIs), both of which can harm reproductive health. Persistent infections may lead to pelvic inflammatory disease (PID), a condition that can cause damage to the fallopian tubes and uterus, reducing fertility. The microbiome also supports the production of healthy cervical mucus, essential for sperm transport during ovulation, and dysbiosis can affect mucus quality, making conception more difficult.

The vaginal microbiome's balance also influences pregnancy health, particularly in implantation and pregnancy maintenance. Microbial imbalances, or dysbiosis, have been linked to an increased risk of miscarriage, preterm birth, and preeclampsia. Infections stemming from dysbiosis can prompt inflammation and immune system dysfunction, both of which present obstacles to a healthy pregnancy.

The influence of a mother's vaginal microbiome extends to her child, particularly in vaginal births. During vaginal delivery, a baby is exposed to the mother's microbiota, which "seeds" the baby's microbiome. This initial exposure is foundational for the infant's immune system and overall health, with beneficial bacteria like *Lactobacillus* and *Bifidobacterium* among the first to colonize the infant's gut. Babies born via vaginal delivery develop a more diverse and beneficial microbiome compared to those delivered by C-section, who are often exposed to skin and hospital-acquired bacteria. This early microbiome diversity supports immune development, helping the body differentiate between harmful and benign microbes, and reduces the likelihood of autoimmune diseases and allergies later in life. Research also shows that a well-seeded microbiome in vaginally born children may offer long-term health benefits, reducing the risk of conditions like asthma, obesity, and type 1 diabetes.

Supporting a healthy vaginal and urogenital microbiome involves several lifestyle practices. Taking probiotic supplements with strains like *Lactobacillus* can help restore balance, particularly after antibiotic treatments or in cases of recurrent infections. A fiber-rich diet that includes prebiotics (e.g., garlic, onions, and asparagus) supports both gut and vaginal microbial health. Avoiding douching and harsh products is crucial, as these can disrupt the natural flora, increasing susceptibility to infections. Finally, maintaining proper hygiene practices, such as wearing breathable cotton underwear and keeping the genital area dry, help foster a balanced and healthy microbiome.

Placental Microbiome

Recent studies indicate that the placenta may host its own unique microbiome, potentially influencing both pregnancy and fetal development. The presence of microbes in the placenta could play a role in maternal and fetal health, with various factors shaping its microbial community. Some research suggests that semen may contain bacteria capable of migrating through the cervix to the uterus, where they may impact the placental microbiome. Depending on its microbial composition, semen could either support a balanced placental microbiome or introduce disruptive bacterial species.

The maternal gut microbiome appears to be a significant contributor to the placental microbiome. Research suggests that bacteria from the mother's gut can translocate through the bloodstream, thereby influencing microbial diversity in the placenta. A balanced maternal gut microbiome, particularly rich in beneficial strains like *Lactobacillus* and *Bifidobacterium*, is associated with healthier pregnancies and a reduced risk of complications.[421] Similarly, the maternal vaginal microbiome contributes to placental microbial populations. During pregnancy, the vaginal microbiome typically undergoes changes, often with increased *Lactobacillus* species that provide protective effects against infections. However, imbalances such as BV can lead to infections in the placenta and elevate the risk of complications, including preterm birth.

Recent research indicates that the microbiome of sperm and semen can significantly influence the vaginal microbiome and, by extension, the health of the placental microbiome. Semen carries a diverse community of microbes, including both beneficial and potentially harmful bacteria. During intercourse, these microbes are introduced into the vaginal environment, where they can alter the microbial balance. This shift in the vaginal microbiome may have implications for pregnancy outcomes and placental health.

When semen introduces specific bacteria, such as *Gardnerella vaginalis* or *Escherichia coli*, it can disrupt the vaginal microbial balance, potentially leading to dysbiosis. Such imbalances may result in infections, like BV (bacterial vaginosis) or UTI (urinary tract infection), both of which can impact fertility by creating an inhospitable environment for sperm or increasing the risk of infections that impair reproductive health. Semen contains special substances that help regulate the immune system (called immunomodulatory factors), which interact with the vaginal and cervical immune defenses. These factors help create a more welcoming environment for sperm by reducing inflammation, preventing the immune system from attacking sperm as foreign invaders, and influencing the balance of beneficial bacteria in the female reproductive tract. Through molecules like cytokines, semen can either promote immune tolerance or elicit an immune response, shaping the growth and composition of specific bacterial populations within the vaginal flora.

Infections and inflammation during pregnancy can also alter the placental microbiome, often through conditions such as chorioamnionitis, an infection of the placenta and fetal membranes. Such infections may disrupt microbial balance, leading to inflammation and an increased likelihood of adverse pregnancy outcomes. Maternal diet plays a crucial role as well; a high-fiber diet rich in prebiotics and probiotics supports a healthy gut and placental microbiome, while diets high in processed foods and saturated fats may encourage dysbiosis, potentially impacting placental health.

Additional factors, such as antibiotic use and environmental exposures, also influence the placental microbiome. Use of antibiotics during pregnancy should be judicious, as they may disrupt both maternal and placental microbial communities. If antibiotics are warranted, use the gut restoration process on page 357. By now, it's probably no surprise to you that environmental exposures, including pollution, chemicals, and stress, have also been linked to microbiome alterations, with some endocrine-disrupting chemicals and pollutants potentially increasing risks for adverse pregnancy outcomes.

Maintaining gut health through a fiber-rich diet and consuming fermented foods (such as yogurt, kefir, sauerkraut, and kimchi) can nourish beneficial bacteria. Probiotic supplements containing strains like *Lactobacillus* and *Bifidobacterium*, among others, can further support a balanced microbial environment. Avoiding unnecessary antibiotics and practicing healthy vaginal hygiene can help maintain a supportive microbial environment in the placenta. Lastly, managing stress and reducing exposure to environmental toxins can contribute to healthier maternal and placental microbiomes, supporting better pregnancy outcomes.

Fetal Microbiome

Emerging research indicates that a baby's microbiome is influenced by the mother's microbiome during pregnancy and birth. The method of delivery—vaginal birth versus C-section—has a profound effect on the infant's microbiome. Babies born via vaginal delivery are exposed to the mother's vaginal and gut bacteria, which helps "seed" the baby's own microbiome, while C-section babies are more likely to acquire skin and hospital-associated bacteria.

The mother's microbiome can affect the baby's gene expression through epigenetic mechanisms, such as DNA methylation and histone modification. This may influence the child's risk of developing obesity, diabetes, asthma,[422] and autoimmune diseases later in life.[423] Babies born by C-section have a more than doubled risk of asthma and allergies,[424] and are associated with a 46 percent increase in obesity risk and a 20 percent increased risk of developing type 1 diabetes, when compared with children delivered vaginally.[425] This is due to differences in early microbiome development.

Breast Microbiome

Breast tissue, particularly in lactating women, contains a microbiome that may influence the composition of breast milk. This microbiome is believed to contribute to the infant's gut microbiome and immune system development. Disruptions in the breast microbiome have been linked to breast infections like mastitis. Furthermore, if the mom has an overgrowth of candida, she can potentially spread that to her baby through breast milk, causing thrush, which is an overgrowth of candida, a type of fungus. Thrush appears as white patches on the tongue, gums, or inside the cheeks and can make feeding uncomfortable for the baby. All of this is important for you as a mom to keep in mind as you prepare your body for pregnancy and lactation.

Eye Microbiome

The eye also has its own microbiome, though it is less diverse compared to other areas of the body. The microorganisms present on the ocular surface help protect against eye infections and maintain healthy vision.[426] Changes in the eye microbiome are associated with conditions like conjunctivitis and dry eye disease.

Nasal Microbiome

The nasal passages host a specific community of microorganisms that play a role in filtering out harmful pathogens from the air we breathe. Disruptions in this microbiome are associated with sinusitis and respiratory infections.

Each of these microbiomes interacts with the body's systems in intricate and profound ways, contributing to overall well-being and playing pivotal roles in the prevention or development of various health conditions. While not all of these microbiomes are directly involved in preconception or fertility, they are deeply interconnected, forming a web of communication and influence throughout the body. Ultimately, the human body functions as a unified system, where the balance or imbalance of one microbiome can ripple through and affect others, demonstrating the interdependence of these microbial communities and their collective impact on reproductive and overall health.

Kimberly's Gut Transformation: A Fertility Success Story

My patient Kimberly had a history of ovarian cysts and was considering freezing her eggs, worried about her ability to conceive in the future. Seeking answers, she underwent a comprehensive lab workup, which revealed a cascade of issues: suboptimal methylation, hypothyroidism, elevated levels of mercury, arsenic, and lead, as well as high levels of inflammation marked by elevated hs-CRP (high sensitivity c-reactive protein, a way to detect inflammation). Most notably, her gut health was in disarray, with significant yeast overgrowth contributing to systemic imbalances.

These findings became the foundation for a targeted plan to address Kimberly's health from the inside out. We focused heavily on optimizing her gut microbiome, which included clearing out the candida. Through dietary changes, strategic supplementation, and a focused effort to detoxify her system, her body began to heal.

When Kimberly decided to start trying for a baby at age thirty-four, her health was in a much stronger place. She conceived naturally, though her first trimester presented challenges with low progesterone levels. We replaced her progesterone with hormone supplementation, and she carried her baby to term.

After the birth of her first child, Kimberly came back in, wanting to set the stage for baby number two. With testing and tuning, her nutrient levels, gut health, and inflammation markers were optimized. Two years later, at age thirty-eight, she welcomed her second child into the world.

Kimberly thought her family was complete, but at forty-one, she received a surprise: She was pregnant again. This time, her body's systems were so well balanced that she didn't require supplemental progesterone, an indication of the profound transformation her health had undergone.

THRIVE

Kimberly's story illustrates the power of addressing gut health and systemic imbalances as the cornerstone of optimizing fertility. By focusing on restoring her microbiome, reducing toxic burdens, and enhancing nutrient absorption, she not only achieved her dream of motherhood but also built a foundation for vibrant health that supported her through three successful pregnancies.

Final Thoughts

Maintaining a balanced gut microbiome is crucial for regulating the reproductive and metabolic endocrine systems, affecting fertility and the health of future generations. Its interaction with hormone levels, influence on pregnancy outcomes, and impact on the epigenetic health of offspring all point back to the importance of a balanced "gut garden" within. Your journey to conception involves cultivating this garden, optimizing not only your own well-being but also setting the stage for the healthiest possible start for your future child. By tending to this internal ecosystem, you're fostering a beautiful legacy of health.

Q&A

Q: What are microbiomes?

A: This simply refers to the community of microorganisms, including bacteria (good and bad), fungi, viruses, protozoa, and archaea (types of microorganisms). Most of these are in the gut, which is why we are speaking about "gut health" extensively. But it's also important to know about these microorganisms in other parts of your body and how to regulate them.

Q: Wait, are you telling me my body is full of—and surrounded by—germs?

A: It's good to remember that not every bacterium is bad! We've been raised to think of "bacteria" as bad and as another name for "germ." *Germ* is a broad term for microorganisms that can cause disease, but this does not mean every bacteria causes disease! It might take some time to think of this differently, but some bacteria (in fact, a huge number!) are actually your friends and help you stay healthy.

Q: Do microbiomes affect my hormones?

A: Yes! A balanced gut microbiome allows your body to clear estrogen metabolites and maintain hormonal equilibrium. When the microbiome is imbalanced, it can lead to hormone dysregulation, particularly affecting estrogens, which play an important role in reproductive health. This interaction between the gut and hormones is so intricate that the microbiome is often referred to as an endocrine organ.

Q: How long does it take to improve gut health for conception?

A: Although gut health improvement is a gradual process, research shows that positive changes in diet can alter the gut microbiome within just twenty-four to forty-eight hours. However, sustained benefits require consistent healthy choices over time. Ideally, dedicating at least three to six months to gut health through a

THRIVE

balanced diet, stress management, and probiotic intake can support a healthier preconception journey.

Q: Is there a quick way of remembering what I need to do to keep a healthy gut?

A: Yes! Remember to follow the 5R Protocol:
Remove
Replace
Reinoculate
Repair
Rebalance

Q: Are there specific foods that help boost beneficial bacteria in my gut?

A: Foods rich in fiber and natural prebiotics are key to nurturing beneficial bacteria. Some great choices include garlic, onions, asparagus, bananas, and artichokes. Adding fermented foods, such as kefir, sauerkraut, and kimchi, introduces probiotics that support a diverse and thriving microbiome, essential for overall health and fertility.

Q: How does my gut health affect my immune system during pregnancy?

A: Your gut health is deeply connected to your immune system, with about 70 percent of your immune cells located in the gut. A healthy microbiome teaches your immune system to differentiate between harmful invaders and harmless substances, reducing the risk of autoimmunity and allergies. This balance becomes especially important during pregnancy to protect both you and your developing baby, so building a strong foundation during preconception sets you up for a healthier pregnancy.

Q: My partner and I both have a busy lifestyle. Are there quick ways to support gut health daily?

A: Absolutely. Start with a diverse, colorful diet, which is an easy way to nourish your microbiome. (Check out chapter 7 on nutrition for more specific information.) Adding a handful of fiber-rich vegetables to meals or incorporating a daily probiotic smoothie can make a big difference. Small changes like swapping processed snacks for whole foods and managing stress with quick mindfulness exercises support gut health, even with a hectic schedule.

Q: Is it true that antibiotics can disrupt gut health? If so, what do I do if I need them?

A: Yes, antibiotics can affect the balance of your gut microbiome by wiping out both harmful and beneficial bacteria. If antibiotics are necessary, consider taking a high-quality probiotic during and after treatment to help repopulate your gut with beneficial bacteria. Also, focus on eating probiotic-rich foods and fiber to help restore your microbiome after a course of antibiotics.

THRIVE

CHAPTER 11

Harmonizing Your Hormones

You might remember learning about "the birds and the bees" at some point in your upbringing. Depending upon who taught you how babies are made (and how much you were really paying attention versus being horrified about the conversation), the details might be a little fuzzy. Sure, the basics are easy to grasp, but what you might not realize—even as you are considering having a baby soon—is that conception is a *highly* complex and finely tuned process. It's incredible, really! And I think it's important that you understand the finer details of conception, mostly so you can be in awe of just how many processes are involved. But also, because the more you understand all the mechanisms required for conception, the more you will gain a new respect for how hard your body is working to reproduce, and I hope it will inspire you to stay the course in making so many changes during the preconception window. So let's delve into the details of conception a bit deeper, with a specific focus on hormones.

Hormonal optimization (not just attaining "sufficient" levels) is essential for both men and women, as it regulates the development, maturation, and function of sperm and eggs, as well as creating a supportive environment for fertilization and implantation. For instance, women often assume if they're having regular periods, everything is fine, but that's not necessarily the case. Like a beautiful symphony, there's an optimal harmony that has to be achieved within our hormones in order for conception to occur.

Key Hormones in Female Fertility

Hormones control every step of the fertility process, from ovulation to implantation. They work together like a team, and if even one is out of balance, it can make conception harder. In this section, we'll break down the key hormones that impact fertility and why keeping them in sync is so important.

- **Follicle-Stimulating Hormone (FSH)**, made in the pituitary gland (a small gland located at the base of the brain), takes a starring role in the early stages of the menstrual cycle by stimulating the growth and maturation of ovarian follicles, which contain the eggs. Balanced FSH levels ensure that eggs are maturing properly, a key factor in successful ovulation.

- **Luteinizing Hormone (LH)**, also made in the pituitary gland, triggers ovulation, the release of the mature egg from the ovary. It also stimulates the production of progesterone, which is necessary for preparing the uterine lining to receive a fertilized egg. Without proper LH levels, ovulation may not occur.

- **Estrogen** is made in several parts of the body—the ovaries, adrenal glands, fat cells, and the placenta (during pregnancy). Estrogen plays a central role in regulating the menstrual cycle and preparing the reproductive organs for conception. It helps thicken the uterine lining, creating a receptive environment for embryo implantation. Estrogen also supports cervical mucus production, which is vital for helping sperm reach the egg.

- After ovulation, **progesterone** (which is made in the ovaries, adrenal glands, gut bacteria, and the placenta during pregnancy) stabilizes and maintains the uterine lining to support implantation and the early stages of pregnancy. It is crucial for sustaining a pregnancy during the first trimester and is produced by the corpus luteum in the ovary. Low levels of progesterone can lead to difficulties in maintaining a pregnancy.

- The thyroid gland makes its own hormones—**thyroid hormones T3 and T4**. Proper thyroid function is essential for regulating metabolism and supporting fertility. Thyroid imbalances, such as hypothyroidism or hyperthyroidism, can disrupt menstrual cycles, interfere with ovulation, and affect the body's ability to sustain a pregnancy.

- Balanced **insulin** levels support hormonal regulation and prevent insulin resistance, which can affect fertility, particularly in conditions like PCOS. High insulin can lead to an imbalance in reproductive hormones, impacting ovulation and egg quality. The pancreas produces insulin in the body. We'll give this subject some extra attention later in this chapter, as blood sugar and insulin are often overlooked in terms of fertility.

- **Prolactin** is produced in the pituitary gland and helps prepare the body for breastfeeding but can disrupt ovulation when elevated outside of pregnancy. High levels of prolactin (hyperprolactinemia) can suppress FSH and LH, leading to irregular or absent ovulation.

- Women produce **testosterone** in the ovaries and adrenal glands. It can also be converted by the body into estrogen. Testosterone helps regulate follicle development (it stimulates the production of FSH receptors in the ovaries, which helps follicles grow). Both high and low levels of testosterone can contribute to fertility challenges.

- **Dehydroepiandrosterone (DHEA)**, which is produced in the adrenal gland, helps improve egg quality. The body converts DHEA into testosterone and androgens (which then can be converted to estrogen), all of which contribute toward follicle growth, and, of course, play important roles, as mentioned above.
- **Anti-Müllerian hormone (AMH)** is produced by the ovaries and helps control the growth of eggs and follicles during the menstrual cycle.
- **Cortisol** can delay or inhibit ovulation. It is created in the adrenal glands. As we've touched on previously, high levels of cortisol, due to stress, creates various challenges for fertility, including making a successful fertilization difficult and affecting egg quality.

Other Hormones to Consider

Just so you can get an idea of how many hormones play a role in conception, I've listed a few more in the appendix, but I don't necessarily recommend testing for these unless your other lab work indicates a reason to do so.

Now, let's switch gears and look at the hormones involved in fertility from the male perspective. Understanding these key hormones can help identify areas for improvement and optimization.

Key Hormones in Male Fertility

Hormones play a major role in sperm production, quality, and overall reproductive health. Just like in women, these hormones need to be in balance for optimal fertility. In this section, we'll cover the key hormones that affect male fertility and why they matter for conception.

- **Testosterone** is essential for sperm production, or spermatogenesis, in the testes (where it is made). It also supports libido and the overall function of the male reproductive system. Low testosterone levels can result in reduced sperm count and poor sperm quality, affecting fertility. This is where maintaining a healthy body weight is so important, because men with a higher BMI tend to experience lower testosterone levels and higher estrogen levels, which can disrupt sperm production and reduce fertility, leading to lower sperm counts, poorer motility, and changes in sperm DNA integrity.[427] And even beyond fertility, research indicates male obesity also impairs the metabolic and reproductive health of future children, indicating that paternal health information is transmitted to the next generation through the sperm, a process influenced by epigenetics.[428]

- **Follicle-Stimulating Hormone (FSH)** in men stimulates sperm production by acting on the Sertoli cells within the testes, which are responsible for nourishing developing sperm. Balanced FSH levels are necessary to maintain a healthy sperm count and motility.

- **Luteinizing Hormone (LH)** stimulates the Leydig cells in the testes to produce testosterone. Proper levels of LH are vital for maintaining adequate testosterone levels, which in turn support healthy sperm production.

- **Insulin** resistance can affect sperm quality in men, just as it affects ovulation in women. Elevated insulin levels are often linked to oxidative stress, which can damage sperm DNA, reducing fertility (more on this later in the chapter).

- **Cortisol**, the body's stress hormone, plays a significant role in both male and female fertility. As we've discussed in previous chapters, chronic stress and elevated cortisol levels can suppress reproductive hormones like FSH and LH, reducing fertility in both men and women. Managing stress is *imperative* for maintaining hormonal balance and enhancing the ability to conceive.

- **DHEA (Dehydroepiandrosterone)** is often referred to as a precursor to sex hormones like testosterone and estrogen. In men, DHEA is produced primarily by the adrenal glands, and it plays a role in the synthesis of testosterone, which is vital for sperm production and overall reproductive health. Low levels of DHEA can lead to insufficient production of testosterone, indirectly affecting sperm count and quality. Additionally, DHEA has been found to support immune function and reduce inflammation, which may positively influence sperm health. DHEA is a foundational element that supports the optimal production of testosterone, FSH, and LH. This hormonal interplay is crucial for maintaining healthy sperm production, and imbalances in DHEA may disrupt this delicate system, potentially contributing to fertility issues. Once again, it's about striking that balance between all the hormones.

- **Estrogen** is also made by males in the testes and adrenal glands, although at lower levels in the body compared to women. For men, estrogen plays an important role in regulating libido, erectile function, and sperm production, maintaining a balance with testosterone and other hormones.

- **Progesterone** in men is essential for sperm maturation and overall sperm quality, and it also acts as a precursor to testosterone. It plays a vital role in ensuring the proper function and development of male reproductive tissues.

- **Thyroid Hormones (T3 and T4)** in low levels can lead to poor semen quality, reduced sperm count, and impaired testicular function. Thyroid hormone imbalances can also affect other hormones like testosterone, LH, and FSH, further influencing reproductive health.

- **Anti-Müllerian Hormone (AMH)** is produced by Sertoli cells in the testes. A dysfunction of Sertoli cell proliferation or maturation can lead to impaired production of sperm.

- **Corticotropin-releasing Hormone (CRH)** is produced in the hypothalamus and, as with females, regulates the stress response by stimulating the release of another hormone, adrenocorticotropic hormone (ACTH) in the pituitary gland in the brain. This then, in turn, affects the production of cortisol and androgens.

- **Adiponectin** is secreted by fat cells (adipocytes) and plays a vital role in regulating glucose levels and fatty acid breakdown. It impacts male fertility by enhancing sperm functionality and supporting steroidogenesis (hormone production) in the testes.

- **Leptin** plays a role in male fertility by regulating the hypothalamic-pituitary-gonadal (HPG) axis, which influences the release of several hormones essential for testosterone production and sperm production.

- **Gonadotropin-releasing Hormone (GnRH)**, produced in the hypothalamus, stimulates the release of LH and FSH from the pituitary gland, both of which are essential for testosterone and sperm production.

- **Insulin-like Growth Factor (IGF)**, which is primarily produced in the liver but also in the testes, supports male fertility by promoting sperm production, enhancing sperm motility, and improving overall sperm quality.

- **Inhibin**, produced by Sertoli cells in the testes, inhibits and regulates the secretion of FSH from the anterior pituitary gland, playing a key role in sperm production.

- **Growth Hormone (GH)** is crucial for male fertility, as it promotes sperm production, enhances sperm motility, and improves overall sperm quality. It also aids in the development and function of the testes.

- **Adrenocorticotropic Hormone (ACTH)**, produced in the pituitary gland, stimulates the adrenal glands to release cortisol and androgens (sex hormones), essential to maintaining the necessary hormonal balance for sperm production.

- **Oxytocin** is produced mainly in the hypothalamus in the brain, as it is with females, but for men it aids in the contractions of the reproductive tract during ejaculation. It also influences testosterone production and sperm quality.

- **Activin** enhances sperm production but promotes the function of Sertoli cells in the testes (where it is made).

- **Kisspeptin**, which is produced in the hypothalamus (a part in the brain which regulates hormone release), regulates the secretion GnRH.

Hormones

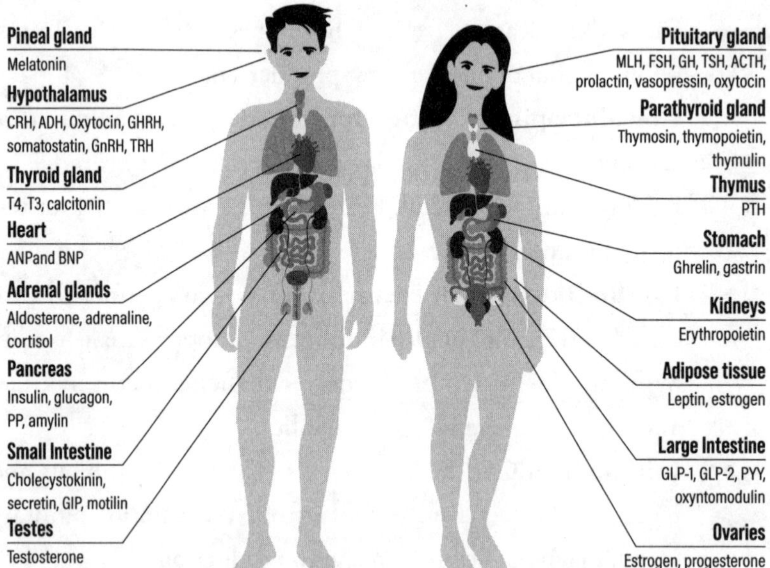

Strategies for Harmonizing Hormones for Conception

Throughout this entire program, we've been working to identify (through saliva testing as well as blood and urine testing, depending upon the hormone) and correct underlying imbalances that may interfere with your body's natural fertility processes. That's why the testing phase was so critical—because it gave us a glimpse into your own unique health profile so we could then tackle your specific issues, whether those are related to gut health, inflammation, detoxification, methylation, stress management, overall nutrient status, or more. The goal is to create an optimal internal environment for conception.

What *Are* Hormones, Anyway?

Have you ever thought about what hormones are—and what they're made of? Basically, hormones are chemical messengers produced by glands in the endocrine system that regulate and control various functions in the body. They are released directly into the bloodstream and travel to specific target tissues or organs, where they trigger specific biological responses.

Think of them like push notifications on your smartphone. Just like push notifications send timely, targeted messages to your phone from different apps, hormones deliver specific signals to different parts of your body when certain actions need to happen. For example, just as a fitness app might send you a notification to move after detecting inactivity, insulin gets "sent" to cells to manage blood sugar after a meal. Each hormone, like a push notification, has a designated "app"—or receptor—it targets, ensuring the right message reaches the right place. If notifications aren't working properly (like hormone imbalances), the system breaks down, leading to missed signals or overactivity.

Hormones are essential for maintaining homeostasis, or balance, within the body. Each hormone has a unique role, and they often work in concert with other hormones to create a complex web of signals that keep the body's systems functioning optimally.

THRIVE

Different types of molecules make up hormones, primarily proteins or lipids (fats), which determines how they interact with their target cells. For example, peptide hormones like insulin are made of amino acids and bind to receptors on the surface of cells to initiate a response, while steroid hormones like estrogen and testosterone are lipid-based and can pass through cell membranes to bind to receptors inside the cell. The body's ability to produce and regulate hormones is vital, as even slight imbalances can have significant effects on health, including fertility, mood disorders, or metabolic problems.

Ultimately, the goal of all hormones is to achieve that equilibrium amid the current environment the body is dealing with. For instance, when your body is going through an acute illness, TSH (thyroid-stimulating hormone) goes up briefly until the infection is resolved. That's just one example of hormones driving many of the body's processes, allowing cells to communicate with each other and respond to changing needs or external stimuli.

The Main Event: Understanding Conception

Now that you've learned about the hormones that regulate fertility, let's look at how conception actually happens.

Each month, a mature egg (oocyte) is released from the ovary and travels into the fallopian tube, where it may meet sperm. Meanwhile, millions of sperm begin their journey, but only a few hundred make it to the egg, and just *one* will successfully fertilize it.

For fertilization to occur, the sperm must undergo changes that help it penetrate the egg's protective layers. Once the sperm enters, the egg immediately blocks any others from getting in, ensuring normal chromosome pairing and preventing genetic abnormalities.

This intricate process, guided by hormones and cellular interactions, is the first step in the creation of new life. For a more thorough explanation, see the appendix.

When His Genes Meet Hers

At the moment of fertilization, the genetic materials from the sperm and egg combine, creating a unique genetic blueprint for the baby. The sperm contributes half of the genetic material, while the egg provides the other half. The egg carries more than just DNA—it also contains cytoplasmic components, which are the proteins, nutrients, and cellular structures inside the cell that support early development. These components provide the energy and building blocks needed for the embryo to grow in its first stages before it can rely on the placenta for nourishment. Key among them are mitochondria, which supply the energy needed for cell division and growth. (This is one of the many reasons why we've talked about boosting the health of your mitochondria.) The cytoplasm also contains maternal RNA, which are genetic instructions from the mother that help control early cell division before the embryo can start using its own DNA. Along with proteins, these maternal RNAs provide the necessary signals to kick-start development in the first few days after fertilization.

All of these cytoplasmic components are essential because the embryo is largely reliant on maternal resources until it can begin to express its own genes and sustain its own development. This makes the egg's cytoplasm crucial in supporting the transition from a fertilized egg to a multicellular organism.

Epigenetic Factors

As you know by now, epigenetics involves changes in gene expression that do not alter the underlying DNA sequence. In the context of conception, keep in mind that all the factors we've been talking about, including parental environment, nutrition, and stress, can lead to epigenetic modifications that influence how genes are *expressed* in the developing embryo. These modifications can affect the embryo's growth, development, and health, potentially having lasting impacts throughout its life—and this is something you have a lot more control over than you could have even imagined!

The maternal environment, including nutrient availability and hormonal balance, can influence the epigenetic landscape of the embryo. For instance, a mother's diet rich in folate and antioxidants may support healthy epigenetic programming, while exposure to toxins or poor nutrition can lead to detrimental changes.

Every time I reflect on the intricate processes behind egg and sperm maturation, or the way a parent's environment can shape a child's future before conception even occurs, I'm in awe. My patients often share this same sense of wonder when they learn just how much intention and care can influence fertility. Understanding these processes isn't just about science—it's about appreciating the incredible gift of new life and taking empowered steps to create the healthiest foundation for pregnancy and beyond.

Endometriosis

Endometriosis happens when tissue resembling the uterine lining grows outside the uterus. This misplaced tissue can attach itself to the ovaries, fallopian tubes, and other pelvic organs, leading to inflammation, scar tissue, and severe menstrual pain. Sadly, it can also lead to infertility. Women who struggle with endometriosis often experience a mix of emotions, ranging from frustration to exhaustion, due to chronic pain, fatigue, and uncertainty about their fertility. Many feel isolated or overwhelmed by the unpredictable flare-ups and the impact the condition has on their daily lives and futures, especially when it comes to trying to conceive.

Endometriosis is highly estrogen-dependent, meaning that high levels of estrogen can worsen the growth of endometrial-like tissue outside the uterus. Estrogen stimulates the growth and thickening of this tissue, which then leads to inflammation, pain, and scarring. But there is hope—in severe cases, surgeons can remove the endometrial tissue, and in less severe cases, hormonal therapies can help.

What causes endometriosis? Recent research suggests that genetic factors and inflammatory responses play key roles in its development.[429] Studies have identified specific genetic variants, such as those in the NPSR1 gene, that increase the risk of developing endometriosis, especially in its more severe forms (stages III and IV).[430] This gene appears to be involved in inflammatory and pain pathways, suggesting that endometriosis may share genetic roots with other chronic pain conditions like migraines and back pain. This could explain why many women with endometriosis also experience widespread pain.

In addition to genetics, environmental factors like exposure to toxins and immune dysregulation have also been linked to endometriosis.[431] Some studies point to *Fusobacterium*, a type of bacteria, as a potential trigger for the inflammatory response seen in endometriosis,[432] especially in cases of pelvic inflammation.[433] This bacterial theory adds another layer to understanding how endometrial-like tissue grows outside the uterus.

Research continues to explore how genetic and environmental factors interact to cause the condition, and newer findings are paving the way for non-hormonal treatments targeting inflammation and pain, such as inhibiting the NPSR1 gene's activity.[434] This growing body of research is providing much-needed insight into both the causes and potential treatments for this often-debilitating disease.

THRIVE

Blood Sugar: Often Overlooked but Critical to Conception

While it's probably not the first thing you think of when you're picturing how conception occurs, blood sugar, or glucose, is critical to your mission, especially in terms of fertility. Glucose is the body's primary source of energy, and it's regulated by insulin—a hormone produced by the pancreas. When you eat carbohydrates, they are broken down into glucose (sugar), which enters the bloodstream. Insulin acts as the key that unlocks cells, allowing them to absorb glucose from the blood and use it for energy or store it for later use, thereby lowering blood sugar levels.

Glucagon is another hormone that plays an important role in this process, and it works in opposition to insulin. When blood sugar levels drop too low, glucagon signals the liver to release stored glucose into the bloodstream to bring levels back to normal. Other hormones like cortisol and adrenaline (stress hormones) also increase blood sugar levels during periods of stress or fasting, ensuring your body has enough energy.

Hormonal imbalances, such as insulin resistance (common in conditions like type 2 diabetes or PCOS), can disrupt this system, causing elevated blood sugar levels and contributing to metabolic issues. This shows how maintaining balanced hormones is critical for proper blood sugar regulation and overall health.

When blood glucose levels are intermittently above optimal ranges, it can lead to insulin resistance, a condition where the body's cells do not respond effectively to insulin. This imbalance has profound implications for fertility in both men and women. High blood sugar levels can also lead to systemic inflammation, another condition that has significant implications for fertility.

When blood sugar levels remain elevated over time, the body's normal metabolic processes are disrupted. High glucose levels in the blood can damage blood vessels and nerves throughout the body, leading to the production of advanced glycation end products (AGEs)—harmful compounds that form when protein or fat combine with sugar in the bloodstream. The formation of AGEs triggers the release of inflammatory cytokines, which are signaling proteins involved in the body's inflammatory response. Inflammation induced by high blood sugar can have several adverse effects on fertility.

- In women, inflammation can directly impact ovarian function, affecting the regularity of ovulation. Chronic inflammation has been linked to conditions like PCOS, which is a common cause of infertility due to irregular ovulation and anovulation (the absence of ovulation). According to the World Health Organization (WHO), "polycystic ovary syndrome (PCOS) affects an estimated 8–13% of reproductive-aged women, and up to 70% of affected women remain undiagnosed worldwide."[435] Although most women go undiagnosed, PCOS *can* be reversed and is not a "forever" diagnosis by any stretch.

- The health of the endometrium (the lining of the uterus) is crucial for the implantation of the embryo. Inflammatory conditions can lead to an inhospitable endometrial environment, making it difficult for the embryo to implant and grow.

- In men, inflammation can decrease sperm quality by affecting sperm count, motility, and morphology. Inflammation can also damage the DNA in sperm, reducing fertility.

- Inflammation can disrupt the balance of reproductive hormones in both men and women. In women, it can lead to excess production of androgens (male hormones), which can interfere with ovulation. In men, it can affect testosterone levels and other hormones critical for sperm production.

Beyond the issues that inflammation causes in fertility, high blood sugar in and of itself can wreak havoc as well. For women with high blood glucose, one of their primary concerns is its impact on hormonal balance. Studies such as those published in the *Journal of Clinical Endocrinology & Metabolism* have found a direct correlation between insulin resistance and PCOS,[436] a leading cause of infertility. PCOS is characterized by irregular menstrual cycles and anovulation, making conception challenging.

THRIVE

Men are not immune to the effects of high blood sugar on fertility. Research in the *American Journal of Physiology-Endocrinology and Metabolism* indicate that insulin resistance can negatively affect sperm quality, including parameters like volume, concentration, and motility. These changes can drastically reduce male fertility and the likelihood of successful conception.

High blood glucose levels can also lead to complications during pregnancy, such as gestational diabetes, which poses risks to both the mother and the developing fetus. According to *Diabetes Care*, maintaining optimal blood sugar levels is crucial for minimizing these risks and ensuring a healthy pregnancy outcome. And there's no better way to prevent issues with blood sugar during pregnancy than to get a handle on it during the preconception period.

Elevated blood sugar levels can have a profound effect on the health and genetic profile of your future child through epigenetic inheritance. Changes in gene expression caused by factors like high blood glucose in parents can be inherited by their children, possibly increasing their susceptibility to various health conditions.

The statistics do seem to suggest that children are being impacted by elevated blood sugar in general. Obesity among children and adolescents in the US is on the rise, averaging to about 19.7 percent, according to research from the Centers for Disease Control and Prevention (CDC) conducted from 2017 to March 2020.[437] The prevalence of obesity also seems to increase with age. During the same time, obesity prevalence was 12.7 percent among US children 2–5 years old, 20.7 percent among those 6–11, and 22.2 percent among adolescents 12–19.[438]

Metabolic syndrome (the precursor to diabetes) and diabetes are also on the rise among children. The incidence of youth-onset type 2 diabetes has seen an annual increase of 6.8 percent (2019).[439] The incidence was even higher than expected in 2021, a fact that seems to be linked to the Covid-19 pandemic.[440] There are even increasing cases worldwide of diabetes in prepubertal children.[441]

How Blood Sugar Issues Become Generational

You might be curious about how epigenetic inheritance works when it comes to high blood glucose. Epigenetic changes in the sperm and eggs can carry altered patterns of DNA methylation and histone modifications to the offspring. High blood glucose levels in either parent can lead to epigenetic alterations in these gametes, affecting gene expression in the embryo and subsequently in the adult.[442] The in-utero environment, influenced by the mother's metabolic state, including her blood glucose levels, can also lead to epigenetic modifications in the developing fetus. These changes can persist into adulthood, influencing health outcomes.

Over time, high blood sugar can result in other health conditions in an individual, but what you might not realize is that children of parents with high blood sugar are also at risk for developing certain health conditions. Children of parents with high blood glucose levels may have an increased risk of developing metabolic disorders, including obesity and type 2 diabetes. This is due to inherited epigenetic modifications that affect metabolism, insulin sensitivity, and energy regulation.

There is emerging evidence that parental blood glucose levels and associated epigenetic changes can impact neurodevelopment, possibly contributing to an increased risk of neurodevelopmental disorders and altered cognitive and behavioral outcomes in children.

Preventive Measures

Given the potential for high blood glucose levels to induce heritable epigenetic changes, managing blood sugar through lifestyle interventions is crucial for prospective parents. Let's take a look at some effective prevention strategies.

You Are What You Eat

What you eat plays an enormous role in your overall health, and especially in the health and harmonization of your hormones. Choose a diet rich in organic whole vegetables, fruits, and lean proteins. Also, eliminate processed foods and foods high in refined sugars in order to help regulate blood sugar levels, as well as lower inflammation.

You've Got to Move It, Move It

Consistent exercise habits can help lower blood sugar levels and reduce inflammation. Exercise improves insulin sensitivity, helping to lower blood glucose levels. Incorporating a mix of cardiovascular, strength training, and flexibility exercises is most beneficial. If you're wearing a continuous glucose monitor (CGM), you can see the power of going for even a ten-minute walk after eating!

Master Your Stress

Chronic stress can exacerbate blood glucose fluctuations and inflammation in the body, so learning how to properly manage, mitigate, and master your stressors will have a positive impact. Techniques such as yoga, meditation, and mindfulness are all helpful, and check out chapter 8 for a refresher.

Gain Valuable Insight with a CGM

A continuous glucose monitor (CGM) is one of the most powerful weapons we have against chronically high blood sugar. Why? Because knowledge is power. Armed with clear data from a CGM, you'll be able to tailor your diet and exercise plans based on your own, unique glucose responses. Foods and activities affect individuals differently; what spikes one person's glucose might have a minimal impact on another's. By understanding your unique responses, you can customize your lifestyle choices to maintain steadier glucose levels.

Support with Supplements

Following is a list of supplements that have been researched for improving insulin resistance and metabolic syndrome, and I've seen many patients benefit from these:

- **Berberine** is an alkaloid that activates AMPK (AMP-activated protein kinase), which regulates energy metabolism. By activating AMPK, berberine helps increase glucose uptake in cells, enhance insulin sensitivity, and reduce glucose production in the liver. Studies have shown that berberine can reduce blood sugar levels and improve insulin sensitivity, similar to the effects of metformin, a common diabetes drug.

- **Magnesium** plays a key role in insulin signaling pathways and glucose metabolism. It helps cells become more responsive to insulin, facilitating glucose uptake. Low magnesium levels are associated with an increased risk of insulin resistance. Supplementing with magnesium improves insulin sensitivity, especially in those who are magnesium deficient.

- **Chromium** is an essential mineral that enhances the action of insulin. It improves insulin receptor activity, allowing glucose to be used more effectively by the cells. Chromium picolinate has been shown to improve insulin sensitivity and reduce fasting blood glucose levels, particularly in individuals with type 2 diabetes.

THRIVE

- **Alpha-lipoic acid (ALA)** is a potent antioxidant that helps reduce oxidative stress, which is a major contributor to insulin resistance. It also enhances insulin sensitivity by increasing glucose uptake in muscle cells. ALA improves insulin sensitivity, reduces blood glucose levels, and has anti-inflammatory effects that are beneficial in managing metabolic syndrome.

- **Omega-3 fatty acids (EPA and DHA)** improve insulin sensitivity by reducing inflammation, a significant factor in the development of insulin resistance. They also reduce triglyceride levels and improve lipid profiles, which are important for managing metabolic syndrome. Omega-3 supplementation helps decrease insulin resistance, especially in individuals with metabolic syndrome or obesity.

- **Cinnamon** contains bioactive compounds like *cinnamaldehyde* that mimic insulin and increase glucose uptake by cells. It slows down carbohydrate digestion and improves insulin sensitivity. Studies show that cinnamon supplementation can lower fasting blood sugar and improve insulin sensitivity, particularly in individuals with type 2 diabetes.

- **Vitamin D** improves insulin sensitivity by enhancing the function of pancreatic beta cells, which produce insulin. It also reduces inflammation that contributes to insulin resistance. Low levels of vitamin D are associated with insulin resistance and metabolic syndrome. Supplementing with vitamin D has been shown to improve insulin sensitivity and lower the risk of type 2 diabetes.

- **Probiotics** help modulate the gut microbiome, which can influence insulin sensitivity and systemic inflammation. Supplementation with certain strains of probiotics (e.g., *Lactobacillus* and *Bifidobacterium*) has been shown to improve insulin sensitivity, reduce inflammation, and improve glucose metabolism.

- **Resveratrol** is a polyphenol found in grapes and red wine. It activates SIRTI and AMPK pathways, which enhance insulin sensitivity and improve mitochondrial function. Resveratrol improves glucose metabolism, reduces oxidative stress, and increases insulin sensitivity, particularly in individuals with obesity and metabolic syndrome.

- **Coenzyme Q10 (CoQ10)** is a powerful antioxidant that supports mitochondrial function and reduces oxidative stress. It helps improve energy production in cells, which is crucial for proper insulin signaling. Supplementation with CoQ10 improves insulin sensitivity and reduces blood sugar levels, particularly in individuals with type 2 diabetes.

- **Curcumin** is the active compound in turmeric and has strong anti-inflammatory and antioxidant properties. It reduces oxidative stress and inflammation, both of which contribute to insulin resistance. Studies show that curcumin improves insulin sensitivity, lowers blood sugar levels, and reduces inflammation associated with metabolic syndrome.

- **Dietary fiber (e.g., Psyllium, Glucomannan)** slows the absorption of sugar into the bloodstream and reduces spikes in blood glucose levels. It also improves gut health, which influences insulin sensitivity. Fiber supplements can reduce insulin resistance, lower fasting blood sugar levels, and improve lipid profiles, which are important for managing metabolic syndrome.

- **N-acetyl cysteine (NAC)** is a precursor to glutathione, the body's most powerful antioxidant. It helps reduce oxidative stress and inflammation, which are key drivers of insulin resistance. NAC improves insulin sensitivity by reducing inflammation and oxidative damage in the body.

- **Bitter melon (*Momordica charantia*)** contains compounds that mimic insulin and help lower blood sugar levels. It improves glucose utilization and reduces the production of glucose in the liver. Bitter melon has been shown to reduce fasting blood glucose levels and improve insulin sensitivity in individuals with metabolic syndrome and type 2 diabetes.

- ***Gymnema sylvestre*** is a herb that helps regulate blood sugar by enhancing insulin secretion and improving glucose uptake in cells. It also helps reduce sugar cravings, which can lead to better glucose control. *Gymnema sylvestre* has been shown to improve insulin sensitivity and reduce fasting glucose levels in individuals with diabetes.

This exploration into the relationship between blood sugar levels and fertility reveals the importance of intentional implementation of health habits that have a synergistic and profound effect in the conception process. While individual experiences may vary, the overarching message is clear: Maintaining balanced blood sugar levels can create a more favorable foundation for fertility and a healthy pregnancy.

A Word on Bioidentical Hormones and Peptides

When preparing for conception, many individuals are advised to explore treatments such as hormone replacement, including bioidentical hormone therapy and peptides. While these treatments can be beneficial for specific conditions, it's critical to approach them with caution during the preconception period. I have one patient who comes to mind immediately when I think about this subject, because when he came to me, he'd been prescribed a wide array of peptides and testosterone replacement. But his physician wasn't monitoring his labs regularly. When I ordered some tests, the results were alarming. His hormones had gotten totally out of whack. Thankfully, we were able to get him straightened out, but I often share his story as a cautionary tale.

As we've been discussing, your body's hormonal balance plays a significant role in fertility and overall reproductive health, and introducing exogenous hormones or peptides can complicate this delicate balance. Therefore, it's essential to first explore the root causes of any hormonal imbalances through comprehensive, precision testing before jumping to treatments.

Like detectives, we aim to discover the *core* of a hormonal issue, allowing for more targeted and safer approaches to treatment. Sometimes—if not most of the time—lifestyle factors, nutrient deficiencies, environmental toxins, or underlying medical conditions are contributing to the imbalance. Precision testing, such as hormone panels, genetic assessments, and gastrointestinal health evaluations, help us uncover these hidden factors. Addressing them naturally through dietary, lifestyle, or targeted nutritional interventions— rather than jumping straight to hormone replacement—is often more conducive to optimizing health for conception.

Moreover, bioidentical hormone therapy and peptides, while often marketed as "natural" or "safe," can still introduce synthetic elements into the body that may disrupt the hormonal environment necessary for conception. During preconception, your body is preparing to create and then support new life, and even small disruptions can affect fertility, egg and sperm quality, or hormonal harmony. Engaging in such therapies without fully understanding the body's baseline state could inadvertently hinder your chances of conception.

I recommend avoiding these types of interventions during the preconception period unless absolutely necessary. Instead, focus on creating a fertile and balanced environment through the methods we've been discussing, and give your body the best chance to conceive naturally.

Final Thoughts

In the grand orchestration of life, few things are as awe-inspiring as conception itself—a process so intricate and finely tuned that it leaves little doubt about the majesty at work. Hormones are the silent conductors of this symphony, guiding every step, every transformation, and every new beginning. These chemical messengers regulate everything from the maturation of eggs and sperm to the moment of fertilization and the complex dance of genetic material that follows.

The Every Baby Well program outlined throughout the book is designed to do more than just improve fertility—it's here to harmonize your body's hormones so that all these delicate processes can occur as they are designed to. We've explored how to optimize everything from stress response optimization to nutritional intake, all with one goal in mind: creating an environment in which your hormones can perform their essential roles seamlessly. By aligning your body's internal systems, you're not only increasing your chances of conception but also giving your future child the healthiest possible start in life.

By focusing on harmonizing your hormones and preparing your body, you are laying the groundwork for the miraculous transformation that is about to take place—one that begins with a single, awe-inspiring moment and extends into the lifelong journey of parenthood.

Q&A

Q: I'm having regular periods. Isn't this a sign that everything is OK and I don't need to really be concerned about the information in this chapter?

A: While regular periods are a good sign, and an indicator that your hormones like estrogen and progesterone are probably functioning well enough to have a cycle, this isn't the whole story. Thyroid imbalances can occur even if menstrual cycles are regular. Insulin resistance can also exist alongside regular periods but can lead to several conditions like PCOS. Also, stress hormones can lead to an increase in cortisol, which causes several other issues with fertility.

Q: I'm a man, and everything seems to be functioning perfectly. Do I need to be concerned about any of this?

A: While signs of a hormone imbalance might be subtler in men, there are several hormones and imbalances that will contribute to fertility issues. Some of these may be easier to see, such as your stress levels, while others are not as noticeable.

Q: What about hormone treatments?

It's critical to approach any hormone treatment with caution, especially during the preconception period. Introducing exogenous hormones or peptides can complicate this delicate balance. Don't just jump to treatments—seek more advice and then make an informed decision.

THRIVE

CHAPTER 12

Taming Inflammation

You've seen the term "inflammation" mentioned many times in this book, and that's because if your body is fighting chronic inflammation, it will negatively impact your ability to conceive a healthy child. If you're inflamed, then the epigenetics you pass onto your child will also be impacted. And that's not all; you'll also have higher chances of complications during pregnancy. So, long story short: Taming chronic inflammation is mission critical.

An analogy I like to use when talking about inflammation has to do with a fireplace. Imagine a lovely, glowing fire in the living room fireplace. It's perfectly contained and as a result, perfectly enjoyable. But then imagine a spark escapes the fireplace and sets the furniture nearby on fire. It quickly spreads and before you know it, the whole living room is engulfed in flames. Now, imagine that you or the fire department couldn't contain it fast enough, so it spreads to other homes and suddenly, the entire neighborhood is on fire. Maybe you recall the Los Angeles fires in 2025 . . . now, that was a seriously terrifying fire. And that's exactly how inflammation can get wildly out of control in your body, causing all kinds of damage in its path.

There are many potential sources for inflammation, and we'll explore a lot of them in various ways throughout this book. But in this chapter specifically, I want to draw your attention to a few common—and unexpected—causes of inflammation that I often see in my practice. These include histamine imbalance, oxalate overload, and autoimmunity. I really want you to know about these key sources of inflammation because they are often overlooked or ignored, and I suspect they contribute to many, if not most, cases of subfertility. Let's dig in!

Questions to Consider

You might be surprised when you look at this list of questions. Most of these may seem to be unrelated or benign, but the answers could be the result of your body telling you something very important.

- Does your skin turn red easily?
- Do you experience bloating in your abdomen?
- Do you get rashes?
- Do you have allergies?
- Do you get migraine headaches?
- Do you have sensitivities to some foods?
- Do you get brain fog?
- Do you experience fluctuating anxiety or insomnia?

If you answered yes to any of these questions, it's possible that underlying inflammation is playing a role in your overall health—and possibly affecting your fertility more than you realize.

Why Inflammation Matters for Preconception

When inflammation becomes chronic, it acts like a low-grade fire throughout the body. Over time, this fire damages cells, tissues, and even DNA.[443] In the reproductive system, inflammation can interfere with hormone signaling, damage egg and sperm quality, impair embryo implantation, and increase the risk of pregnancy complications.[444]

In fact, broader fertility trends reflect just how important this is. In 2023, the general fertility rate in the United States dropped by 3 percent from the previous year, reaching a historic low according to the CDC's National Center for Health Statistics. From 2014 to 2020, the rate consistently decreased by 2 percent annually.[445] Although many factors are involved, hidden inflammation is one of the underlying forces silently affecting fertility across populations.

Learning how to detect and calm inflammation gives you a profound opportunity: It allows you to optimize your body's ability to create new life—and to pass on healthier genetic and epigenetic patterns to your child.

Dr. Jeff Bland and the Root Cause of Disease

One of the first lectures I attended after residency to pursue additional training (around 2004) was taught by Dr. Jeff Bland, the father of functional medicine. During that weekend-long lecture, he spoke about inflammation—and how it is linked to nearly every major disease: diabetes, cancer, osteoporosis, heart disease, autoimmunity, dementia, and more.

The information was so data-rich and compelling, it felt as if I were drinking from a firehose! That lecture completely changed my approach to medicine. Instead of just treating symptoms, I began looking for the root causes of disease—and restoring true balance. Dr. Bland continues to be one of my favorite teachers, mentors, and humans to this day.

Detecting Inflammation

There are many ways to detect excess inflammation. It's incredibly helpful to monitor a few markers during your preconception work so that progress can be measured not just by how you feel, but by what's happening biologically.

Here are some of the lab markers I commonly check for inflammation:

- C-Reactive Protein (CRP)
- High-sensitivity C-Reactive Protein (hs-CRP)
- Erythrocyte Sedimentation Rate (ESR)
- White Blood Cell Count (WBC)
- Ferritin (can rise with inflammation)
- Fibrinogen
- Platelet Count
- Albumin (can decrease during inflammation)
- Procalcitonin (specific for bacterial infections)
- Complement Components (C3, C4)
- Autoimmune Antibodies (e.g., ANA, RF, and more)
- Cytokine Panels (IL-1β, IL-6, IL-10, TNF-α, IL-17, IL-23)

Markers specific to gut inflammation include:

- Calprotectin
- Lactoferrin
- Zonulin (marker of gut permeability)

Advanced testing markers include (see more in the appendix):

- Lipid Peroxidases
- 8 hydroxy 2' deoxguanosine
- Myeloperoxidase
- LpPla2
- Glutathione

We'll explore a few of these in more detail throughout the book, but know that your functional medicine practitioner can help you order any of these labs if needed. (For an even deeper dive into specialized inflammation and oxidative stress markers, see the appendix material for this chapter.) It's important to check for several of these markers and, if elevated, find the root causes and take action until they are reduced into the normal range.

Hidden Drivers of Inflammation in Preconception

In my clinical practice, there are three major drivers of inflammation that are often overlooked that I want you to know about as you prepare your body for pregnancy:

- Histamine Imbalance
- Oxalate Overload
- Autoimmune Processes

Let's take a closer look at each.

Histamine Imbalance: If you've ever had seasonal allergies, you're probably very familiar with a class of over-the-counter medications called antihistamines. (I live in Austin, Texas, and some people refer to it as the allergy capital of the world because we have such dense pollen, especially in the winter!) The reason these medicines work to slow down your allergic response to pollen in the air is because they block your body from overproducing a chemical known as histamines (hence "anti" histamines). But the mere fact that your immune system is having an overreaction to the pollen indicates that you likely have a histamine imbalance. And as it turns out, a histamine imbalance has a direct impact on reproductive health! It's an area of research that is still emerging.

When thinking about histamines, there are two conditions that can have a profound influence on hormonal balance, menstrual cycles, implantation, and pregnancy outcomes. They are histamine intolerance (HIT) and mast cell activation syndrome (MCAS).

Histamine Intolerance (HIT): In simple terms, histamine intolerance (HIT) happens when your body has trouble breaking down histamines, and as a result, too many build up.[446] Histamine is normally a good thing—your body uses it to fight off germs, help with digestion, and regulate things like blood flow. It's also found in certain foods, especially things such as aged cheese, wine, smoked meats, and fermented foods. But if you don't break down histamine properly (usually because the enzyme that clears it out—called histamine-n-methyltransferase (HNMT), which is inside the cells and high in the brain, liver, kidney and bones, and DAO, which is outside cells and mostly in the gut—isn't working well), histamine can pile up and cause a bunch of annoying symptoms. Some reasons why they may not be working well are genetic predispositions and nutrient deficiencies such as B6, B12, magnesium, and folate. Here are some symptoms you might experience:

- Headaches or migraines
- Hives or itchy skin
- Stuffy nose or sneezing
- Stomach pain, bloating, heart burn, or diarrhea
- Feeling dizzy or lightheaded
- Flushing or feeling hot

It can look a lot like allergies—but it's not caused by pollen or pets. It's more about how your body is handling (or not handling) something that's already inside you.

Evelyn's Battle with Histamines: Evelyn was a thirty-three-year-old patient who struggled with cyclical migraines, severe PMS, and irregular menstrual cycles. Her lab work revealed low DAO levels and a MTHFR mutation that impaired her ability to break down histamine effectively. We implemented a low-histamine diet, added DAO supplementation and vitamin C, and incorporated a limbic retraining program to help regulate her stress response. Over the next several months, her symptoms dramatically improved—her cycles became regular, her migraines and PMS lessened significantly, and she conceived naturally six months after starting the protocol.

Mast Cell Activation Syndrome: Mast cells are special immune cells in your body—they're like little emergency alarm systems. When they detect a threat (such as an infection or injury), they release chemical signals, such as histamine, to trigger swelling, alert your immune system, and help you heal. Mast cells are prevalent in the female and male reproductive tract and play a role in fertility and even labor.[447] In Mast Cell Activation Syndrome (MCAS), the mast cells start sounding the alarm. They go a little haywire—releasing too many chemicals such as histamine, tryptase, prostaglandins, cytokines inappropriately or excessively—which makes you feel sick even though nothing major is wrong. Because mast cells are in lots of places (skin, gut, lungs, brain), MCAS symptoms can show up almost anywhere, such as:

- Flushing, hives, rashes
- Abdominal pain, diarrhea, nausea
- Racing heart, low blood pressure
- Dizziness
- Breathing problems (like asthma)
- Brain fog
- Fatigue
- Anxiety or weird allergy-like reactions
- Muscle aches
- Insomnia
- Headaches
- Musculoskeletal pain
- Bladder pain
- Sensitivity to many substances

THRIVE

Being aware of the influence of histamines on these mechanisms can be crucial for optimizing preconception health and fertility both for you and your partner. It's important to get to the root of the reason the body is sounding the alarm. Possible triggers include temperature extremes, strong scents, pollution, mold, and other toxins (metals, pesticides, PFAS, BPA). Food additives, high histamine foods, alcohol, and acute infections or low-grade chronic infections can keep the mast cells in a constant state of reactivity. Chronic physical or emotional stress can also activate mast cells. For some people medications such as NSAIDS, opioids, contrast dyes, and some antibiotics can provoke mast cells.

The Fungal-Histamine Connection: There is a link between fungal overgrowth and histamine dysregulation, which is often an underappreciated driver. Certain fungi, including the *Candida* species, directly produce histamine as a metabolic byproduct, can trigger immune responses that activate mast cells, and impair the function of DAO. As mentioned in this book elsewhere, fungi alter the gut microbiome balance, which in this case also reduces the population of the types of bacteria that help regulate histamine levels.

Histamines, Hormones, and Fertility: Histamine itself is not the villain. It acts as both a neurotransmitter and immune modulator. In reproduction, it has some positive roles: enhancing blood flow, immune regulation (supporting embryo acceptance), and uterine contractility (supports the uterine contractions necessary for implantation). However, it's the build-up of histamine that leads to negative aspects such as inflammation, which I touched on earlier. There is also the risk of an immune imbalance where overactive histamine responses may trigger immune attacks on the embryo. Too much histamine increases blood vessel permeability, which can potentially hinder embryo attachment (vascular permeability).

So it's about getting the balance right. Let's take a closer look at how histamine interacts intimately with reproductive hormones:

- **Estrogen stimulates histamine release** and inhibits the enzyme DAO (which breaks down histamine).
- **Progesterone counteracts histamine**, calming inflammation.

Because of this, women with hormonal imbalances (especially estrogen dominance) often experience worsened histamine symptoms around ovulation and menstruation.

During pregnancy, the placenta produces large amounts of DAO—naturally lowering histamine levels. However, if DAO is low from the beginning, the risk of miscarriage or pregnancy complications can rise.

Symptoms that suggest a histamine-hormone issue might include:

- Severe menstrual cramps
- Cyclical migraines
- Fluctuating anxiety
- Fertility challenges without obvious cause

For a deeper dive into histamine genetics, mast cell stabilization strategies, and advanced supplement protocols, refer to the appendix material for this chapter.

Wyatt's Mast Cell Story: Wyatt was thirty-seven years old when he came to me after experiencing unexplained low sperm motility and difficulty conceiving with his partner. Through deeper evaluation, we uncovered signs of Mast Cell Activation Syndrome (MCAS), which was contributing to chronic inflammation in his body. His treatment plan included natural mast cell stabilizers like quercetin and luteolin, methylation support, and DAO supplementation. After five months of targeted therapy, his sperm motility improved significantly, and he and his partner were able to conceive naturally.

HIT vs. MCAS Treatment Comparison: Just to help you understand some of the nuances between histamine intolerance and mast cell activation syndrome, here is a chart with a closer look at the comparison.

Category	Histamine Intolerance (HIT)	Mast Cell Activation Syndrome (MCAS)
Dietary Changes	Low-histamine diet (avoid aged/fermented foods, alcohol, leftovers)	Low-histamine, low-oxalate, low-salicylate diet (individualized)
DAO Support	DAO enzyme supplements, vitamin C, vitamin B6, copper	Supportive only if concurrent HIT (DAO, Vitamin C)
Antihistamines (H1 Blockers)	Loratadine, Cetirizine (used symptomatically)	Loratadine, Cetirizine, Hydroxyzine, Fexofenadine (often daily)
Antihistamines (H2 Blockers)	Famotidine, Ranitidine (optional if gut symptoms present)	Famotidine, Nizatidine, Ranitidine (for GI and systemic support)
Mast Cell Stabilizers	Not typically required unless symptoms overlap with MCAS	Cromolyn sodium, Ketotifen, luteolin, sodium cromoglycate
Anti-inflammatory Nutrients	Quercetin, vitamin C, omega-3s	Quercetin, luteolin, curcumin, omega-3s
Other Pharmaceuticals	Occasionally cromolyn sodium or Ketotifen if overlap with MCAS	Montelukast, low-dose Naltrexone, sometimes Omalizumab or antihistamine combos
Gut Support	Treat SIBO, dysbiosis, support mucosa with L-glutamine, probiotics	Address gut permeability, mold, parasites, chronic infections
Lifestyle Strategies	Stress reduction, sleep hygiene, avoid histamine-releasing triggers	Pacing yourself, trigger tracking, EMF and toxin reduction, trauma-informed care

Preconception Support for Inflammation

You can immediately begin combating inflammation by following this simple table, highlighting a daily supplement routine.

Time of Day	Supplement	Details
Morning	Vitamin C + quercetin	500 mg + 500 mg to stabilize mast cells. *Quercetin has antioxidant and anti-inflammatory effects, combined with vitamin C's antioxidant properties.*
Before meals	DAO enzyme	Take before breakfast, lunch, and dinner, especially if consuming high-histamine foods as DAO enzyme can break the histamine down.
Afternoon	Magnesium + Zinc + Glutathione	200 mg + 15 mg. This combination supports overall health by enhancing immune function and promoting antioxidant activity (also great for improving sleep). Magnesium and zinc work very well together, especially combined with the strong antioxidant properties of liposomal glutathione.
Evening	Vitamin C + quercetin	500 mg + 500 mg to stabilize mast cells again.
Throughout	Hydration + stress response optimization	Stay hydrated; practice stress response optimization techniques that work for you.

Oxalate Overload: A Hidden Barrier to Fertility

In the intricate world of fertility, one surprising (and often overlooked) contributor to inflammation and reproductive dysfunction is oxalate overload. Oxalates are naturally occurring compounds found in many healthy foods—such as spinach, almonds, beets, and sweet potatoes. In healthy metabolism, oxalates are broken down or excreted efficiently, thus small amounts are handled easily by the body. But in certain individuals, when oxalates accumulate (due to high dietary intake, poor gut health, nutrient deficiencies, or genetic factors), they can:

- Damage tissues (such as kidneys, joints, bladder, reproductive organs) through crystal formation
- Trigger immune responses and inflammasome activation
- Create or increase oxidative stress that injures DNA, mitochondria, and cell membranes
- Disrupt calcium and mineral balance crucial for cellular health
- Cause gut permeability ("leaky gut")

Symptoms of oxalate overload may include:

- Chronic joint and muscle pain
- Digestive issues (bloating and discomfort)
- Urinary discomfort
- Vaginal irritation (without infection)
- Fatigue, despite rest
- Brain fog or difficulty concentrating
- Skin rashes or hives

These symptoms are often attributed to other conditions (or dismissed entirely), so oxalate overload often goes undetected unless specifically considered and tested.

In the context of fertility, high oxalate levels have been associated with:

- Ovarian dysfunction
- Endometrial inflammation

- Impaired embryo implantation
- Increased miscarriage risk
- Poor sperm quality and DNA fragmentation

Because oxalates can deposit in reproductive tissues, they may contribute to unexplained infertility. For a deeper dive into oxalate metabolism, advanced testing, and step-by-step therapeutic protocols, refer to the appendix material for this chapter.

How Fungi Contribute to Oxalate Burden

One of the most intriguing and clinically significant connections is the relationship between fungal overgrowth and oxalate metabolism. Fungi can increase oxalate levels through multiple pathways. *Candida*, for example, directly produces oxalates as metabolic byproducts.[448] Fungi also possess enzymes that convert certain compounds into oxalates,[449] and fungal overgrowth reduces the beneficial bacteria that help degrade oxalates in our intestinal tracts. The most alarming reality is there is a bidirectional relationship—fungal overgrowth that increases oxalate production and absorption, while elevated oxalates may support continued fungal growth.

Managing Oxalates

Reducing oxalates too quickly can cause "oxalate dumping," a sudden release of stored oxalates that can temporarily worsen symptoms. A slow, steady approach is best.

General strategies include:

- Moderate (not extreme) reduction of high-oxalate foods such as almonds, beets, sweet potato, chocolate, and kale.
- Calcium citrate intake with meals to bind oxalates in the gut and prevent absorption.

- Magnesium supplementation to support cellular function and reduce inflammation, taken at bedtime or another time of day when you haven't recently eaten. (Potassium citrate or magnesium citrate can bind calcium, reducing its availability for oxalate binding.)
- Optimizing hydration (at least 2.5–3 liters of water per day)
- Supporting gut health
- Supplementing vitamin B6 and probiotics

Moderating oxalates intelligently—not fearfully—is an essential part of restoring healthy inflammatory balance and optimizing reproductive health. For a full clinical guide to oxalate metabolism, fertility impacts, and therapeutic protocols, see the appendix material for this chapter.

Autoimmunity and Fertility: The Hidden Threat

Perhaps the most overlooked driver of inflammation affecting fertility is autoimmunity—especially the early, silent forms of it that evade traditional diagnosis.[450] Autoimmunity occurs when the immune system mistakenly attacks the body's own tissues. Reactivity exists on a spectrum. At one end are full-blown autoimmune diseases such as lupus and Hashimoto's thyroiditis, while at the other end there is optimal immune function. In between is the area of autoimmune dysregulation. Even without a formal diagnosis, many individuals experience "subclinical autoimmunity"—a state of immune imbalance that can interfere with fertility years before any disease is officially diagnosed.[451] In this state:

- Immune systems are improperly activated.
- Tissues experience low-grade inflammation.
- Reproductive health quietly suffers.

Autoimmunity and Subclinical Inflammation

Although there may not be any symptoms, you could still have a positive lab test that lets you know there is an underlying issue brewing. Signs that you might have subtle autoimmune activity include:

- Low energy
- Brain fog
- Unexplained joint or muscle pain
- Skin rashes
- Digestive problems
- Infertility without clear cause

How Autoimmunity Disrupts Fertility

Subclinical autoimmune activation can affect fertility at multiple levels:

- **Ovarian Health:** Inflammation can damage ovarian follicles, impairing egg quality and ovulation.[452]
- **Endometrial Receptivity:** The endometrial lining must be finely balanced between defense and acceptance. Inflammation skews this balance, reducing the chance of embryo implantation.[453]
- **Sperm Function:** Autoimmune factors can damage sperm motility, morphology, and DNA integrity.[454]
- **Hormonal Signaling:** Chronic inflammation interferes with the delicate communication between the brain, ovaries/testes, and reproductive tract.[455]
- **Placental Development:** Early immune imbalance increases the risk of miscarriage, preeclampsia, and growth restriction.[456]

Interestingly, a 2023 study showed a 24.4 percent prevalence of antinuclear antibody (ANA) positivity in women with unexplained infertility, compared to 8.5 percent in fertile women.[457] I think the data is clear; autoimmunity, even subclinical, needs to be addressed prior to receiving the "green light" for conception.

Detecting Subclinical Autoimmunity

Here are some key tests that can help assess any hidden autoimmune activity:

- **High-sensitivity C-reactive protein (hs-CRP):** Elevated even when traditional CRP is normal.
- **Antinuclear antibodies (ANA):** Even low-titer positives can signal risk.
- **Double stranded DNA antibodies:** This is basically an antibody to your own DNA. It's the main marker for lupus, for example, and just because you have it doesn't mean you have lupus. But catching the marker early means you can reverse it before the disease process begins, and I've even had patients with full-blown lupus who have been able to reverse it. We can discover all this information through a regular blood test; it's the autoimmune blood test that reveals this along with ten other markers.
- **Anti-thyroid antibodies (TPO, TG, TR):** Linked to infertility even if thyroid hormones are normal. Again, this is typically reversible by following the suggestions we're talking about in this chapter.
- **Antiphospholipid and Anticardiolipin antibodies:** These are when the autoimmune attacks the cell membranes, and this is a huge area of risk for fertility because it can cause blood clots, recurrent miscarriages, stillborn, and preeclampsia

among other things, due to placental insufficiency. I know firsthand this can be reversed—because I had it!

- **Full autoimmune panel** (smooth muscle, Sjogren's, RNP [ribonucleoprotein antibodies], and so forth). See the appendix for more detail.
- **Gut permeability markers:** Zonulin, LPS, or bacterial toxin markers suggesting leaky gut—an ignition point for autoimmunity.

For an expanded list of autoimmune and inflammatory testing options, refer to the appendix material for this chapter.

Healing Autoimmunity Before Conception

The extraordinary news is this: Autoimmune processes are reversible—especially at early stages. Your body is built to heal. You can calm your immune system, heal your gut, clear hidden infections, balance your hormones, and restore reproductive health.

Key strategies include:

- **Anti-inflammatory nutrition:** Rich in colorful vegetables, clean proteins, and healthy fats.
- **Gluten- and dairy-free:** Gluten and animal dairy are key drivers in autoimmunity. It is essential and foundational to avoid them meticulously. Vibrant zoomer or enterolab tests are the most reliable ways of testing how big the impact will be.
- **Methylation support:** Optimizing folate, B12, B6, and other methylation nutrients to modulate immune tolerance.
- **Microbiome restoration:** Repairing gut integrity to prevent immune triggers.
- **Environmental detoxification:** Reducing exposure to toxins such as endocrine disruptors, mold, heavy metals, and

enhancing detoxification pathways to lower the body stores of toxins. See chapter 6.

- **Remove hidden infections:** Treat with nutraceuticals, pharmaceuticals, and/or alternative therapies.

- **Stress regulation:** Lowering cortisol dysregulation that fuels inflammation.

- **Targeted supplementation:** Using omega-3s, curcumin, resveratrol, glutathione, and other natural immune modulators.

Addressing autoimmunity before conception gives your future child the greatest possible gift: a healthier start at the genetic and epigenetic level.

Hidden Autoimmunity

Mark and Zoe got married at thirty-four years old and came into my office wanting to optimize their health before trying for their first child, rather than gambling that everything would be OK. They were already doing a lot of things right, and felt good, but they just lacked the data from testing. Zoe's lab work came back positive for DSDNA, a marker for lupus, but she didn't have any serious symptoms. Over the next six months, we also found she had gluten sensitivity, elevated heavy metals, some nutrient deficiencies, and elevated candida. We're working through it all now, and I'm very optimistic!

Inflammation and Epigenetics

Chronic low-grade inflammation doesn't just impact your ability to conceive; it can also alter gene expression through epigenetic mechanisms. Here are just a few ways this can occur:

- **Impacts on Eggs and Sperm:** Oxidative stress and inflammation associated with oxalate burden can alter epigenetic marks in both eggs and sperm.[458]

- **Embryonic Development:** Altered epigenetic programming in gametes can influence early embryonic development and placental development.[459]
- **Offspring Health Programming:** Epigenetic changes transmitted through the germline may influence health outcomes in offspring, including metabolic function, inflammatory regulation, and potentially even reproductive capacity.[460]

The health of your future child is on the line. Healing underlying immune dysregulation before conception is one of the most powerful gifts you can give your next generation.

Final Thoughts

Inflammation is not just an obstacle to conception. It's a messenger—a signal from your body that something needs attention, healing, and balance. By tuning in to these signals early, you're not just improving your own fertility journey—you're shaping the epigenetic future of your family tree. Taming inflammation is not about suppressing symptoms with quick fixes. It's about reclaiming the extraordinary healing intelligence built into your body—supporting it, guiding it, and unleashing its ability to create life.

Through understanding hidden drivers like histamine imbalance, oxalate overload, and autoimmune activation, you now have powerful tools to:

- Calm chronic inflammation
- Optimize egg and sperm health
- Enhance implantation success
- Reduce pregnancy complications
- Pass on healthier genetic expressions to the next generation

Taming inflammation isn't about eliminating it altogether—your body needs inflammation for healing and defense! The focus is on regaining healthy control, ensuring inflammation rises when needed and resolves efficiently afterward. Your body's ability to heal and rebalance is extraordinary. With knowledge, testing, and targeted strategies, you can extinguish the hidden fires that threaten fertility—and build something beautiful in their place.

Q&A

Q: How can I tell if inflammation is affecting my fertility?

A: Symptoms such as irregular cycles, pelvic pain, bloating, fatigue, headaches, and skin issues can all be subtle signs. Specialized lab testing—such as hs-CRP, cytokine panels, gut health assessments, and markers for histamine or oxalate imbalance—can reveal deeper causes.

Q: What are some everyday habits that contribute to inflammation?

A: High-sugar diets, chronic stress, poor sleep, exposure to environmental toxins, gut dysbiosis, and eating a lot of processed or inflammatory foods can all quietly stoke inflammation over time.

Q: Is it enough to just take an anti-inflammatory supplement such as cucurmin?

A: While supplements like curcumin can help, they aren't a substitute for addressing root causes such as infections, food triggers, gut health issues, and hormone imbalances. A comprehensive approach is key.

Q: Can calming inflammation really improve my fertility even if I don't have a diagnosis?

A: Absolutely. Reducing inflammation improves egg and sperm quality, enhances implantation, balances hormones, and creates a more receptive environment for pregnancy—whether you have a formal diagnosis or not.

THRIVE

Q: How long does it take to see improvements after working on inflammation?

A: Many people notice changes within a few weeks, but true cellular and epigenetic healing often takes three to six months. Patience and consistency are crucial in this journey.

CHAPTER 13

Fertility GPS: Navigating Your Reproductive Journey

I had been working with Bob, one of my patients, for years to optimize his health and help him overcome some chronic issues he'd been struggling with. Despite his busy work schedule and the weight of his responsibilities at his company, Bob was diligent about following the protocol, and his lab work was improving steadily.

During this process, he met the woman of his dreams, and they were head over heels for each other. He was forty-seven years old, and he felt he had been so focused on building his business that he'd been ignoring his biological clock, but suddenly it was ticking quite loudly. Bob knew he was ready to be a father.

After Bob got married, his wife came to see me, and it didn't take long for her to become "super fertile" just from doing a little work (I'm telling you—it can happen fast!). They quickly got pregnant with their first child—a boy—and they were thrilled. After she gave birth and they'd settled comfortably into their role as parents, they thought they'd try for one more. About eighteen months later, his wife was pregnant again, this time with a girl. They were on cloud nine.

During her second pregnancy, they received news that rocked their world—Bob had prostate cancer. Suddenly, he needed to divert some of the attention he was giving to his family and career to his own healing. All the roles that he played in life came into sharp focus. He knew he had to step back from his position at his company for a time, and his wife was able to lean into their community so Bob could take care of himself. I'm happy to report that he did make a complete recovery from cancer.

I share this with you at the start of this chapter on fertility because I want to set the tone for this conversation by reminding you that you are not the roles you play in life. You might hold a position as a CEO, a business owner, or an employee. You might be a daughter or a son or a friend, neighbor, leader, teacher, wife, or husband—but those are just roles you play. They do not define *you*. You are something far beyond all of this—even beyond the physical body that you're in. Keep that in mind as you prepare to invite a new baby into your family.

It's easy to get caught up in the mechanics of reproduction—even to the point of obsession, which can certainly take all the fun out of it. It's also easy to lose your identity in your pursuit of parenthood, especially if this will be your first child. I've had patients tell me they simply won't know who they are if they cannot become a mother. And I've had patients tell me they were "meant to be" a family of five, and they wouldn't be at peace until they had that last child. But those points of view put so much unnecessary pressure on everyone, often making the desire for children the sole defining factor of one's identity and self-worth.

I encourage you to remember that regardless of whether this journey culminates in bringing new life into this world, you are an exquisite work of art. You are precious. You are more than just your body or your roles—you are a soul. And never forget—your identity is not defined by your ability to conceive or the number of children you have, but by the unique, irreplaceable person you are at your core.

The Truth About Women's Age and Fertility

It's completely understandable if concerns about fertility are weighing heavy on your mind. Even if you haven't experienced fertility challenges firsthand, the increasing prevalence of infertility can make it difficult not to worry. It's only natural to find yourself wondering about your ability to conceive and sustain a healthy pregnancy in today's world. According to the WHO, one in six people worldwide experience infertility at some point in their lives.[461] Infertility is defined as the failure to achieve pregnancy after twelve months or more of regular, unprotected sexual intercourse, and it can result from a range of male and female factors[462]—many of which we've already addressed in various ways throughout this book.

I've designed this chapter to help you navigate the complex and often overwhelming landscape of fertility. The insights and unique perspectives I'll share here draw upon key principles discussed throughout this book—in other words, the decisions you make throughout your preconception journey have a direct impact on your fertility. Most importantly, woven throughout this discussion is something I often find to be missing regarding this topic—*hope.*

I think the mainstream conversation around women's fertility has caused so much unnecessary fear, and it's all centered upon the dreaded biological clock. For decades, women have been fighting against a deeply ingrained belief that if they wait too long before getting pregnant, their child will be disabled in some way, or that it's basically impossible for older women to have a normal, healthy child. There's even a label they've been given after a certain age (which is typically thirty-five)—"AMA," or advanced maternal age. Another not-so-subtle label is "geriatric pregnancy." In my opinion, this puts far too much weight on the age of the mother, which is only one small factor in the big picture of what it takes to create a healthy child. And in truth, it's a non-factor once you learn how to optimize your health.

All this worry and obsession with maternal age has led to a massive increase in the percentage of women choosing to freeze their eggs at a younger age, so they can use those eggs in IVF later when they are ready. According to the US Department of Health and Human Services, "Between 2012 and 2021, ART use has more than doubled and the number of infants born who were conceived through ART has increased by 50%. In 2021, an estimated 2.3% of all infants born in the United States were conceived using ART. Approximately 413,776 ART cycles were performed at 453 reporting clinics resulting in 112,088 pregnancies in the United States. Of these pregnancies, 86,146 ART-conceived infants were born in 2021."[463] Are women worried? I think the statistics say a resounding *yes*.

In recent years, a growing number of companies have even begun offering egg freezing as an employee benefit, framing it as their way of empowering women to prioritize their careers without compromising their future family plans. Major tech companies such as Apple and Meta led the charge in 2014, offering up to $20,000 for female employees to freeze their eggs.[464] Since then, other companies, including Google, eBay, and Uber, have followed suit, with many offering similar financial support for fertility preservation.[465] This benefit is often positioned as a way for women to "have it all" and delay motherhood while advancing their careers. However, it raises a complex question: Is this truly an empowering step forward for women in the workplace, or does it subtly reinforce the expectation that the ideal employee remains unencumbered by pregnancy or family responsibilities? While egg freezing can offer women more control over their reproductive timeline, critics argue that the focus should be on making workplaces more accommodating to parenthood rather than encouraging employees to delay it.[466]

You might have already gone the route of egg freezing, or plan to. It can be your backup plan, but I still prefer that you get your own body as healthy as possible and try to get pregnant naturally and keep those eggs as a backup plan. If you haven't yet frozen eggs and feel the urge to do so, go through the Every Baby Well program first so you can optimize the eggs that you do freeze.

Going back to the subject at hand—the collective fear around having a baby later in a woman's reproductive years—I'd like to point out something that easily gets lost. Children of moms who are thirty-five–plus years old are *not the only ones* who are born with genetic abnormalities or develop chronic health challenges. The truth is, these things can happen to a child born to a mother of *any* age. I know that Down syndrome comes to mind for many women thinking of having a baby in their late thirties or forties because many researchers have made the correlation. But I want to get you thinking differently about this by applying all the new information we have about the power of epigenetics. In other words, *don't let a few stats deter you from having a child into your forties.*

I hope you're sitting down because I'm about to say something that might shock you. After spending years working with couples to help them have the healthiest possible babies, and after closely reviewing the latest research on this topic, the age by which I suggest most women be finished having babies is forty-six. That's not a typo—it's true! I believe that, up until around that age (and barring any physiological barriers such as a fallopian tube issue in women or azoospermia, when there are no sperm present in the semen in men), you can absolutely prepare your body to carry and birth a beautiful, healthy, vibrant baby. So if you've been letting your age or the non-stop ticking of your biological clock stress you out, take a deep breath and let it go. (I recently had a patient who was told by her internist that she probably missed the window for fertility at age thirty-one. I will be sending her doctor a copy of this book!)

I know there are many years of conditioning that have gotten us to the place where we worry so much about having a baby past the age of thirty-five, but it is time to start deprogramming ourselves. There are many times in our lives when we discover that a closely held belief isn't serving us, or wasn't even true to begin with, and we have to do the work to hold up that belief, look at it objectively, and then choose to leave it behind. This is one of those times. Visualization techniques or adjusting your internal monologue to reflect your new belief can help. Whatever it takes, I hope you will do the work to change your mindset around what a "healthy" age is for conceiving a child. The truth is—there isn't any one age. It's truly all about the steps you and your partner are taking to optimize your health. In fact, when I'm working with women to generally improve their health, a by-product is a boost in their fertility. (I always warn them!)

The Big Drop

Historically, the average woman has birthed around five children or more, a trend seen across many countries including the US, UK, Russia, India, and China. (In my travels, I discovered that in Tanzania most families have a goal of at least six children.) However, starting in the 1950s, this pattern began to shift. Since 1965, the average has *halved*. Today, the average number of children born to a woman throughout her lifetime has dropped to fewer than 2.5 children globally.[467]

Researchers attribute this to several key factors. The empowerment of women through increased education and employment opportunities has given women greater control over family planning. Additionally, improvements in child mortality rates mean that parents no longer feel the need to have a large number of children to ensure that some survive. Rising costs associated with raising children have also played a significant role in reducing family sizes. But there's no doubt about it—this unprecedented global shift reflects profound social and economic changes that continue to shape fertility trends around the world.

You might still be wondering about the natural decline in fertility that women experience as they age. Yes, this does occur, largely due to the aging of our eggs. Egg depletion, or the decline in the number and quality of eggs (oocytes) as women age, is a natural process that starts before birth and continues throughout life, culminating in menopause. It might surprise you to learn that by the time a female is born, most of her eggs have already been depleted! And the process accelerates as she ages. While this process cannot be entirely stopped, some strategies may help slow down egg depletion and improve overall ovarian health.

A key factor in this process is *mitochondrial health*, which helps maintain the quality of oocytes. Mitochondria, which you probably know by now are the "powerhouses" of the cell, are directly responsible for generating the energy needed for cellular functions, including those vital for egg maturation and development. Studies have shown that mitochondrial function declines with age, leading to a reduction in mitochondrial DNA (mtDNA) and increased damage from oxidative stress, all of which contribute to diminished egg quality and ovarian reserve.[468]

Exciting research, however, indicates that we have more control over this aging process than we previously thought. That's why targeting mitochondrial health is a huge part of navigating your fertility journey; it can seriously help rejuvenate aging oocytes and extend reproductive longevity. Lifestyle modifications that reduce oxidative stress can support mitochondrial function and thus improve fertility outcomes if you're conceiving later in life.[469] Addressing mitochondrial dysfunction is thus a promising strategy for potentially mitigating the effects of time on reproductive health.

Many of the strategies we've been discussing throughout this book are designed to help boost your mitochondrial health. But a few of them seem to have the biggest impact on slowing down the depletion of your egg reserves:

- **Eat a healthy diet.** You've read it a few times by now, but your diet is critical. A nutrient-dense diet rich in antioxidants, such as vitamins C and E, folic acid, and omega-3 fatty acids, may protect eggs from oxidative stress, which is a big factor in aging. Flip back to chapter 7 for more specific information on fertility-friendly foods.

- **Get some exercise.** Regular moderate exercise can improve overall health and hormonal balance, contributing to better ovarian function. However, extreme exercise may negatively impact fertility, so moderation is key.

- **Avoid smoking.** I think it goes without saying, but *do not smoke or vape.* Smoking and vaping accelerate the depletion of ovarian follicles and can lead to earlier menopause. Cigarettes (and vape pens) contain chemicals that can damage oocytes and lead to premature aging of the ovaries.

- **Eliminate alcohol and caffeine.** Even moderate alcohol and caffeine intake may negatively impact ovarian health. I highly recommend eliminating these substances during your preconception window.

- **Optimize your weight.** Both underweight and overweight women may experience hormonal imbalances that can affect ovarian reserve and function. Maintaining a healthy weight can improve reproductive health and slow ovarian aging. Flip back to chapter 3 to find information on your ideal BMI.

- **Feed your mitochondria with coenzyme Q10 (CoQ10).** CoQ10 is an antioxidant that plays a role in cellular energy production, and its levels decrease with age. Research suggests that supplementation with CoQ10 may improve mitochondrial function in eggs, potentially improving egg quality in older women. One of the forms of CoQ10 I recommend is MitoQ, which I discussed in detail in chapter 9.

- **Take other supplements to rejuvenate mitochondria.** Phosphatidyl choline, L-carnitine, D-ribose, B vitamins, NAD+ (nicotinamide adenine dinucleotide), alpha-lipoic acid, liposomal glutathione, vitamin c, resveratrol, berberine, green tea, magnesium, omega-3 fatty acids, curcumin, quercetin, N-acetylcysteine, and melatonin are all recommended.

- **Supplement with DHEA (Dehydroepiandrosterone).** DHEA is a hormone that may improve ovarian function and egg quality in women with diminished ovarian reserve. Some studies have found that DHEA supplementation can increase the number of oocytes retrieved during IVF cycles, although more research is needed. I only recommend supplementing if your bloodwork shows you're deficient.

- **Consider inositol.** Myo-inositol and D-chiro-inositol are compounds that can improve insulin sensitivity and are often used to support women with PCOS. There is some evidence that inositol supplementation can also improve egg quality in older women. There's more information on this in chapter 9.

- **Reduce your exposure to environmental toxins.** Exposure to pollutants, endocrine disruptors, and other environmental toxins can accelerate egg depletion. Limiting exposure to harmful chemicals in everyday products, such as plastics (containing BPA), pesticides, and heavy metals, may help preserve ovarian health.

- **Optimize your stress response.** Chronic stress may impact hormonal balance, potentially affecting ovarian function. Practices such as yoga, meditation, and mindfulness can help manage stress and support hormonal health.

While egg depletion is a natural part of aging that cannot be completely halted, lifestyle modifications, dietary changes, and certain supplements may slow down the process and help maintain better egg quality. By taking these steps, you can actively support your reproductive health and give yourself the best chance for a healthy conception, no matter where you are in your conception journey.

Preventing Pregnancy Issues Now

All the recommendations I'm making to help boost your fertility can also help prevent some serious health-related pregnancy complications. And it's a good thing, because those complications are on the rise. According to the NIH, "The prevalence of chronic hypertension in pregnancy in the United States doubled from 2007–2021."[470] That's an alarming statistic, given how serious hypertension during pregnancy can be, putting both the mother and unborn baby at risk of death. Research indicates that the rate of preeclampsia diagnoses has been steadily increasing as well.[471] Preeclampsia is a pregnancy-related condition characterized by high blood pressure and signs of damage to organs, most often the liver and kidneys. It usually occurs after twenty weeks of pregnancy in women who had never had high blood pressure before. Preeclampsia can also be life-threatening for both the mother and the baby if not managed properly.

The Pregnancy Mortality Surveillance System, which is run by the CDC, reported that "pregnancy-related deaths in the United States increased from 7.2 deaths per 100,000 live births in 1987 to 24.9 deaths per 100,000 live births in 2020."[472] Why the rise? Well, I believe there are multiple factors at play. But certainly, certain factors put you at a greater risk—for instance, obesity. Plus, there are many subclinical conditions such as inflammation that can suddenly become a big problem once your body is dealing with the physical stress of pregnancy.

Again, this is why following the Every Baby Well program is so essential. It's better to discover and heal any condition that's festering under the surface *now* than run the risk of compromising your health or the health and viability of your unborn baby once you're pregnant.

The Truth About Men's Age and Fertility

So far, we've been focused on women's fertility, but you might also be wondering how age impacts male fertility. There isn't nearly as much conversation about this, and people generally believe that men can father healthy children throughout most of their lifetime. Though men can produce sperm throughout their lives, sperm quality does decline over time, and age-related factors can affect overall reproductive health. This decline isn't as rapid or predictable as it is in women, but it's important to understand the changes that occur in sperm as men age.

Sperm count, motility, and morphology all tend to decrease with age, starting around the mid-forties. Additionally, as men get older, sperm may accumulate more DNA damage, which can affect the ability to conceive and the health of future offspring. Studies show that older paternal age can be linked to an increased risk of genetic abnormalities and certain developmental disorders in children.

In 2022, researchers published a meta-analysis study in the journal *Human Reproduction Update*, aimed to examine global trends in sperm count (SC) and total sperm count (TSC) among men across all continents. Previously, the same researchers had discovered there was a clear decline in sperm count in North America, Europe, and Australia, and their aim was to discover whether the same thing was also happening in South/Central America, Asia, and Africa, and whether the global decline has continued into the twenty-first century. Their findings were alarming, to say the least.[473]

The study confirmed a significant global decline in SC and TSC between 1973 and 2018. On average, sperm concentration decreased by 51.6 percent, and total sperm count declined by 62.3 percent among unselected men (men not specifically chosen for fertility status).[474] The rate of decline has accelerated in recent years. From 1973 to 2000, the decline was 1.16 percent per year, but from 2000 onward, the decline has more than doubled to 2.64 percent per year.[475]

So, guys, don't just assume that your fertility is assured! However, as we've been discussing throughout the book, you can take steps to support your reproductive health and mitigate some of the age-related decline in sperm quality. Targeting overall health, reducing oxidative stress, and improving mitochondrial function in sperm cells are all important strategies. Here are some science-backed ways to optimize sperm health and fertility as you age:

- **Reduce exposure to environmental toxins.** Just like for women, limiting exposure to environmental toxins, including pesticides, heavy metals, and endocrine disruptors, can help protect sperm from damage. Avoiding plastics containing BPA and reducing exposure to industrial chemicals may preserve sperm health.

- **Eat a healthy diet.** A diet rich in antioxidants, such as vitamins C and E, zinc, selenium, and omega-3 fatty acids, can help reduce oxidative stress in sperm cells, improving motility and reducing DNA fragmentation. You'll find more detailed nutritional guidance in chapter 7.

- **Get exercise.** Regular moderate exercise supports overall health, improves testosterone levels, and enhances sperm motility. However, like with women, too much exercise—especially long-distance running or extreme endurance training—can negatively impact fertility. Stick to a balanced routine.

- **Avoid smoking.** Smoking has been linked to a significant decline in sperm quality. The toxins in cigarettes can damage sperm DNA, reduce motility, and lower sperm count, so quitting smoking is crucial for maintaining healthy sperm.

- **Limit alcohol and caffeine.** Excessive alcohol and caffeine consumption have been shown to negatively affect sperm parameters. For optimal fertility, it's best to eliminate these substances, especially during the preconception period.

- **Optimize your weight.** Being either overweight or underweight can lead to hormonal imbalances and affect sperm quality. Maintaining a healthy BMI can optimize testosterone levels and improve fertility.

- **Consider taking coenzyme Q10 (CoQ10).** Like in women, CoQ10 supplementation may improve sperm motility and concentration due to its role in energy production and antioxidant properties. I recommend MitoQ for its high bioavailability, as discussed in chapter 9.

- **Focus on folate.** Folate isn't just important for women—it plays a role in male fertility too. Men with a higher folate intake have been shown to have better sperm quality, with lower rates of DNA damage. I recommend the 5MTHF folate.

- **Improve your stress response.** Chronic stress can lead to hormonal imbalances and reduce sperm quality. Practices such as meditation, yoga, and mindfulness can help optimize stress levels, supporting reproductive health.

While men do not experience the same dramatic decline in fertility as women, sperm quality does diminish with age and studies show there is a global sperm crisis, where sperm counts overall are trending downward. By making proactive lifestyle changes, improving your diet, and incorporating key supplements, you can help maintain healthy sperm and support optimal fertility outcomes. Sperm testing through SpermQT may demonstrate the positive effects of implementing these strategies.

Whether you are a man or a woman, creating a strong connection with your body during the preconception period can be transformative. I recommend working on tuning into your intuition and learning to listen to the subtle signals your body sends. Your body constantly communicates through cues like changes in energy levels, mood shifts, and physical sensations, and by tuning in to these signals, you can gain insight into your reproductive health. This two-way communication can help you identify when your body is in balance or when adjustments may be needed to support optimal fertility.

Practices that we've talked about in earlier chapters, like mindful breathing, meditation, or body-awareness exercises, can help deepen this intuitive connection. By regularly checking in with how your body feels, you will start to understand its rhythms more clearly, allowing you to catch potential imbalances early. Trusting this intuition, paired with scientific tools like fertility trackers, can give you a fuller picture of your reproductive health and guide you toward a more natural, harmonious approach to conception.

Controlling Our Fertility

When birth control became widely available, our world changed in many ways because women were given the power to send a very clear signal to their bodies—and that signal is: *Do not get pregnant.* Some women send that signal for most of their reproductive lifetime—college, grad school, out in the workforce building a career, discovering who she is and what her goals are in life. And then suddenly, she meets "the one," they desire a family, and overnight she goes from telling her body absolutely, categorically *do not get pregnant* to telling her body—*get pregnant* now! Imagine how confusing that might be on a cellular level.

If you've been on birth control pills or even a hormonal intrauterine device for any length of time, I encourage you to give your body a little extra grace in preparing to conceive. The sooner you get off hormonal birth control, the better, *but* (and this is a very important "but") you need to give yourself plenty of time to do your lab work and follow the steps in this book before you even think about having unprotected sex with your partner. Remember, just because your body *can* get pregnant doesn't mean you *should* yet. Our goal is to optimize your and your partner's health to create the healthiest baby possible from an epigenetic perspective, and this process takes some time.

Of course, I understand you want to be able to have intimacy with your spouse. But until you have the green light to conceive, find a nonhormonal method of contraception, such as condoms. I know they aren't ideal, and there's evidence that some condoms contain PFAS.[476] But there are plenty of companies making condoms that don't contain forever chemicals and are just as effective.[477]

At-Home Ovulation Tests

Tracking your ovulation patterns can be a very helpful navigational tool on this fertility journey, and as I touched on in chapter 4, at-home ovulation kits can take the guesswork out of predicting your most fertile days. They can give you a comprehensive view of your fertility window in real time.[478]

These kits track LH and progesterone levels through daily urine tests. These hormones are crucial for understanding when ovulation is about to occur and whether your body is successfully transitioning through the luteal phase post-ovulation. It uses an easy-to-read color-coded system in the app, providing clear guidance on whether you're in your fertile window, approaching ovulation, or past it.

Sperm QT: Tracking Male Fertility

Fertility is a team effort, and understanding the man's reproductive health is just as important as tracking the woman's cycle. Sperm QT, which we discussed in chapter 4, is a user-friendly app and at-home sperm test designed to help men monitor key aspects of their sperm health, including motility, count, and morphology—all crucial factors for conception. Beyond that, Sperm QT "analyzes the sperm's genes to measure its ability to find, bind, penetrate, and fertilize an egg."[479]

With Sperm QT, you can easily self-track changes in sperm quality over time. The app provides personalized insights based on lifestyle factors like diet, exercise, and sleep, offering practical suggestions to optimize sperm health naturally. Additional sperm tests are becoming available as well, such as PSfertility. I'll keep you up

THRIVE

to date through the Every Baby Well website and preconception program on how well they work, and how to implement them into your plan.

My Controversial Stance on IVF

As I shared in the introduction, I faced infertility issues. I know first-hand how the pressure can be immense. I vividly recall getting so excited each month, and then feeling so let down when my period would arrive. I understand that fertility roller coaster and how gut-wrenching it can be.

When we were trying for our second child, I was working at a trauma hospital as a medical resident, and I was stressed out to the max. But I just knew my son needed a sibling. At one appointment my doctor looked at my labs and said, "This is not going to happen, Ann. You guys need to do IVF. There's no way you'll get pregnant." I resigned myself to the fact that he was probably right, so we decided to head in that direction. As soon as my next period started, I planned to get on birth control, which is the first step in egg harvesting. I waited and waited, until finally one morning, I decided to do a pregnancy test. It was positive! My husband was so shocked that he asked me to do another one.

Looking back, if I had it to do over again, I would not consider IVF so quickly. In recent years, the demand for fertility treatments like IVF has surged. According to the American Society for Reproductive Medicine, the number of babies born via IVF increased from 89,208 in 2021 to 91,771 in 2022, now making up 2.5 percent of all births in the US.[480] Additionally, the number of IVF cycles performed rose by over 6 percent during this period, reflecting a growing reliance on assisted reproductive technologies (ART).[481] While this growth shows that more people are seeking fertility solutions, I believe IVF should be considered a *last resort* for most couples.

One of the primary reasons I take this stance is that longitudinal studies have shown that IVF-conceived children can have a higher risk of birth defects, cancer, cardiovascular risks, and developmental issues than those conceived naturally. In one 2017 study, after accounting for factors such as preterm birth, maternal age, and pregnancy complications, researchers concluded that children conceived with fertility treatments have about twice the risk of developing tumors compared to naturally conceived children.[482] This increased risk was observed across both benign and malignant tumors, suggesting a potential link between the mode of conception and long-term health outcomes.[483]

A 2020 study looked at whether children conceived through fertility treatments such as IVF or ovulation induction are more likely to have long-term gastrointestinal health issues compared to those conceived naturally. Researchers tracked over 240,000 children and found that hospitalization rates for GI problems were higher among those conceived through fertility treatments, even after accounting for factors like birth weight, maternal health, and preterm delivery.[484] The findings suggest that IVF may be an independent risk factor for long-term digestive issues in children.[485]

Another study titled "Long-Term Effects of ART on the Health of the Offspring" examines the potential long-term health consequences for children conceived through ART, including IVF. The authors highlight several areas of concern:

- ART-conceived children may have a slightly increased risk of birth defects compared to naturally conceived children.
- Some studies suggest a higher prevalence of cancer among ART-conceived individuals, though findings are not consistent across all research.
- There is evidence indicating that ART-conceived children might be more susceptible to high blood pressure and other cardiovascular issues later in life.

- An increased risk of metabolic issues, such as insulin resistance and obesity, has been observed in some ART-conceived individuals.
- The procedures involved in ART, including hormonal treatments and the artificial environment during gamete and embryo manipulation, may lead to genomic and epigenetic alterations, potentially contributing to long-term health complications.[486]

But that's not all. An article titled "An umbrella review of meta-analyses regarding the incidence of female-specific malignancies after fertility treatment" reviews the potential long-term risks of fertility treatments (FT), such as IVF and ovulation induction, specifically concerning female-specific cancers such as ovarian, endometrial, breast, and cervical cancer. It found a statistically significant increase in the risk of ovarian cancer and borderline ovarian tumors among women who underwent FT, particularly IVF.[487] For ovarian cancer, the odds of developing the disease were about 1.21 times higher overall and 1.65 times higher with IVF specifically.[488] The use of certain fertility drugs, like clomiphene citrate (CC) and human menopausal gonadotropins (hMG), was also associated with an increased risk of these tumors.[489]

All this information emphasizes the need for ongoing research to fully understand these potential risks for the child as well as the mother, and to develop strategies to mitigate them. It also suggests that the underlying causes of infertility in parents may play a role in the observed health outcomes of ART-conceived children.

That leads me perfectly into my next point: I believe infertility often acts as a signal from the body. I think it's Mother Nature's way of telling you to "stop" and address underlying health issues before conceiving a child. There are often epigenetic factors that need to be resolved, and attempting to bypass these natural signals through IVF risks passing unresolved issues on to the baby. These issues could stem from nutrient deficiencies, hormonal imbalances, or chronic inflammation, all of which can influence both the mother's and the baby's long-term health. For instance, the health of the mother's mitochondria, which produce the energy necessary for cellular functions, plays a crucial role in egg quality and embryo development. If mitochondrial dysfunction is not addressed, it can lead to issues not only with conception but also with the child's health later in life. Essentially, IVF is a shortcut that allows couples to bypass the body's natural signals that it isn't ready to conceive, potentially leading to long-term health concerns for the baby.

Moreover, rushing into IVF may ignore the deeper root causes of infertility. Whether it's insulin resistance, chronic stress, or an autoimmune condition, there are often reversible factors at play that can be addressed through lifestyle changes, dietary improvements, and targeted therapies. I have found that when couples take six to eighteen months to optimize their health before pursuing IVF, many are able to conceive naturally, avoiding the need for invasive procedures altogether. This timeframe allows both partners to focus on reducing oxidative stress and addressing other underlying factors that contribute to fertility struggles. Through lifestyle changes, a reduction in exposure to toxins along with detoxification, improved nutrition, and precise medical testing, many fertility issues can be corrected naturally, giving you the best chance for a healthy (and far less expensive!) conception.[490]

That said, there are certain cases where IVF is a good option. For instance, if there is a physical issue like blocked fallopian tubes or azoospermia (where a man does not produce sperm), IVF or intrauterine insemination (IUI) can provide a solution. In these scenarios, IVF doesn't bypass nature's warnings but addresses a mechanical barrier to natural conception. However, for most people, IVF should *not* be the first option. Optimizing health and focusing on natural conception can provide a much safer path to starting a family, with fewer risks to future generations.

It's Supposed to be FUN: Finding the Joy in Preconception

The journey toward conception often comes with a mix of excitement and anxiety, but it's easy for the process to become more about stress than joy. Many couples find that the spontaneity of their relationship takes a back seat to ovulation tracking, and intimacy starts to feel like a task rather than a connection. For women, the monthly cycle of hope and disappointment can become an emotional roller coaster, leading to feelings of pressure and wondering if pregnancy will ever happen.

And these negative emotions can work against your goal of conceiving. As we've talked about, stress and anxiety can impact hormone levels and disrupt the delicate balance required for conception. That's why an essential part of your fertility journey is learning to let go, relax, and rediscover the fun. Finding moments of joy with your partner, whether through spontaneous date nights, playful activities, or simply appreciating each other outside the realm of baby-making, can help create a positive environment that is more conducive to conception. By embracing a lighter, more playful approach, you can turn the preconception phase into a time of connection and growth rather than a stressful countdown. Here's a list of ideas to help you maintain joy in the fertility journey:

- **Plan date nights unrelated to baby talk.** Set aside time each week for a date where the rule is to avoid talking about fertility or the baby-making process. Use this time to reconnect over activities you both enjoy—like trying a new restaurant, taking a dance class, or simply having a movie night at home.
- **Create a "just for fun" bucket list.** Make a list of activities or experiences you'd like to try together before becoming parents, or, if you already have kids, before inviting a new child into the family. It could include planning weekend

getaways, hiking new trails, or learning a new hobby. Focus on experiences that bring you closer and add adventure to your relationship.

- **Practice mindfulness/spirituality together.** Engage in activities like yoga, meditation, prayer, or deep breathing exercises as a couple. If you attend church, synagogue, or another house of worship, consider joining a small group or starting a study of the scriptures to complete as a couple. Not only do these types of activities help reduce stress, but they also allow you to focus on the present moment and appreciate the journey rather than just the destination.

- **Take a break from the apps.** Constantly tracking ovulation can make the process feel clinical and stressful. Take a month off from apps and calendars and allow for spontaneous intimacy, focusing on connecting with each other rather than hitting the perfect fertility window.

- **Set up a "monthly celebration" ritual.** Instead of dreading the arrival of a new cycle, create a ritual that celebrates each month you have together. This could be cooking a special dinner, writing down what you're grateful for, or planning a little indulgence, like a spa day or a weekend trip.

- **Make intimacy playful.** Bring the fun back into the bedroom by exploring new ways to connect that don't center around the goal of conception. Use this time to rediscover what you enjoy about each other and add a sense of playfulness to your intimate moments.

- **Celebrate the little wins.** Focus on small successes in your health and relationship. Maybe you've both adopted a healthier diet and lifestyle, are exercising more, or have found new ways to communicate better. Recognizing these wins, no matter how small, can help shift the focus from stress to gratitude and joy.

THRIVE

Communication Tools

Since I'm focusing on helping you navigate your fertility as a couple, I want to spend a little time getting you to think about your communication during preconception. This is a journey you're taking together, and strengthening the foundation of your partnership is the first stop before you can really form your specific "parentship" for this child you'll be inviting into your lives. With that in mind, here are some communication tools you can start to use right now to help you navigate toward a successful conception.

- **Schedule regular check-ins.** The process of trying to conceive can come with ups and downs, which can be emotionally taxing. To keep communication clear and honest, schedule regular check-ins with each other. These conversations can be a time to express how you're feeling about the process, discuss any frustrations, and share successes or changes in goals. Clear communication helps prevent misunderstandings and ensures that both partners feel heard and supported.

- **Practice active listening.** It's important to listen deeply and empathetically when your partner shares their thoughts and emotions about fertility. Avoid jumping to solutions or dismissing their feelings; instead, listen to understand. Reflect back what you heard and validate their experience. This strengthens emotional intimacy and creates a supportive environment where both partners feel safe expressing their fears, hopes, and concerns.

- **Be open about your emotions.** Trying to conceive can stir up a wide range of emotions—hope, excitement, frustration, and even grief at times. It's important to be open and honest about how you're feeling, even if it's hard to admit you're struggling. Suppressing emotions can lead to resentment and misunderstandings, so commit to creating a safe space where you can both share your emotional journey without judgment.

- **Use "we" language.** Instead of framing fertility as an individual struggle, use language that emphasizes the partnership—phrases like "we're working on this together" or "we'll get through this" can reinforce the idea that you're a united team. This shift in language can help both partners feel more connected and reduce feelings of isolation during difficult moments.

- **Seek outside support together.** If the emotional burden of fertility becomes overwhelming, don't hesitate to seek help from a therapist, counselor, or fertility support group. Engaging in therapy as a couple can provide you both with new tools to communicate effectively, manage stress, and maintain emotional balance during this time.

By fostering strong teamwork and communication, you can reduce the stress of the fertility process and ensure that both partners feel supported. Working together—both physically and emotionally—will help you navigate the highs and lows of conception while reinforcing the strength of your relationship.

Final Thoughts

As you continue your preconception journey, remember that you are not defined by the outcome alone. Your body is resilient, and your potential is limitless. Fertility is a dynamic process, one that requires patience, hope, and an understanding of your body's natural rhythms. By approaching it with both intuition and the science-backed strategies we've explored throughout this chapter, you can trust that you are navigating the path in the best possible way.

Fertility is not just about timing or mechanics—it's about embracing the fullness of who you are. Whether the road to parenthood happens quickly or takes longer than anticipated, you are on a voyage of growth and transformation that goes far beyond biology. Take heart in knowing that each step brings you closer to your family, in whatever form that may take, and celebrate the strength and courage it takes to walk this path. Trust that your body and mind are working together, helping you move forward toward the outcome that is meant for you.

Q&A

Q: What is the most important mindset shift to adopt when starting my fertility journey?

A: The most important mindset shift is to remember that your identity is not defined by your ability to conceive or how many children you have. You are not just the roles you play—partner, parent, professional—you are a whole, irreplaceable human being. This perspective brings peace and helps reduce the emotional pressure.

Q: Is it really possible to have a healthy baby later in life, despite everything I've heard about maternal age?

A: Yes, absolutely. While maternal age is a factor, it is only one piece of the puzzle. When you focus on optimizing your health—especially mitochondrial health, reducing oxidative stress, and following personalized protocols—you can dramatically improve your chances of having a healthy baby later in life.

Q: What role does a man's fertility play in the overall conception journey, and why is it often overlooked?

A: Male fertility is half the equation, yet it's often underestimated or ignored in the preconception conversation. Sperm quality—count, motility, and morphology—declines with age and can be affected by lifestyle, toxins, and oxidative stress. This chapter highlights that sperm health matters just as much as egg quality and offers clear, science-backed ways men can optimize their fertility. Tools such as SpermQT now make it easier than ever to track and improve sperm health at home, making fertility a true team effort.

THRIVE

Q: How does birth control history affect fertility, and what do I do if I've been on it for a long time?

A: Long-term birth control use can send confusing signals to the body. After stopping hormonal contraception, it's important to give your body time to re-regulate and heal. Lab testing can help uncover and address any underlying imbalances before trying to conceive.

Q: How can couples maintain emotional connection and joy during what can be a stressful preconception journey?

A: It's essential to actively protect your relationship from the stress that can come with trying to conceive. That means setting aside time for fun, laughter, and intimacy that isn't centered around ovulation calendars. Practicing rituals like "just for fun" date nights, monthly celebrations, and mindfulness together can shift the energy from pressure to presence. Remember: Conception is a team journey, and joy is a powerful fertility booster.

Believe

Introspect

Renew

Thrive

Hope

Section V Introduction

Welcome to the *Hope* section of your journey—a time brimming with promise and possibility as you prepare to bring new life into the world. This is where all the effort and intention you've poured into optimizing your health come together, aligning your body, mind, and spirit for conception. The path to parenthood can often be marked by longing and resilience, but through focused preparation, it can be transformed into a journey of profound growth and hope.

I've been privileged to witness the life-changing impact of the Every Baby Well program in my patients' lives. My patient Hannah is a beautiful example of this. Her first pregnancy had been filled with complications, followed by a severe case of postpartum depression. When she later found herself struggling to conceive, Hannah came to me feeling hopeful but defeated. We began a comprehensive preconception program tailored specifically for her, and just four months into our work together, she became pregnant naturally. This pregnancy was completely different—smooth, healthy, and joyful. Hannah told me she felt incredible throughout, hardly needing any visits because everything went so well. Now, five weeks postpartum, she was fully present and relishing every moment with her new baby, feeling healthier and happier than ever. "I feel like myself, and it's wonderful," she shared, glowing with confidence and joy.

Another couple's story shows how profound the power of preparation can be. Years ago, Beth came to me after struggling to conceive, only achieving pregnancy through IVF due to her husband's very low sperm count. Determined to optimize their health, Beth and her husband embarked on a transformative detox journey, moving out of a moldy home, overhauling their lifestyle, and embracing the program fully. This time, they conceived not just one but two children naturally. Their story serves as a reminder that focused preparation can open doors that once seemed closed, leading to unexpected, wonderful outcomes.

Stories like Hannah's and Beth's highlight the profound impact a dedicated preconception program can have, allowing couples to overcome health challenges and experience the joy of family. As you read the chapters in this section, I hope you'll feel inspired and encouraged, knowing that each step you take brings you closer to the "green light" moment where readiness and hope intersect at last. You are laying the groundwork not just for conception but for a legacy of health and love, beginning with your commitment and continuing in every precious life you welcome into the world.

CHAPTER 14

All Systems Go: Green Light for Baby

Welcome to the "All Systems Go" phase—the moment when all your body's systems, like a finely tuned engine, are primed and ready for the journey ahead.

Years ago, I took a road trip to Mount Rainier in Washington State with a friend. Between us, we had six kids packed into a Suburban, along with snacks, games, and our excitement for the trip. We were relying on a GPS system, which was still a somewhat new concept at the time, and we carefully followed its instructions, turn by turn. We made our way through winding roads and small towns, and after what seemed like hours, we finally reached the park's entrance—only to find it closed! There we were, the car full of restless kids, snacks running low, and a bit of frustration setting in as we realized we needed to reroute to a main entrance. That experience taught me a valuable lesson about setting a clear course and staying open to whatever unexpected adventures or detours the adventure might bring.

We often invest so much thought and intention into the trips we take, ensuring we're equipped for wherever the road may lead us. As you embark on this deeply meaningful journey, I hope you'll carry that same spirit of mindfulness and openness, trusting that each step forward is guided by care, purpose, and love.

From the beginning of this program, you've had a "red light" and have held off on conception to ensure that every part of your being—physically, mentally, emotionally, and spiritually—is in peak condition. Just as you'd prepare every detail of a vehicle before a long trip, you've optimized each system of your body, giving your future baby the healthiest environment to begin life. You and your partner have put so much energy into this mission, and I hope you are feeling empowered, encouraged, excited, and—most of all—accomplished. Making it to this point is no small thing; it's actually quite a feat.

This chapter marks an important turning point in your journey. Now it's time to reassess, fine-tune, and ensure that your bodies, spirits, and minds are in the best possible state to conceive a child together. I'm sure you're already feeling the positive effects of all your hard work, and this is when you get to *see* the results reflected in updated lab work as well. Allow yourself to be proud of your perseverance. And now, let's get you to the "green light"!

Retest and Reassess

Sometimes when we've worked so hard at accomplishing a goal and we're so close to the finish line, there's a temptation to stop a bit early and call the job done. Especially when you've been so dedicated and changed so much about your lifestyle, that temptation can be very strong. But I want to encourage you to dig deep and find it within yourself to truly complete this process. That means retesting to see the fruits of your labor. It's such a gift that you're giving to your future child, and I want to see you succeed fully. Let's talk a little more about what this final—and key—part of the process looks like.

It starts by going back and looking at your initial test results and refreshing yourself on what you were working on and why. If your initial testing revealed any abnormalities—whether in the autoimmune panels, toxin levels, mitochondrial function, inflammation levels, hormones, nutrient levels, gut health, or other key areas—you'll want to retest to make sure your body has been responding to what you've been doing to fix any issues. Are your toxin levels down? Have any autoimmune markers now returned to normal? Are there any lingering nutrient deficiencies? Has the health of your gut microbiome improved? Your job is to look back at the tests you completed at the start of this program and order new test kits and make appointments for bloodwork. Yes, it takes a little time to get those results, so stay the course in the interim. (And continue to be vigilant when it comes to contraception!)

This phase is essential but remember—your test results will never be perfect, so that's not the goal. But you do want to ensure there's been significant improvements and there aren't any red flags that require additional tweaking. If something still isn't optimal, don't worry! You're on the right path. Minor adjustments—whether through supplements or further lifestyle changes—can fine-tune your body into peak conception mode. Sometimes it can take a little longer, perhaps even twelve to eighteen months, and it might even require hiring a coach to come alongside you or joining the program to get some additional assistance.

As you prepare to welcome a new life into your world, it's helpful to remember the power of epigenetics. Every positive change you've made not only supports your well-being but also contributes to the health blueprint you'll pass on to your child. Our lifestyle choices can shape gene expression, meaning the steps you've been taking can help minimize any unwanted health tendencies from being carried forward. By first "parenting yourself" and nurturing your own health, you're giving your future child the gift of a resilient start, setting them up for vitality and wellness from the very beginning. Embrace this final phase of preparation, knowing it's as much a part of your legacy as it is a step toward conceiving your baby.

When we say, "I want a baby," it's easy to forget the profound reality of what that truly means. You're not only inviting a new life into the world but creating a vessel for a soul to enter, one that connects to generations past and shapes those yet to come. This journey also carries the weight of legacy, a continuum of souls interwoven through time, with each child as a new chapter in a story that spans far beyond us.

Reflecting on Your Readiness

As you approach the "green light" for conception, let's pause to reflect on the incredible shifts you've made. This lifestyle journey has been a time of transformation, both inside and out. Right now, I encourage you to explore how you're truly feeling, acknowledging the positive changes and examining any areas that still need support. Use the following prompts to write your responses, letting your thoughts flow freely to capture your progress and record your anticipation of the next steps to take.

1. Describe your energy levels throughout the day. How has your energy shifted since starting these lifestyle changes? When do you feel most energized, and are there times when you notice dips or sluggishness?

2. How do you feel about your focus and mental clarity? Has your ability to concentrate or stay engaged improved? Describe moments when you feel particularly clearheaded or "in the zone."

3. How would you describe your digestion now compared to before starting the Every Baby Well program? What sensations do you feel after meals, and how does your body seem to be responding to different foods?

4. Throughout this program, you've adopted a lot of healthy habits. Are there any unhealthy habits you still need to replace? Do

you have any lingering habits involving alcohol, vaping, smoking, or recreational drug use, such as marijuana? Are you still relying on caffeine, sugar, or stimulants to keep your energy up? If so, could you explore more sustainable alternatives or routines to boost your energy?

5. Describe your sleeping patterns and any recent improvements. How easy is it for you to fall asleep and stay asleep? How many hours of sleep are you averaging per night? How do you feel upon waking in the morning—refreshed and ready or still tired?

6. Reflect on your new relationship with food. What foods do you naturally gravitate toward now, and how has this shifted over time? Describe any cravings you experience—are they fewer or more manageable?

7. How would you describe your mood and emotional balance? Have you noticed greater stability in your mood, even in times of stress? What emotions do you experience most often, and how does your mental health feel throughout the day?

8. Describe any improvements in your physical strength and resilience. How does your body feel during physical activity? What changes have you noticed in your endurance, flexibility, or stamina?

9. Reflect on your pelvic floor health and any improvements you've noticed. Are you incorporating pelvic floor exercises regularly, and how have they impacted your physical comfort or strength? How does your pelvic floor feel during activities like exercise or daily movements—stable, supported, or in need of further strengthening?

If you've answered with a sense of excitement, recognizing so many positive changes that you've adopted, you're likely in an excellent place to move forward confidently. If certain areas still need attention, let this exercise serve as a gentle guide, helping you continue to make the changes necessary to truly nurture and care for yourself. Celebrate your progress—you're creating a strong foundation for conception and a healthy pregnancy.

Revisiting Your Starting Point: Reflecting Together

As you near the "green light" for conception, I encourage you to closely look over the checklist (starting on page 19) you've been working on to see if there are any areas that still need some attention and focus. Plus, it's valuable to revisit some of the inner work you did earlier in this journey, particularly those areas you explored in chapter 2. Taking the time to assess your current state across the different areas of your life—nutrition, exercise, emotional well-being, relationship, finances, and spirituality—can not only strengthen your own readiness for conception but also foster a deepened sense of partnership and alignment. Just as these factors play a key role in your individual health, they're equally impactful in the shared foundation you're building for your future child.

Use the following prompts to explore how far each of you has come and determine where you might still need to support each other as you enter this new phase.

Physical Health and Nutrition

- How would each of you describe the changes in your diet and physical health since beginning this journey?
- What are some nutrition goals you can set as a team to ensure continued, mutual support?
- Are there any lifestyle habits, such as consistent meal prepping or cooking together, that could reinforce your joint commitment?

Emotional and Mental Well-Being

- Reflect together on how you manage stress and emotional challenges. What strategies are you each using, and how do they impact your relationship?

- How can you continue to support each other in managing stress and ensuring a calm and peaceful environment as you prepare for conception?

Relationship and Communication

- Assess the current state of your relationship. Are there areas where you feel more connected, and are there any "cracks" in the foundation that need attention?
- Open up to each other about any concerns or goals related to parenting styles, balancing responsibilities, and aligning on shared values. How can you strengthen these areas now?
- We "parent ourselves" with an inner monologue, which very quickly can become our dialogue with our children. Have you both worked to keep your self-talk positive and uplifting?

Spiritual and Shared Beliefs

- What are your individual spiritual values, and how have they grown or evolved? Discuss how you'll approach this area of parenting and explore where each of you may need more understanding or alignment.
- Are there any practices, like prayer or meditation, that you've established together as a couple to reinforce a spiritually supportive environment for your family?

Financial and Lifestyle Readiness

- Talk openly about your financial situation and goals. What areas of financial planning have been solidified, and where might you still need to budget, save, or adjust?

- Review your shared goals for the future—things like living arrangements, childcare plans, and work-life balance—and make sure you're both comfortable with the adjustments that may come with growing your family.

By having open communication about these areas, you're building a solid, resilient foundation for your family—one that will eventually support everyone. These conversations are a testament to the work you've done so far, and they're a powerful way to strengthen the loving and intentional environment you're creating for your future family.

Continue Your Lifestyle Changes—Both of You!

As you prepare for conception, it's vital to maintain the new healthy habits you've already adopted. Work together to continue your new way of thinking and behaving in the areas of nutrition, exercise, supplementation, stress management, and sleep optimization. Your preconception routine isn't just about getting pregnant—it's about creating the healthiest possible environment for your future baby to thrive.

Consider this an ongoing journey, one that continues throughout conception, pregnancy, and beyond. Keep cheering each other on and encouraging one another within your new lifestyle together. This is a shared effort, and both of you play an equally important role in the health of your future child.

Fine-tuning Your Supplement Routine for Conceiving

As you move forward into the next phase of your preconception journey, you'll want to keep taking all the supplements you've now gotten used to in your routine, with just a few exceptions.

- **Glutathione:** Since glutathione at high doses is a major detoxifier, it could cause your body to release stored toxins into your bloodstream, which could theoretically expose a developing embryo to higher toxin levels, potentially posing risks during conception or early pregnancy. Although it may be safe in pregnancy since you make it endogenously, it hasn't been studied to supplement it during pregnancy, and therefore I don't recommend it.

- **Detox Supplements:** Whether you were working to detox from heavy metals or environmental toxins such as mold, now is the time to taper off detox supplements such as Liposomal Glutathione, Zeo Binder, Liver Detox Protect, and PectaSol.

- **Neo40:** If you're not already taking it, I recommend adding Neo40 to your supplement routine. It's designed to enhance the body's nitric oxide levels, which play a crucial role in cardiovascular health. Developed from research at the University of Texas Health Science Center's N-O Discovery Program, Neo40 helps maintain optimal blood pressure levels, promotes cardiovascular and heart health, and aids in better blood flow.

- **Vein Support by Every Life Well:** This supplement promotes healthy veins, capillaries, and overall circulation. Its primary ingredient, diosmin—a citrus-derived flavonoid—has been utilized for decades to support vascular health and microcirculation. Vein Support also includes a micronized purified flavonoid fraction (MPFF), which enhances vein tone. Research suggests that the components in Vein Support may support healthy veins, capillaries, and blood flow; promote healthy lymphatic drainage; enhance antioxidant activity; and support blood glucose metabolism as well as cognition.

HOPE

Alternatives to the Glucose Test

As you continue preparing for conception, I want to put on your radar the traditional glucose test that's typically recommended during the second trimester of pregnancy. This test, called the Oral Glucose Tolerance Test (OGTT), involves consuming a highly concentrated sugary liquid and then having your blood sugar measured at regular intervals. It can be harsh on your body because the products that many doctors use for this test contain unhealthy ingredients, including artificial food coloring.[491]

I recommend avoiding this test altogether; instead, wear a CGM (continuous glucose monitor) for two weeks or more and report those numbers to your obstetrician or midwife. Not only does this eliminate the need for ingesting questionable ingredients, but it also provides far more comprehensive data. Instead of one quick snapshot of how your body responds to a sugar overload, you'll get a detailed picture of how your body processes glucose throughout the day in response to your normal diet, exercise, and even stress levels.

In case your practitioner insists on an in-person glucose test, there is a cleaner option available, called the Fresh Test.[492] This product is a non-GMO, BPA-free, dye-free alternative to the standard glucose solution. It contains no artificial additives, making it a healthier option. Discuss this with your provider as a potential compromise if wearing a CGM isn't an option.

Regardless of the method you choose, it's important to keep tabs on your blood sugar levels during pregnancy. Stable blood sugar not only helps prevent gestational diabetes but also reduces the risk of complications such as preeclampsia and macrosomia (excessive fetal growth), which can lead to challenging deliveries. Even if you've never had blood sugar issues before, pregnancy introduces a cascade of hormonal changes that can affect how your body processes glucose. That's why monitoring it closely during this critical time is essential for both your health and the well-being of your baby.

With that said, since you have optimized your blood sugar during the preconception period, using a CGM, it is likely that your habits and lifestyle changes have reduced your risk for developing gestational diabetes, but it's still important to check.

I have been developing some specific guidance for diet and lifestyle during pregnancy—and yes, it applies to both mom and dad, since you're in this together—so be on the lookout for that book and program soon!

Final Thoughts

With your tests reviewed, lifestyle changes solidified, a deep alignment established between you and your partner, and supplements tailored to your needs, you're officially ready to embrace the conception phase. The groundwork you've laid is more than just preparation—it's a playbook for creating the best environment for nurturing your baby and for that child to grow and thrive. This phase is a time of patience and trust, knowing that your body is in its most optimal state to welcome new life.

Remember, the journey to conception can take time, and it's perfectly normal for it to happen on its own timeline. Continue caring for your body, mind, and spirit, and focus on the joy and excitement of this process. You're moving forward with intention, creating the healthiest start for both of you and your future baby—and for generations of your family to come! The green light is finally on—and it's time to step into your next chapter of life with confidence.

Q&A

Q: I've made all these changes, but how do I know I'm truly ready to conceive?

A: You're ready when you've retested any markers that were initially out of range and confirmed improvement. Your lifestyle changes likely now feel sustainable, and you are probably in a place of overall vitality—steady energy, restorative sleep, balanced hormones, and a well-functioning gut. If you've been following the road map in this book, your body is as prepared as it can be to support a healthy pregnancy.

Q: Do I continue all my supplements or adjust them before trying to conceive?

A: Some supplements should be continued, while others may need to be adjusted or discontinued. Keep essential prenatal nutrients like folate, choline, and omega-3s in your routine, but certain detoxifying or high-dose supplements may not be appropriate once you're actively trying.

Q: Do both partners need to keep up with lifestyle changes, or is it just the woman's responsibility?

A: Fertility is a shared journey! The quality of sperm plays a crucial role in conception and the health of your baby. Both partners will want to continue nutrient-dense eating, avoiding toxins, and managing stress to optimize reproductive health. This is about building a foundation for your future child together.

Q: I'm nervous about the glucose test during pregnancy. Are there alternatives?

A: Yes! Many women prefer to monitor their blood sugar at home using a continuous glucose monitor (CGM), hgA1C blood test, or a glucometer with finger sticks instead of drinking the glucose challenge drink. Talk with your provider about these alternatives to ensure they align with your pregnancy care plan.

Q: How do I maintain this new lifestyle once I conceive?

A: Keep your focus on whole foods, clean water, quality sleep, and stress reduction. Minimize exposure to environmental toxins and continue moving your body in ways that feel good. Pregnancy is a continuation of all the work you've done—think of it as a transition rather than a drastic shift.

HOPE

CONCLUSION
YOUR NEXT CHAPTER

As you move forward, remember your preconception journey is rooted in progress, not perfection. It's easy to feel the pressure to get everything exactly right, but real growth comes from holding your goals loosely and celebrating each small step you take. Life rarely unfolds in a straight line; it's a circuitous path with detours, unexpected turns, and sometimes even U-turns. Embracing this rhythm, rather than resisting it, lets you discover joy in the process, knowing that each decision, however small, contributes to a healthier future for yourself, your partner, and your child.

The rewards of your commitment to this journey are profound. By making choices that prioritize your health and well-being, you're laying the groundwork for a healthy baby, equipped for a strong and vibrant start in life. Anticipate these rewards and let them fuel your motivation. Knowing that your efforts today contribute to your child's lifelong health brings deeper meaning to each step you take. Celebrate the progress and trust that you're creating the best possible environment for your future family.

I believe the next generations of souls joining us are going to be highly collaborative, focused on unity. We've seen so much division in recent years, and I feel intuitively that is all about to change. I know it might seem strange to think about the souls who want to come in, but it's a concept that's been so heavy on my heart. As you prepare your body to conceive and carry a child, think about the healthy body you are helping create for that soul so they can thrive and flourish! It's really a beautiful way of thinking about your future child.

I hope this book has become a grounding space for you, one that gently pulls you out of the noise and overwhelm and guides you into a place of clarity and calm. In these pages, I hope you have found a centered, intuitive sense of purpose—a clear and steady knowing that brings peace as you prepare for your next chapter. This is a place from which to welcome new life—grounded, connected, and fully present for the profoundness of what lies ahead.

I am so grateful and honored that you have invested
the time and energy into reading this book. I hope it has
had a meaningful impact on your journey toward conception.
I am always adding more information to my website,
Every Baby Well. There, you'll also find information
about how to hire a preconception coach and how to
become one too. I'd love to see you there!

Be well,
Ann Shippy, MD

Scan here to learn more at Every Baby Well:

LETTERS OF INSPIRATION

first reached out to Dr. Shippy about three years ago because I didn't have a primary doctor and wanted someone who aligned with my approach to health. I wasn't dealing with any major issues, but I wanted to optimize my health and work with a doctor who could integrate food, supplements, and holistic tools. What I love about Dr. Shippy is that she goes beyond the basics—she doesn't just check your thyroid or run standard bloodwork. She does a deep dive into things such as heavy metal toxicity, gut health, liver function, and how your body is actually using nutrients.

When I started working with her, I was also thinking about starting a family, so we spent about six months cleaning everything up before I got pregnant. My diet and lifestyle were already really clean, but we took it further—making sure my body was in the absolute best place to conceive and carry a healthy baby. We worked on my thyroid and gut health and even ran tests to ensure the nutrients I was eating were reaching the placenta. Along the way, she helped me fine-tune my supplements and incorporate stress-management tools. I had an extremely healthy pregnancy—no sickness, no major symptoms, and I felt amazing all the way through. I was walking miles up until the day I gave birth.

Now I have a healthy daughter and we're working on preparing for baby number two. Dr. Shippy has been incredible at helping me take stock of where I am post-pregnancy and get my body ready again. She also worked with my husband, which was really important to us because it takes two to create a healthy baby. I truly believe the work we did together made all the difference in my first pregnancy, and I wouldn't do another one without her. She's not just guessing or following trends—she tests and tailors everything specifically to what my body needs, and that level of care is priceless.

—Briana

———————

I first met Dr. Shippy when I was eighteen or nineteen, during a time when my family was in a health crisis. We had unknowingly moved into a house with toxic black mold, and while doctor after doctor failed to figure out what was wrong, Dr. Shippy was the first to suspect mold toxicity. That discovery changed everything. We lost our home and belongings, but she guided us through healing and gave us real answers when no one else could. Over the years, she has been the person I turn to for anything beyond what a mainstream doctor could help with—from chronic fatigue to severe acne to a time I was hospitalized with pneumonia after multiple misdiagnoses. My family and I truly feel that she has saved our lives more than once.

When I became a mom, her care became even more impactful. During my first pregnancy, I had terrible digestive issues—persistent burping, gut discomfort, and strange food reactions. My OB had no real solutions, but Dr. Shippy helped me resolve it. Before my second pregnancy, I wanted to check in on my health after nursing and sleep deprivation, so we ran a NutrEval panel and a gut health assessment. With just a few tweaks to my supplements, I felt stronger, and this time around, I had none of the gut issues I experienced with my first pregnancy.

Dr. Shippy's expertise, care, and insight have set me and my family on a path to lasting health, shaping not only my well-being but also my children's future. I don't need to see her as often these days—which is a great thing—but I always know she's there when I do. She has been a true gift in my life.

—Danielle

My heart broke when my first child was diagnosed with developmental delays and sensory processing disorder at eighteen months, which we discovered was mitochondrial dysfunction. After years of dedicated therapy and treatment, I was overjoyed to see my child recover from all the diagnoses and begin to thrive.

While wrestling with this challenge, I endured the devastation of four miscarriages in a single year. Even New York's top specialists were stumped. A holistic dentist, to my surprise, found a parasite infection. After treatment and proper nutrition, I was blessed to conceive our second child without complications at thirty-seven.

After moving to Texas, our second child lost the power of speech after a vaccine, suffered a terrifying seizure, and developed neurological issues. We discovered toxic mold in our house and frantically fled to a hotel.

That's when we found our saving grace—Dr. Shippy. She uncovered parasites our other doctors had missed and put my struggling child on a comprehensive protocol. I watched with immense relief as the symptoms gradually disappeared.

Dr. Shippy gave us a road map that conventional medicine never could—healing our home, bodies, and future before another pregnancy. Her preconception guidance helped me restore my cycle, rebalance my body, and conceive naturally at forty-two. When I developed frightening and rare preeclampsia after delivery, Dr. Shippy's protocol normalized my blood pressure in just a week. Under her care, our third child has been remarkably healthy from day one.

Later, when some of my children showed signs of neurological autoimmunity, Dr. Shippy's personalized approach gave us hope again. After we discovered hidden mold in our newest home, she patiently guided us through testing and detox. She also transformed my husband's mitochondrial dysfunction with targeted IV treatments.

Dr. Shippy's approach gets to the root causes that other doctors miss. Her functional medicine tool kit has been nothing short of life-changing. I cannot comprehend where we'd be without her compassionate care and insight. The tools she has given us have been essential in breaking a cycle of distressing generational health issues.

—Holly

I have been a patient of Dr. Shippy's since 2013, thanks to my mom, who was also her patient and recommended her to me. Initially, I was simply looking for more energy and ways in which I could optimize my health. Dr. Shippy was able to reveal that my eating habits were not serving me, and she introduced several targeting supplements that made a real difference.

A year later, at thirty-four years old, I got married and my husband and I decided very quickly to have our first child. But we spent a year trying to get pregnant with no success. I was just about to go down the IVF path when Dr. Shippy encouraged me to work with her first. Together, we focused on detoxing and took a close look at my thyroid. She put me on specialized thyroid medication and added more targeted supplements to help improve my egg quality. We also found that I had the MTHFR mutation. Dr. Shippy put me on methylated B vitamins, which was critical for health and fertility.

Around that time, my husband also started seeing Dr. Shippy. He's a pretty healthy eater already, but she helped him clean up his diet further and got him on the right supplements.

After we both made these changes, within three months, I got pregnant naturally at thirty-five! Dr. Shippy was so helpful in guiding me through my entire pregnancy, and we were delighted to have a healthy baby!

Post-partum, Dr. Shippy was incredibly supportive with nutritional advice. I knew I wanted another baby, so she helped me rebuild my nutrition stores to make sure I was ready. I got pregnant again and had another baby three years later!

At that point, I felt like our family was complete, but I was still seeing Dr. Shippy to maintain my energy and vitality. Then, very unexpectedly, I got pregnant again and had a perfect baby boy! I honestly feel like Dr. Shippy got me so fertile that at forty-one, I had a surprise baby! What a wonderful gift.

Looking back to when I first started working with Dr. Shippy, some of the initial test results really surprised me. We did heavy metal testing and found my mercury levels were very high, yet I didn't eat a lot of high-mercury fish such as tuna. We did some detox and chelation, which was something I wasn't expecting to have to do. We retested later, and that's when we knew I was ready to have a baby.

Dr. Shippy now sees all my kids. They were all born by C-section, so she has been monitoring their microbiomes. I have celiac genes, and so we've been looking at their propensity for that as well as their methylation genes (they all have MTHFR mutations). But with her guidance, they're all very healthy.

Had I not known, through Dr. Shippy's care, the importance of a good foundation for pregnancy—and how to get there—I do not think I would have gotten pregnant naturally. We really are so grateful to her for encouraging us not jump to IVF. I know several women who did choose IVF, and now they're facing health issues, including breast cancer, which is just devastating.

I'm so thankful for Dr. Shippy's wisdom, support, and everything I've learned from her throughout this journey.

—Ryann

APPENDIX

Chapter 4: Taking Your Body Inventory

Genetic Testing: A Personalized Approach

It was once thought that our genes determined our medical destiny, our health was out of our control, and that *nature* was in the driver's seat. But now, more than ever, it is clear that much of our health is in our control and our genetics generally play a much more supportive role. We know that the environment—not only our physical environment but also the environment we create for our body by what we eat, how we move, what we think, and other important daily habits—determines the vast majority of our health and disease risk.[493]

This is good news. It means that we have a choice, and the choices we make about how we live really matter when it comes to wellness. How empowering is that—especially during this important time in your life, when you're preparing to birth a *new* life?

That's not to say we don't still need to run some DNA testing, because genetic tests still give us valuable insight. There are several options out there for this type of testing. I like Counsyl because I feel they offer the most extensive recessive gene testing. Their test looks at a range of genes that play crucial roles in various aspects of health, particularly those relevant to reproductive health and prenatal care.

Counsyl's test looks at over one hundred genes associated with inherited disorders such as cystic fibrosis, sickle cell anemia, and Tay-Sachs disease, which can impact the health of the baby if both parents are carriers. By identifying carriers of these genetic variants, Counsyl testing helps you understand your risk of passing on these conditions to your child.[494]

There's also GrowBaby, a genetic test for moms-to-be. It offers powerful insights that support maternal health from preconception onward to optimize the chances of a healthy pregnancy and a healthy baby. Variations in certain genes can impact health outcomes that affect maternal and baby health throughout the pregnancy journey. GrowBaby reports on forty-two SNPs involved in eleven biological processes associated with maternal health risks and fatal phenotypes.[495]

IntellxxDNA is another option. I had an opportunity to sit down with Sharon Hausman-Cohen, founder of IntellxxDNA, and during that fascinating conversation, we discussed several genomic factors that can impact fertility and pregnancy outcomes. Here are some of the main ones to be aware of:

- The GP6 gene (glycoprotein 6) is involved in platelet activation and sticky platelets, and having variants of this gene can increase the risk of fetal loss by three to five times.[496] On the upside, this can often be addressed with low-dose aspirin to improve the likelihood of delivering a healthy baby. Of course, I encourage you to discuss this with your doctor to see if this is the best option for you.

- Less common gene variants in factor 2 and factor 5 (prothrombin gene) can also significantly increase the risk of recurrent miscarriages, as well as preeclampsia (a pregnancy condition characterized by high blood pressure and protein in the urine) and fetal growth restriction (when the baby is smaller than expected based on the number of weeks of pregnancy). For these genetic factors, low-dose heparin has been shown to be more effective, increasing the live birth rate by fifteen times. With research related to specific genes progressing so rapidly, it can be helpful to have a healthcare provider who is aware of the latest developments so they can help find the best solutions for you.

- Certain inflammatory pathways (the body's defense response to pathogens and other harmful stimuli) such as IL-6, IL-1, and TNF-alpha also have genetic variants that can be associated with autoimmune disorders and recurrent pregnancy loss. Managing these inflammatory factors through supplements like N-acetylcysteine (NAC)[497] and omega-3s may be beneficial.

Understanding your specific genetic profile can help guide more personalized and effective treatment approaches to improve fertility and pregnancy outcomes, rather than a one-size-fits-all approach. Identifying and addressing the root genetic causes can make a significant difference. So once you've completed genetic testing, seek genetic counseling to find out the latest treatment options for your specific genetic profile.

Toxic Mold Testing

Effects of Mycotoxins on the Fetus

As I mentioned in the chapter on testing, mycotoxins can have serious effects on a fetus. If the father has an elevated level of mycotoxins, that can damage the DNA of the sperm and also create epigenetic influences that change the gene expression in the fetus. And if the mother has elevated levels, those same changes can occur, in addition to the risk of the mycotoxins crossing into the placenta and thus having a direct impact on the fetus as it grows. Here's a deeper look into those effects:

- *Teratogenic effects*: Mycotoxins such as aflatoxins, ochratoxin A, and zearalenone can interfere with fetal development, leading to congenital abnormalities.

- *Neurodevelopmental issues*: Mycotoxins can cross the placental barrier and disrupt brain development, potentially leading to cognitive deficits, learning disabilities, and behavioral issues in a child.

- *Growth restriction*: Mycotoxins may reduce placental efficiency, leading to intrauterine growth restriction (IUGR) and low birth weight.

- *Fetal mortality*: High exposure levels can result in miscarriage or stillbirth, as mycotoxins can disrupt critical developmental pathways or damage the placenta.

- *Endocrine disruption*: Certain mycotoxins, such as zearalenone, mimic estrogen, leading to hormonal imbalances that may interfere with normal fetal sexual development.

Effects of Mycotoxins on the Mother

- *Immune suppression*: Mycotoxins such as aflatoxins and fumonisins suppress the immune system, increasing the risk of infections during pregnancy, which can further endanger fetal health.

- *Increased oxidative stress*: Mycotoxins induce oxidative stress, leading to cellular damage in maternal tissues, the placenta, and fetal organs. This oxidative damage can contribute to complications like preeclampsia or miscarriage.

- *Hormonal imbalances*: Endocrine-disrupting mycotoxins can alter reproductive hormone levels, potentially affecting implantation and placental development.

- *Pregnancy complications*: These include **preterm labor** (mycotoxin exposure can increase inflammation and trigger premature labor); **preeclampsia** (mycotoxins may disrupt endothelial function and increase oxidative stress, both of which are associated with preeclampsia); and **toxic accumulation** (mycotoxins can accumulate in maternal tissues, posing long-term health risks, including liver and kidney damage, which can indirectly impact pregnancy).

- *Placental transfer*: Many mycotoxins cross the placental barrier, directly exposing the fetus to toxic effects. This can lead to DNA damage, apoptosis (cell death), or interference with nutrient and oxygen exchange.

- *Disruption of cellular processes*: Mycotoxins interfere with critical cellular pathways, including protein synthesis, mitochondrial function, and immune regulation.

- *Epigenetic changes*: Mycotoxins can alter the epigenome, potentially causing long-term developmental issues or predisposing the fetus to chronic diseases later in life.

As you can see, mycotoxins are not to be trifled with, and I encourage you to test for their presence in your body. There are a couple of different tests I prefer for mycotoxins. One is by RealTime Laboratories. It's a urine test with a glutathione challenge. (I do it with and without the glutathione, based on how well someone is detoxifying, and estimate the toxins stored in the body.) The RealTime mycotoxin test detects sixteen different mycotoxins. Testing is done using ELISA, a highly sensitive detection method using antibodies prepared against mycotoxins.[498]

The other one is the MycoTOX Profile by Mosaic Diagnostics. It is a urine-based assay designed to assess levels of eleven different mycotoxins, including aflatoxin M1, ochratoxin A, zearalenone, and trichothecenes.[499] I will often run both tests to get a full picture. That way, we can pinpoint any hidden mold-related issues and create a plan to support your body's detoxification process effectively. It's all about getting the clearest insight possible.

- **Aflatoxin M1** is a mycotoxin produced by the mold species *Aspergillus.* Aflatoxin can have adverse effects on the central nervous system, liver, and kidneys, and it can cause a variety of cancers, especially that of the liver.[500] Found in contaminated grains, nuts, and dairy, this mycotoxin can also cause liver damage, immune suppression, and neurodevelopmental harm.
- **Ochratoxin A** is a mycotoxin produced by various fungi and can cause placental disruption and kidney disease.[501]
- **Zearalenone** has frequently been detected in cereals and grain-based products. When cows consume foods contaminated with this mycotoxin, it can be detected in their milk, which also gets it into the human food chain. Zearalenone can bind to estrogen receptors in cells and accumulate in the body. This disruption of hormonal balance can lead to various reproductive system disorders and developmental abnormalities, including prostate, ovarian, cervical, or breast cancers.[502]
- **Trichothecenes** are one of the major classes of mycotoxins and are produced by toxic black mold (which isn't always black in appearance). Poorly ventilated areas can therefore be vulnerable, and trichothecenes can be found in cereal and grain crops. Long-term exposure can cause immune-system impairment and developmental diseases, as well as body pain and temporary bleeding disorders. A subvariant, T-2 trichothecene, is even used in biological warfare.[503]

I know that's a lot of information to take in on a subject you might not have been expecting to learn about, but testing for mycotoxin exposure is incredibly important during your preconception journey.

Autoimmune Panels

Here is a breakdown on some of the impact that autoimmune disorders can have on pregnancy and fertility:

- *Impact on fertility*: Certain autoimmune disorders can affect fertility by disrupting the normal functioning of the reproductive system. These conditions may lead to hormonal imbalances, irregular menstrual cycles, or decreased ovarian reserve, all of which can impact a couple's ability to conceive.

- *Pregnancy complications*: Women with certain autoimmune disorders may be at increased risk of pregnancy complications, such as miscarriage, preeclampsia, or preterm birth. These conditions can also affect fetal development and potentially contribute to epigenetic changes that influence the health of your child.

- *Epigenetic implications*: Autoimmune disorders can trigger inflammatory responses and immune system dysregulation, which may impact epigenetic processes. Epigenetic modifications associated with autoimmune conditions could potentially affect gene expression patterns in reproductive cells and embryos, leading to long-term health consequences for your children, grandchildren, and beyond. You may not have a diagnosis of autoimmune disease, but you might have this process going on in your body, and it can affect the health of your child.

- *Preconception screening*: Conducting an autoimmune panel before conception can help identify any underlying autoimmune conditions that may require management or treatment to optimize fertility and pregnancy outcomes, regardless of if you have a diagnosis of an autoimmune disease. We often can spot the process going on years before it becomes a disease. Addressing the autoimmune state—when the body starts attacking its own healthy tissues—before conception can potentially reduce the risk of pregnancy complications and support a healthier reproductive environment for conception and fetal development.

- *Sperm antibodies*: These antibodies, also known as antisperm antibodies (ASA), are proteins produced by the immune system that see sperm as an invader and set out to destroy them. ASA have been detected in 10 to 15 percent of women, or in 15 to 20 percent of men, who have otherwise unexplained infertility.[504]

Chapter 5: Pollution Solutions

Toxic Mold

Here is some additional information on how toxic mold can impact fetuses. A study titled "Effects of Mycotoxins on Child Development" explores how mycotoxins adversely affect child and fetal development. The authors explain how mycotoxins, particularly aflatoxins and ochratoxins, can disrupt normal developmental processes by inducing oxidative stress, impairing protein synthesis, and altering DNA expression. These disruptions can result in congenital abnormalities, low birth weight, and developmental delays in children.[505] The authors emphasize that exposure to mycotoxins during critical periods of fetal development poses significant risks, including neurodevelopmental defects and epigenetic changes that may have long-term health implications.[506]

Still another relevant study titled "The Presence of Mycotoxins in Human Amniotic Fluid" investigates the occurrence of mycotoxins in amniotic fluid samples collected from pregnant women between fifteen and twenty-two weeks of gestation. Analyzing eighty-six samples, the researchers detected mycotoxins in over 75 percent of cases, with nivalenol (33.7 percent), aflatoxins (31.4 percent), ochratoxin A (26.7 percent), and deoxynivalenol (27.9 percent) being the most prevalent.[507] Notably, 73 percent of samples from fetuses with genetic defects contained these toxins.[508] The study underscores the potential risk mycotoxins pose to fetal development and highlights the importance of reducing your preconception exposure to mycotoxins as well as detoxifying from previous exposures.

Truly, this is a topic that could very easily be its own book! In the testing chapter, we talked about the importance of being tested for mycotoxin exposure because if you've been exposed, it's important to detoxify from the mycotoxins before conceiving a child, as mycotoxins can pose significant risks to fetal development if exposure occurs during pregnancy. Also, some mycotoxins can cross the placental barrier, potentially leading to birth defects or developmental issues.[509]

Common Toxins to Avoid

Toxin	Effects on Health and Fertility	Sources and Examples	Substitutions or Solutions
Perchlorate	Disrupts thyroid function, potential developmental issues	Contaminated water, rocket fuel, fireworks, fertilizers, bleach	Use water filters, support clean industries, avoid contaminated foods, ensure proper industrial waste disposal

Benzidine	Carcinogenic, potential reproductive toxicity	Dyes, industrial chemicals, rubber, plastics, textile industry	Use benzidine-free products, proper protective equipment, ensure proper ventilation
Naphthalene	Respiratory issues, potential carcinogen	Mothballs, air fresheners, tar, industrial solvents, tobacco smoke	Use naphthalene-free products, proper ventilation, avoid mothballs, use natural air fresheners
Hexa-chlorobenzene	Reduced fertility, potential carcinogen	Pesticides, industrial chemicals, contaminated soil and water, fungicides	Use safer alternatives, proper protective equipment, support organic farming ensure proper disposal
Phenol	Skin irritation, potential reproductive toxicity	Disinfectants, industrial chemicals, antiseptics, personal care products	Use phenol-free products, proper protective equipment, choose natural disinfectants and antiseptics
Chlordane	Neurotoxicity, potential carcinogen	Pesticides, contaminated soil, termite control chemicals	Use safer alternatives, support organic farming, ensure proper disposal of old chemicals

Lindane	Neurotoxicity, potential carcinogen	Pesticides, lice treatments, scabies treatments, agricultural applications	Use safe alternatives, support organic farming, choose natural lice and scabies treatments
Formaldehyde	Respiratory issues, potential carcinogen	Household products (furniture, carpets), building materials, cosmetics, disinfectants	Use formaldehyde-free products, ensure good ventilation, buy solid wood furniture
Glyphosate	Hormonal disruption, potential carcinogen	Herbicides, genetically modified crops, contaminated food (soy, corn)	Use glyphosate-free products, buy organic foods, grow your own produce
Lead	Reduced fertility, miscarriage, developmental delays	Old paints, contaminated water, leaded gasoline, plumbing pipes, soil, imported toys	Use water filters, remove old paint, replace lead pipes, test soil, avoid imported toys
Manganese	Neurotoxicity, reduced fertility	Welding fumes, industrial emissions, contaminated water, batteries	Use proper protective equipment, air purifiers, water filters, avoid manganese-containing products

Mercury	Neurotoxicity, impaired fetal brain development	Fish (swordfish, shark, king mackerel, tilefish), dental amalgams, industrial emissions, thermometers	Consume low-mercury fish (salmon, shrimp), or avoid fish altogether during preconception, use mercury-free dental fillings
Carbon monoxide	Reduced fertility, developmental delays	Vehicle exhaust, gas appliances, tobacco smoke, industrial emissions	Use carbon monoxide detectors, ensure proper ventilation, avoid smoking, maintain gas appliances regularly
Chlorpyrifos	Neurodevelopmental issues, reduced fertility	Pesticides, non-organic fruits and vegetables	Use organic pesticides, wash produce thoroughly, buy organic fruits and vegetables
Chromium VI	Carcinogenic, reduced fertility	Industrial emissions, stainless steel production, leather tanning, welding fumes	Use proper protective equipment, support cleaner technologies, ensure good ventilation

Dichloro-diphenyltri-chloroethane (DDT)	Hormonal disruption, potential carcinogen	Pesticides (banned in many countries but persists in the environment), contaminated food	Support organic farming, wash produce thoroughly, avoid areas with high DDT contamination
Ethylene oxide	Miscarriage, developmental toxicity	Sterilization processes, industrial chemicals, medical equipment	Use alternative sterilization methods, ensure proper protective measures
Xylene	Neurotoxicity, potential reproductive toxicity	Paints, solvents, industrial emissions, adhesives	Use xylene-free products, ensure good ventilation, choose safer alternatives
Arsenic	Reduced fertility, miscarriage, developmental delays	Contaminated water, industrial processes, rice, seafood	Use water filters, avoid areas with high industrial contamination, choose arsenic-free rice
Benzene	Reduced fertility, increased risk of leukemia	Industrial emissions, tobacco smoke, gasoline fumes, household products	Avoid smoking, use benzene-free products, reduce gasoline exposure, ensure proper ventilation
Bisphenol A (BPA)	Hormonal disruption, increased risk of miscarriages	Plastics (bottles, containers), canned food linings, receipts, dental sealants	Use BPA-free products, fresh or frozen foods, avoid receipts, use BPA-free dental sealants

Brominated flame retardants	Hormonal disruption, developmental issues	Electronics, textiles, furniture, building materials	Use brominated flame retardant-free products, choose natural fiber textiles, buy flame-retardant-free furniture
Cadmium	Reduced fertility, developmental issues	Industrial emissions, tobacco smoke, contaminated food (shellfish, organ meats)	Avoid smoking, use air purifiers, consume low-cadmium foods, buy organic meat
Ethylbenzene	Neurotoxicity, potential reproductive toxicity	Industrial solvents, paints, inks, fuels, tobacco smoke	Use ethylbenzene-free products, ensure good ventilation, avoid smoking
Hexane	Neurotoxicity, potential reproductive toxicity	Industrial solvents, adhesives, paints, coatings	Use hexane-free products, ensure good ventilation, proper protective equipment
MTBE (Methyl tertiary-butyl ether)	Potential carcinogen, groundwater contaminant	Gasoline additive, industrial emissions, contaminated water	Use alternative fuels, support cleaner technologies, filter drinking water

Nonylphenol	Hormonal disruption, potential reproductive toxicity	Industrial detergents, cleaning products, personal care products	Use nonylphenol-free products, choose natural cleaning products, support environmentally friendly detergents
Styrene	Reduced fertility, neurotoxicity	Plastics (polystyrene), synthetic rubber, insulation materials, food containers	Use styrene-free products, choose natural insulation materials, avoid styrene-containing food containers
Toluene	Neurotoxicity, miscarriage	Paint thinners, adhesives, industrial solvents, nail polish	Use low-toxicity products, ensure good ventilation, choose toluene-free nail polish
PFOA (Perfluoro-octanoic acid)	Hormonal disruption, developmental issues	Non-stick cookware, water-resistant fabrics, food packaging, fire-fighting foams	Use PFOA-free products, switch to cast iron or stainless steel cookware, avoid water-resistant treatments

Silica	Respiratory issues, potential carcinogen	Construction materials (concrete, brick), industrial emissions, sandblasting, ceramics	Use silica-free products, proper protective equipment, ensure good ventilation, wet cutting techniques
Tetrachloro-ethylene (PERC)	Neurotoxicity, potential carcinogen	Dry cleaning, industrial solvents, metal degreasing, textile processing	Use PERC-free products, eco-friendly dry cleaning, proper ventilation, safer alternatives for degreasing
Hydrogen sulfide	Respiratory issues, potential reproductive toxicity	Industrial emissions (petroleum refining, natural gas extraction), sewage treatment plants, manure storage	Use proper protective equipment, ensure good ventilation, support cleaner technologies, reduce exposure
Acrolein	Respiratory issues, potential reproductive toxicity	Combustion of organic matter, industrial emissions, tobacco smoke, vehicle exhaust	Reduce exposure to smoke and exhaust, use air purifiers, support clean air initiatives
Carbon tetrachloride	Liver toxicity, potential reproductive toxicity	Industrial solvents, refrigerants, cleaning agents, fire extinguishers	Use safer alternatives, proper protective equipment, ensure good ventilation

Mirex	Reduced fertility, potential carcinogen	Pesticides, flame retardants, electrical equipment	Use safer alternatives, proper protective equipment, ensure proper disposal of old equipment
Pentachlo-rophenol (PCP)	Carcinogenic, potential reproductive toxicity	Wood preservatives, industrial chemicals, treated lumber, utility poles	Use PCP-free products, safer wood preservatives, ensure proper disposal, use untreated or naturally treated wood
TCDD (Dioxin)	Hormonal disruption, developmental issues	Industrial processes (paper bleaching, herbicide production), contaminated food (meat, dairy)	Avoid contaminated foods, support clean industries, buy organic meat and dairy products
Endosulfan	Neurotoxicity, hormonal disruption	Pesticides, contaminated food, agricultural runoff	Use organic pesticides, wash produce thoroughly, support organic farming

Propylene glycol	Skin irritation, potential reproductive toxicity	Solvents, personal care products (creams, lotions), food additives, antifreeze	Use propylene glycol-free products, choose natural personal care products, avoid antifreeze exposure
Acetone	Respiratory issues, potential reproductive toxicity	Industrial solvents, nail polish removers, paint thinners, cleaning agents	Use acetone-free products, ensure good ventilation, choose safer alternatives for cleaning and nail care

Chapter 6: Clean Slate: Detox for Baby-Building

The Essential Process of Detoxification

We are seriously asking our bodies to move mountains every day when we are putting toxins on our skin, in our food, our air, water— and if we really understood what we are asking our bodies to do, we wouldn't even ask because it sounds ridiculous! And on top of that, we're asking our bodies to produce healthy babies, and then we're asking our babies to do it all over again! When you think about it this way, I think it helps put into perspective the intricacy of what our bodies go through to filter everything out and then function at a high level. This is why I'm putting such a heavy focus on reducing your exposure to toxins.

Right now, let's pull back the curtain and gain a better understanding of how our bodies work to adapt to our internal and external environments through the multi-faceted process of detoxification.

Detoxification is the biological process by which the body removes toxins, which are harmful substances that can be *endogenous* (produced within the body) or *exogenous* (originating outside the body, such as pollutants, drugs, or chemicals). The detoxification process is essential for maintaining homeostasis (a stable internal environment) and preventing damage to cells, DNA, mitochondria, and tissues.

Detoxification occurs at multiple levels, including cellular, tissue, organ, and systemic, but the process begins at the cellular level, where specific biochemical pathways are activated to neutralize and eliminate toxins.

Cellular Processes of Detoxification: Phase I Detoxification (Bioactivation and Transformation)

The first phase of detoxification primarily involves a group of enzymes called cytochrome P450 (CYP450). These enzymes are located in the smooth endoplasmic reticulum of cells, particularly in the liver, which is the main organ of detoxification.[510]

In this phase, toxins are modified through oxidation, reduction, or hydrolysis. These reactions often convert lipophilic (fat-soluble) toxins into more reactive intermediates, which can sometimes be more toxic than the original substance.[511]

Phase I detoxification can result in the generation of reactive oxygen species (ROS), which can cause oxidative stress if not adequately neutralized by antioxidants.[512]

Cellular Processes of Detoxification: Phase II Detoxification (Conjugation Reactions)

Phase II detoxification involves conjugation reactions, where the reactive intermediates from Phase I are linked to hydrophilic (water-soluble) molecules to form less toxic, more easily excretable compounds.[513] The key conjugation reactions include:

- **Glutathione Conjugation:** Glutathione, a tripeptide composed of glutamine, cysteine, and glycine, is a critical antioxidant that neutralizes reactive intermediates by conjugation, forming water-soluble glutathione conjugates.[514]
- **Glucuronidation:** This pathway involves the addition of glucuronic acid to the toxin, facilitated by UDP-glucuronosyltransferase (UGT) enzymes, making the toxin more water-soluble.[515]
- **Sulfation:** Sulfotransferase enzymes add a sulfate group to the toxin, increasing its solubility.[516]
- **Acetylation:** N-acetyltransferase enzymes attach an acetyl group to the toxin, which aids in its excretion.[517]
- **Methylation:** Methyltransferase enzymes add a methyl group to the toxin, which can also facilitate its elimination.[518]

Cellular Processes of Detoxification: Phase III Detoxification (Transport and Excretion)

After conjugation, the detoxified metabolites need to be transported out of the cells. ATP-binding cassette (ABC) transporters, a family of membrane proteins, actively transport these conjugates out of the cells and into the extracellular space.[519]

The final phase of detoxification involves the excretion of these metabolites. They are typically excreted through the urine by the kidneys, in bile via the liver, or in sweat and feces.[520]

Antioxidant Defense Mechanisms

During detoxification, especially in Phase I, reactive intermediates and ROS can be generated, leading to oxidative stress.[521] The body has several antioxidant systems to mitigate those and find balance. We need some ROS, but not too much, so the body works to find balance through these mechanisms:

- **Glutathione Peroxidase:** Catalyzes the reduction of hydrogen peroxide and organic hydroperoxides, using glutathione as a substrate.[522]
- **Superoxide Dismutase (SOD):** Converts superoxide radicals into less harmful molecules like hydrogen peroxide.[523]
- **Catalase:** Converts hydrogen peroxide into water and oxygen, preventing oxidative damage.[524]

Nutritional Factors

Several nutrients and dietary components can support detoxification:

- **Sulfur-containing foods:** Garlic, onions, and cruciferous vegetables enhance glutathione production.[525]
- **Flavonoids:** Found in fruits and vegetables, flavonoids can induce Phase II detoxification enzymes.[526]
- **Fiber:** Dietary fiber supports the elimination of toxins through the digestive system by binding to them and facilitating their excretion.[527]

Cellular Processes of Detoxification in Detail

Now that you have a general understanding of how your body detoxifies, let's take a bit of a closer look.

Phase I Detoxification (Bioactivation and Transformation): Cytochrome P450 Enzymes (CYP450)

The CYP450 enzyme family includes over fifty different enzymes, each with varying substrate specificities. These enzymes are heme-containing proteins that catalyze oxidation reactions, introducing an oxygen atom into the chemical structure of the toxin (usually a xenobiotic, which is a foreign compound).[528]

While Phase I reactions often make toxins more polar, they can also generate reactive intermediates, such as epoxides or free radicals. These intermediates can bind to cellular macromolecules, including DNA, proteins, and lipids, potentially leading to cellular damage or mutations if not promptly neutralized.[529]

Various substances, including certain foods, medications, and environmental chemicals, can induce or inhibit CYP450 enzymes. For example, grapefruit juice contains compounds that inhibit CYP3A4, an enzyme responsible for metabolizing many drugs, which can lead to increased drug levels and potential toxicity.[530]

Phase II Detoxification (Conjugation Reactions): Conjugation Pathways

- **Glutathione** is a powerful antioxidant that plays a critical role in the detoxification of several toxins, including heavy metals, mycotoxins, pesticides and herbicides, environmental pollutants, and pharmaceuticals and certain drugs. Glutathione does this by binding to reactive molecules, including free radicals and heavy metals, neutralizing them and making them easier to excrete via bile or urine. It's a crucial process for eliminating oxidative stress from the body and helping protect the liver and other organs from damage. Glutathione-S-transferase (GST) enzymes catalyze the conjugation of glutathione (GSH) to reactive intermediates. This process not only neutralizes the toxic intermediates but also renders them more water-soluble, facilitating their excretion. Glutathione conjugates are typically excreted via bile or urine.[531] Glutathione also plays a critical role in protecting cells from oxidative stress by directly scavenging ROS and regenerating other antioxidants, such as vitamin C and E, back to their active forms.[532]

- **Glucuronidation**, another key detoxification pathway, also helps to neutralize and eliminate various toxins by making them more water-soluble for excretion. This detoxification process helps to maintain healthy hormonal balance and clear environmental and dietary toxins. Hormones, drugs, environmental toxins, mycotoxins, BPAs, alcohol metabolites, and bilirubin (a breakdown product of red blood cells that's processed by the liver) are all substances detoxified through glucuronidation. This pathway involves the conjugation of glucuronic acid, a derivative of glucose, to hydroxyl, carboxyl, or amino groups of toxins. The UGT enzymes responsible for this reaction are particularly active in the liver. Glucuronidation is a major pathway for the detoxification of endogenous substances, such as bilirubin and steroid hormones, as well as exogenous toxins like drugs and environmental chemicals.[533] Many drugs undergo glucuronidation before being excreted. Deficiencies in UGT enzymes can lead to toxic accumulation of drugs or other substances.[534]

- **Sulfation** involves adding a sulfate group to a compound, which makes it more water-soluble. This process is important for the detoxification of steroids, bile acids, and food additives and preservatives, among other harmful substances. Sulfation is essential for maintaining hormone balance and neutralizing various drugs and environmental toxins, preventing their accumulation in the body. Sulfation involves the transfer of a sulfate group from 3'-phosphoadenosine-5'-phosphosulfate (PAPS) to hydroxyl or amine groups of toxins. This reaction is catalyzed by sulfotransferase enzymes. Sulfation is crucial for the metabolism of various hormones, neurotransmitters, and xenobiotics.[535] While sulfation and glucuronidation pathways often work in tandem, sulfation typically handles smaller, more hydrophilic molecules, whereas glucuronidation is preferred for larger or more lipo-philic substances.[536]

- **Acetylation** is a detoxification process in the liver and other tissues that's primarily facilitated by a group of enzymes called N-acetyltransferases. This pathway helps metabolize a range of substances and inactivate certain toxins and drugs, which help eliminate them from the body. Acetylation goes after substances like:

  - *Aromatic amines*: Found in tobacco smoke and some dyes, these compounds undergo acetylation to be safely eliminated from the body.

  - *Heterocyclic amines*: These are carcinogenic compounds formed during the cooking of meat at high temperatures (e.g., grilling and frying).

  - *Sulfonamides*: A class of antibiotics that are detoxified through acetylation.

  - *Caffeine*: Acetylation is one of the pathways involved in the metabolism of caffeine.

  - *PABA (para-aminobenzoic acid)*: Found in some sun-screens and certain medications, PABA is detoxified via acetylation.

  - *Certain endogenous compounds*: Acetylation is also involved in metabolizing neurotransmitters and other internal compounds such as serotonin and histamine.

Acetylation involves the transfer of an acetyl group from acetyl-CoA to amines or hydrazines, a reaction catalyzed by N-acetyltransferase enzymes. This pathway is particularly important in the metabolism of aromatic amines, such as those found in some drugs and environmental carcinogens.[537]

There is significant genetic variability in acetylation capacity among individuals, categorized as "slow" or "fast" acetylators. Slow acetylators may be at increased risk for certain drug toxicities or cancers due to prolonged exposure to active metabolites.[538]

- **Methylation** is a crucial detoxification pathway that involves adding a methyl group to toxins, making them more water-soluble for excretion. This process is not only essential for eliminating toxin buildup but also for supporting DNA repair, regulating gene expression, and maintaining overall health. Methylation involves the transfer of a methyl group from S-adenosylmethionine (SAM) to hydroxyl, amine, or thiol groups on toxins. Methyltransferase enzymes regulate various physiological processes, including the inactivation of catecholamines (e.g., dopamine, epinephrine) and the detoxification of heavy metals like arsenic. A number of toxins and substances are detoxified through the process of methylation:
  - *Heavy metals* such as mercury, arsenic, and lead undergo methylation to be safely detoxified and excreted.
  - *Hormones,* including excess estrogens, testosterone, and catecholamines (such as adrenaline and dopamine), are metabolized via methylation to maintain hormonal balance.
  - *Neurotransmitters* like dopamine, norepinephrine, and serotonin rely on methylation for proper breakdown and elimination.
  - Methylation helps convert *homocysteine* into methionine, preventing its accumulation, which could otherwise contribute to cardiovascular issues.
  - When it comes to *toxins from smoking and alcohol,* harmful substances such as formaldehyde and acetaldehyde (an alcohol metabolite) utilize methylation for detoxification.

    ○   *Medications* like methotrexate rely on methylation for metabolism and clearance.

Beyond detoxification, methylation plays a crucial role in *epigenetic regulation* by methylating DNA and histones, thereby influencing gene expression. Aberrant methylation patterns are associated with diseases, including cancer.

Impairments in methylation can lead to toxin buildup and associated health risks, underscoring the importance of supporting methylation pathways through adequate intake of nutrients like folate, B12, and betaine.[539]

Phase III Detoxification (Transport and Excretion): Transporter Proteins

ATP-binding cassette (ABC) transporters play a critical role in cellular detoxification by actively pumping conjugated toxins out of cells. These transporters use energy derived from ATP hydrolysis to move substances across cellular membranes against their concentration gradient. Key types of ABC transporters involved in detoxification include P-glycoprotein (P-gp, also known as MDR1), multidrug resistance-associated proteins (MRPs), and breast cancer resistance protein (BCRP). They are essential for eliminating drugs, bile salts, and other metabolites from the body. However, their function can be influenced by several factors, both positively and negatively. A number of factors can enhance ABC transporter function:

- **Sufficient ATP availability:** ABC transporters require ATP to function. Supporting mitochondrial function and ATP production with nutrients like CoQ10, magnesium, and B vitamins is essential.
- **Optimal cellular health:** Healthy cell membranes maintained with omega-3 fatty acids, phospholipids, and

antioxidants (e.g., vitamins C and E) are vital for transporter integrity.

- **Detoxification support:** Enhancing detoxification pathways with glutathione and N-acetylcysteine (NAC) reduces the toxic burden on cells, improving transporter efficiency.
- **Gene expression support:** Nutrients like folate and B12 can support the gene expression of proteins involved in ABC transporter production.

Other factors inhibit ABC transporter function:

- **Toxins:** Exposure to heavy metals (e.g., mercury, lead), pesticides, and solvents can damage transport proteins or overwhelm the system.
- **Drug interactions:** Certain medications, including chemotherapy agents, antidepressants, and antivirals, may inhibit ABC transporter function, contributing to drug resistance or toxicity.
- **Oxidative stress:** High oxidative stress levels impair transporter functionality; antioxidants like glutathione, vitamin C, and selenium can mitigate this.
- **Chronic inflammation:** Inflammation downregulates ABC transporter expression and function; anti-inflammatory diets and supplements like curcumin and fish oil help counteract this.
- **Nutrient deficiencies:** Deficiencies in magnesium, zinc, and B vitamins impair ATP production, reducing ABC transporter efficiency.
- **Excretion mechanisms:** ABC transporters facilitate the removal of toxins through various excretory pathways. In *renal excretion*, water-soluble metabolites are filtered by the kidneys and excreted in urine through glomerular filtration and active tubular secretion. In *biliary excretion*, larger conjugates, especially those involving glucuronidation, are excreted

into bile and eliminated in feces. Enterohepatic circulation may recycle some substances. In *pulmonary excretion*, volatile substances such as alcohol or anesthetic gases are expelled via the lungs. And in *dermal excretion*, the skin excretes toxins through sweat glands, contributing to detoxification and maintaining skin health.

ABC transporters are crucial for maintaining cellular health and systemic detoxification. Ensuring optimal nutrient intake, minimizing toxic exposures, and supporting mitochondrial function are essential strategies for keeping these transport systems functioning effectively.[540]

Detoxification and Oxidative Stress: Balancing ROS and Antioxidants

While ROS are generated as by-products of Phase I detoxification, they are also produced during normal cellular metabolism, particularly in the mitochondria during oxidative phosphorylation. In controlled amounts, ROS serve as signaling molecules. However, excessive ROS can damage cellular components, leading to oxidative stress.[541]

The body maintains a delicate balance between ROS production and antioxidant defenses. Key antioxidants, like glutathione, superoxide dismutase, catalase, and peroxidases, are crucial for neutralizing excess ROS and preventing oxidative damage.[542]

The Nrf2 (nuclear factor erythroid 2-related factor 2) pathway is a major regulator of the antioxidant response. Upon exposure to oxidative stress or electrophilic chemicals, Nrf2 dissociates from its inhibitor (Keap1) and translocates to the nucleus, where it induces the expression of various detoxifying and antioxidant enzymes, including those involved in glutathione synthesis, Phase II detoxification, and ROS scavenging.[543]

Chapter 9: Smart Supplements: Powering Up for Parenthood

Liposomal glutathione is something that I just love and am so grateful for because it truly helps me get toxins out of people without detox symptoms. I have seen it work wonders to the point of saving the lives of many patients, friends, family, and even myself! It's such a miracle, and I want you to love it as much as I do! I always say it's my "desert island" supplement, because I would choose it over almost anything else. If you're curious about why it's so amazing, here is a list of some of the toxins that glutathione is capable of detoxifying:

Heavy Metals

- **Mercury:** Glutathione binds to mercury and helps in its excretion, which is particularly important in preventing neurotoxicity.
- **Lead:** By chelating lead, glutathione helps reduce its toxic effects on the nervous system and cardiovascular system.
- **Arsenic:** Glutathione facilitates the excretion of arsenic, which is commonly found in contaminated water and certain industrial exposures.
- **Cadmium:** Found in tobacco smoke and certain industrial processes, cadmium is detoxified through glutathione conjugation.
- **Aluminum:** Though the detoxification process is more complex, glutathione plays a supportive role in removing excess aluminum from the body.

Environmental Toxins

- **Pesticides and Herbicides:** Glutathione helps detoxify organophosphates and other chemical agents used in agriculture (e.g., glyphosate, DDT, atrazine).

- **PCBs (Polychlorinated Biphenyls):** These industrial chemicals, found in electrical equipment and other environmental pollutants, are detoxified in part through glutathione.
- **Dioxins:** Highly toxic compounds formed during combustion processes (e.g., waste incineration), glutathione aids in mitigating their impact.
- **Phthalates:** These plasticizers, found in plastics and personal care products, are detoxified with the help of glutathione.
- **Bisphenol A (BPA):** A common environmental toxin found in plastics, glutathione can assist in reducing BPA's harmful effects.

Industrial Chemicals and Solvents

- **Benzene:** A carcinogenic solvent found in industrial processes, gasoline, and cigarette smoke, glutathione helps neutralize its toxic effects.
- **Toluene:** Common in paint thinners, adhesives, and other industrial products, toluene is detoxified by glutathione conjugation.
- **Formaldehyde:** Used in building materials and certain household products, formaldehyde is detoxified in part by glutathione.
- **Hexane:** A solvent found in adhesives and other industrial products, detoxification of hexane is supported by glutathione.
- **Xylene:** Found in paints and gasoline, glutathione plays a role in its detoxification.

Pharmaceutical and Drug Toxins

- **Acetaminophen (Tylenol):** Glutathione is critical in detoxifying NAPQI, the toxic metabolite of acetaminophen overdose.

- **Chemotherapeutic Drugs:** Many chemotherapy agents, particularly those that induce oxidative stress (e.g., cisplatin, cyclophosphamide), are detoxified with glutathione's help.
- **Alcohol:** Ethanol metabolism produces acetaldehyde, a highly toxic compound that is neutralized by glutathione.
- **Antibiotics:** Some antibiotics, especially those that can cause oxidative stress (e.g., metronidazole, sulfonamides), are detoxified through glutathione pathways.

Metabolic Toxins

- **Reactive Oxygen Species (ROS):** Glutathione neutralizes superoxide, hydrogen peroxide, and hydroxyl radicals, protecting cells from oxidative stress.
- **Lipid Peroxides:** Glutathione helps detoxify oxidized lipids, which are by-products of fat metabolism and can damage cellular membranes.
- **Peroxynitrite:** This is a potent free radical formed from the reaction between nitric oxide and superoxide, often implicated in chronic inflammation and tissue damage. Glutathione helps reduce its harmful effects.
- **Advanced Glycation End Products (AGEs):** Formed from the reaction between sugars and proteins or fats, AGEs contribute to aging and chronic diseases; glutathione helps mitigate their accumulation.

Pollutants and Airborne Toxins

- **Particulate Matter (PM2.5):** Found in air pollution, these fine particles can cause oxidative stress and inflammation, which glutathione helps neutralize.

- **Ozone:** Exposure to high levels of ozone can lead to oxidative damage in the lungs, which glutathione helps protect against.
- **Cigarette Smoke Toxins:** Glutathione detoxifies numerous harmful compounds in cigarette smoke, including acrolein and other aldehydes.
- **Exhaust Fumes:** Nitrogen oxides and other pollutants from vehicle exhaust are detoxified by glutathione, particularly in the lungs.

Mycotoxins (Mold Toxins)

- **Aflatoxins:** Produced by molds that contaminate food, aflatoxins are carcinogenic, and glutathione plays a crucial role in their detoxification.
- **Ochratoxin A:** Found in water-damaged buildings and some contaminated foods, this mycotoxin is detoxified through glutathione conjugation.
- **Trichothecenes:** These are highly toxic mycotoxins that can suppress the immune system and are detoxified in part by glutathione.

Plastic and Synthetic Toxins

- **Polystyrene:** Found in packaging and insulation materials, glutathione helps to reduce the oxidative damage caused by polystyrene exposure.
- **Styrene:** A chemical used in the production of plastics and synthetic rubber, it is detoxified through glutathione pathways.

Food Additives and Contaminants

- **Artificial Sweeteners:** Some studies suggest that glutathione can help detoxify potentially harmful metabolites of artificial sweeteners like aspartame.
- **Preservatives:** Glutathione may support the detoxification of chemical preservatives like sodium benzoate and sulfites, which can cause oxidative stress.
- **Artificial Dyes and Flavors:** Many synthetic food additives and coloring agents are linked to oxidative stress and are mitigated by glutathione.

Biotoxins

- **Snake Venoms:** Glutathione helps detoxify certain components of snake venom, reducing the oxidative damage they can cause.
- **Bacterial Toxins:** Lipopolysaccharides (LPS) from gram-negative bacteria can cause severe immune reactions and inflammation, which glutathione helps mitigate.
- **Ciguatoxins:** Found in contaminated fish, these toxins can cause ciguatera poisoning, and glutathione assists in reducing the oxidative damage.

Endogenous Toxins from Dysbiosis (an imbalance in the gut microbiome)

- **Ammonia:** Overgrowth of certain gut bacteria can lead to the production of ammonia, which is toxic at high levels and detoxified through glutathione.

- **Indoxyl Sulfate and p-Cresol:** These are toxins produced by gut bacteria from protein fermentation, and they are detoxified via glutathione conjugation in the liver.

Radiation-Induced Toxins

- **Ionizing Radiation:** Radiation exposure (from X-rays, CT scans, or radiation therapy) produces free radicals, which are neutralized by glutathione.
- **Uranium and Radon:** Radioactive toxins that can damage cells through oxidative stress are mitigated by glutathione's antioxidant properties.

Chapter 11: Harmonizing Your Hormones

Other Hormones to Consider

Often we just think about estrogen, progesterone, and testosterone as our primary hormones, but there are many, many hormones that help our bodies do all the necessary functions, and that play a role in fertility and reproduction. When we understand even a little about how fine-tuned our bodies are, it just gives us even more appreciation for what our bodies can do. Here are some other hormones to appreciate!

Corticotropin-releasing hormone (CRH) is responsible for regulating how the body responds to stress, as well as managing other vital physiological functions. It is produced by the hypothalamus in the brain.

- **Adiponectin**, a hormone produced by fat tissue, enhances insulin sensitivity, reduces inflammation, and improves lipid metabolism.

- **Leptin**, a hormone produced by fat cells, helps regulate body weight by signaling the brain to reduce appetite and increase energy expenditure. It regulates the hypothalamic-pituitary-gonadal (HPG) axis, influencing the secretion of several hormones essential for ovulation and reproductive health.

Gonadotropin-releasing hormone (GnRH), which is produced in the hypothalamus, triggers the release of reproductive hormones, like LH and FSH, from the pituitary gland. This helps regulate your reproductive system.

- **Insulin-like growth factor (IGF)** plays a significant role in female fertility by improving the yield and quality of oocytes, enhancing embryo quality, and contributing to follicle maturation in the ovaries. It is produced in the liver and in the ovaries.
- **Inhibin** is a hormone produced by the granulosa cells in the ovaries that primarily acts to inhibit the secretion of FSH from the anterior pituitary gland.
- **Growth hormone (GH)** is produced by the pituitary gland and supports ovarian function, enhances ovarian angiogenesis, and improves oocyte quality.
- **Adrenocorticotropic hormone (ACTH)** is produced by the pituitary gland and stimulates the adrenal glands to release cortisol and androgens (sex hormones).
- **Oxytocin**, which is often called the "love hormone," is produced mainly in the hypothalamus in the brain and plays a significant role in fertility by regulating uterine contractions during labor, aiding in sperm transport within the female reproductive tract, and facilitating ovulation and

follicle development. Interestingly, it also enhances bonding between parents and their newborns.

- **Activin** is produced in several tissues, including the gonads, pituitary gland, and placenta, promotes oocyte maturation, and regulates granulosa cell function, essential for female fertility.
- **Kisspeptin**, which is produced in the hypothalamus, stimulates the release of GnRH.

Chapter 12: Taming Inflammation

Expanded Testing Options for Inflammation

If you suspect your body is fighting chronic inflammation, here is an expanded list of lab tests that can help identify what's going on.

Inflammatory Cytokines

- IL-1β (primary pro-inflammatory cytokine)
- IL-6 (inflammation and immune regulation)
- IL-8 (neutrophil activator)
- IL-10 (anti-inflammatory cytokine)
- TNF-α (tumor necrosis factor-alpha)

Specialized Inflammatory Pathway Tests

- NF-κB Activity
- NLRP3 Inflammasome Activation
- COX-2 Expression

Gastrointestinal Inflammation Markers

- Calprotectin
- Lactoferrin
- Zonulin

- β-defensin
- Short-Chain Fatty Acids (SCFAs)

Oxidative Stress and Antioxidant Status

- Glutathione (reduced/oxidized ratio)
- Superoxide Dismutase (SOD)
- Nitrotyrosine
- Lipid Peroxidation Products
- Total Antioxidant Capacity

Vascular Inflammation Markers

- Advanced Lipid Testing (including LDL particle size)
- Myeloperoxidase (MPO)
- PLAC Test (Lp-PLA2)
- Endothelin-1
- Asymmetric Dimethylarginine (ADMA)
- Oxidized LDL
- Matrix Metalloproteinases (MMPs)

DNA Damage and Oxidative Stress

- 8-hydroxy-2'-deoxyguanosine (8-OHdG)
- Lipid Peroxidase (markers of membrane oxidative damage)

Expanded Genetics Related to Histamine and Mast Cell Activation

- MTHFR (A1298C and C677T variants affecting methylation)
- DAO (Diamine Oxidase) gene (AOC1)
- HNMT (Histamine-N-methyltransferase) gene variants
- MAO (Monoamine Oxidase) variations
- Histamine Receptor (H1R, H2R, H3R, H4R) sensitivity
- KIT mutations (mast cell disease predisposition)

In-Depth Histamine Stabilization Supplement Options

There are other supplements that have been shown to help support your body's histamine stabilization. Of course, vitamin C and DAO supplements are your frontline supplements, but other options include:

- Luteolin
- Rutin
- Curcumin (especially liposomal forms)
- Omega-3 Fatty Acids (EPA/DHA)
- Glutathione and NAC
- Pycnogenol
- Resveratrol
- Palmitoylethanolamide (PEA)
- Pterostilbene
- Baicalin (Chinese Skullcap)
- Milk Thistle
- Boswellia
- Black Seed Oil
- Melatonin (low-dose for mast cell stabilization)
- Alpha Lipoic Acid (ALA)

Expanded Strategies to Tame Inflammation

If you're looking to go deeper on ways in which you can tame inflammation in your body, here are some strategies to look into:

- Limbic Retraining Programs (such as DNRS, Gupta Program, Primal Trust)
- Neurofeedback Therapy (for mast cell stabilization and vagal tone)
- Vagus Nerve Stimulation techniques (breathing, cold exposure, devices)

Oxalates: Expanded Information

Here is some additional insight into the relationship between oxalate overload and inflammation, as well as more ways to combat it:

Mechanisms by Which Oxalates Promote Inflammation

- Activation of inflammasome pathways (especially NLRP3)
- Direct mitochondrial injury and oxidative stress
- Triggering mast cell degranulation
- Induction of local tissue inflammation (kidneys, joints, reproductive tissues)

Advanced Oxalate Management Strategies

- Gradual dietary oxalate reduction (avoid sudden dumping)
- Calcium citrate 200–400 mg with meals
- Magnesium glycinate or citrate supplementation
- Vitamin B6 (P5P form) 50–100 mg daily
- Gut healing strategies (probiotics, glutamine, SCFAs)

HIGH HISTAMINE FOODS

FOODS HIGHEST IN HISTAMINES

- Fermented foods: sauerkraut, wine, pickled items, kombucha, alcohol, yogurt, Kim Chi
- Vinegar and vinegar containing foods
- Processed/aged meats
- Soured foods (sour cream, sourdough bread)
- Aged cheeses
- Canned foods

MEATS
Dried and smoked meats —
- Sausage
- Salami
- Prosciutto
- Bacon
- Chorizo
- Pancetta
- Avoid ground meat unless freshly ground

FISH (MOST FISH)
- Tuna
- Mackerel
- Sardines
- Anchovy
- Shellfish (clams, mussels, oysters)
- Crustaceans (scallops, crab, shrimp)
- Salmon

VEGETABLES
- Eggplant
- Spinach
- Green beans
- Mushrooms
- Peas
- Squash
- Soybeans (edamame)
- Pumpkin

BEVERAGES
- Green tea
- Black tea
- Kefir
- Kombucha
- Alcohol

CONDIMENTS
- Ketchup
- Soy sauce
- Vinegars

FRUITS
- Avocados (ripe)
- Citrus fruits
- Strawberries
- Bananas
- Pineapple
- Pears
- Tomatoes
- Olives
- Papaya
- Plums
- Dried fruits

GRAINS
- Generally low in histamine but high inflammation

NUTS
(See Histamine liberators)
- Cashews
- Walnuts
- Sunflower seeds

LEGUMES
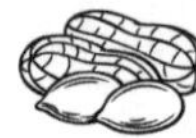
- Peanuts
- Lentils
- Beans

SWEETENERS
- Honey and sugar are low in histamines; however, they can spike blood sugar, triggering inflammation, activating the immune system, and leading to histamine release.

OTHER
- Artificial colors/preservatives

HIGH HISTAMINE FOODS

HISTAMINE LIBERATORS AND DAO BLOCKERS

Histamine liberators
Foods that can promote the release of histamines in other foods.

Histamine blockers
Foods that prevent DAO from breaking down histamine Inflammatory foods.

When following a low histamine diet, you should also avoid both, which include:

HISTAMINE LIBERATORS

- Avocados (ripe)
- Citrus fruits
- Chocolate, cocoa
- Nuts (macadamia, pine nut, pistachio, Brazil, almond)
- Papaya
- Beans

DAO BLOCKERS

- Alcohol
- Black tea, green tea, mate tea
- Energy drinks (always avoid)

LOW HISTAMINE FOODS

VEGETABLES

- Artichokes
- Arugula
- Asparagus
- Basil
- Bean sprouts
- Beets
- Bok choy
- Broccoli
- Broccolini
- Brussels sprouts
- Cabbage – Chinese
- Cabbage – Green and Red
- Cabbage – Napa
- Carrots
- Cauliflower
- Celery
- Celery root
- Collards
- Cucumber
- Daikon radishes
- Dandelion greens
- Dill
- Escarole
- Fennel
- Garlic
- Ginger

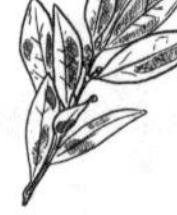

- Green split peas
- Jicama
- Kale
- Kohlrabi
- Leafy greens
- Leeks
- Lettuces: Butter, endive, red leaf, green leaf, iceberg, radicchio, romaine, mesclun, mustard greens
- Mint
- Okra
- Onions
- Parsnips
- Peppers
- Potatoes
- Radishes
- Rhubarb
- Rutabaga
- Scallions (green onions)
- Shallots
- Squash (except pumpkin)
- Sweet potatoes
- Swiss chard
- Turnip
- Watercress

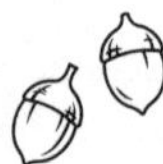

HERBS

- Chives
- Cilantro
- Parsley
- Sage
- Saffron

NUTS/NUT BUTTERS
(see Histamine liberators)

The following nuts are less likely to aggravate histamine intolerance. Notice of how you feel after consuming.

- Pistachios
- Macadamia nuts/macadamia butter
- Hazelnuts/hazelnut butter

LOW HISTAMINE FOODS

FRUIT

- Apples
- Apricots
- Avocado (not ripe)
- Blackberries
- Blueberries
- Cantaloupe
- Cherries
- Coconut (fresh)
- Cranberries (fresh)
- Currants (fresh)
- Dragon fruit
- Honeydew melon
- Kiwis
- Loquats
- Mangoes
- Nectarines
- Passion fruit
- Peaches
- Pears
- Persimmons
- Pomegranate
- Raspberries
- Rhubarb

GRAINS

- Rice
- Quinoa

SWEETENERS/OTHER

- Monk fruit
- Stevia
- Carob

MEATS/AMIMAL PRODUCTS

Freshly cooked beef/pork/poultry/fish (It is best to consume fresh, grass-fed, flash frozen)

If in doubt, ask grocer, purchase from farmer's market.

- Beef
- Bison
- Chicken
- Duck
- Lamb
- Liver
- Pork
- Quail
- Rabbit
- Salmon (frozen) – gutted and frozen within 30 minutes of catch (Vital Farms)
- Turkey

CONDIMENTS

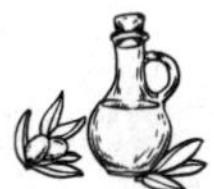

- Olive oil
- Coconut oil
- Distilled vinegar

BEVERAGES

- Herbal teas
- Rooibos tea
- Dairy-free milks (avoid cashew, walnut)
- Coffee – can trigger histamine release be aware

Oxalates in Food

What is an "oxalate"?

Oxalate, also referred to as "oxalic acid," is a naturally occurring compound found in many plants and other foods we eat. It is considered an anti-nutrient because it can inhibit our body's ability to absorb essential vitamins and minerals.

Why is it best to avoid high oxalate foods?

Too much oxalate leads to oxalate crystals, which can cause renal damage, activate the immune system, upset the GI tract, and deplete glutathione.

Why else are oxalates dangerous?

High oxalate levels have also been linked to inflammation, autoimmune disorders, and mitochondrial dysfunction.

Do not eat these foods very often.

Vegetables & Herbs

Asparagus
Beets and beet greens*
Celery
Collards
Dandelion greens
Eggplant
Escarole
Kale
Leeks*
Okra*
Parsley*
Potatoes
Pumpkin
Rhubarb
Rutabagas
Sorrel
Spinach*
Squash, yellow, summer
Sweet potato*
Swiss chard*
Turnip
Turnip greens
Watercress
Yams

Legumes, Nuts, Seeds

Black beans
Cashews
Chili beans
Hazelnuts
Navy beans
Nut butters
~~Peanuts~~
Pecans
Peanut butter
~~Sesame seeds~~
~~Soybean curd (tofu)~~
~~All soy products~~

Fruits

Apricots
Avocado
Grapes (Concord)
Currants
Dewberries
Figs (red)
Dried Figs
Dried Gooseberries
Dried Pineapples
Kiwi
Raspberries
Tangerines

Grains

~~Graham flour~~
~~Grits, white corn~~
~~Kamut~~
~~Oatmeal~~
~~Popcorn~~
~~Rice bran~~
Rice flour (brown or white)
~~Spelt~~
~~Stone ground flour~~
~~Wheat bran~~
~~White flour~~
~~Wheat germ~~
~~Whole wheat flour~~
~~Yellow dock~~

Other

Cocoa (chocolate)
Tea
~~Beer~~
Stevia
Ginger
~~Soy sauce~~ (unless GF)
~~Potato chips~~
Black pepper (ground)

Dr. Shippy does **not** recommend consuming the foods with a line through them.

*Extremely high in oxalate

Moderate Oxalate Foods

Eat these foods only in moderation.

Vegetables

Brussels sprouts
Carrots, cooked or raw
Corn
~~Eggplant~~
Fennel
Winter squash
Green beans
Mushrooms
Parsnips
Potato, boiled

Legumes, Nuts, Seeds

Black beans
Cashews
Chili beans
Green beans,
 pod, runner
Hazelnuts
Navy beans
Pecans
~~Sesame seeds~~
~~Soybean curd (tofu)~~
~~All soy products~~

Fruits

Apples with skin
Blackberries
Lemon peel
Mandarin oranges
Orange peel
Prunes
Strawberries
Tomatoes

Grains

White rice
~~Bulgur~~
~~Cornmeal~~
~~Semolina~~

Other

Tea (black, green, white)
Wine

Dr. Shippy does **not** recommend consuming the foods with a line through them.

Low Oxalate Foods

Focus on eating primarily these foods.

Vegetables

Artichoke
Bell peppers (green are lowest, red, orange, yellow are slightly higher)
Bok choy
Broccoli
Cabbage
Cauliflower
Chives
Cucumber
Garlic, cooked
Lettuce (iceberg or romaine)
Mushrooms
Onions, cooked
Peas
Pickles
Radish
Sauerkraut
Yellow zucchini
Squash

Fruits

Apples, peeled
Apricots
Bananas
Blueberries
Cantaloupe
Cherries
Cranberries, dried
Grapefruit
Grapes
Honeydew melon
Lemon
Lime
Mango
Nectarines
Olives
Papaya
Peaches
Pears
Pineapple
Plantain
Plums
Raisins
Watermelon

Meat, Poultry, Seafood

Bacon
Beef
Chicken
Eggs
Ham
Pork
Turkey
Vension
Wild game
Shellfish
Fish (except sardines)

Dairy

~~Butter~~
~~Buttermilk~~
~~Cheese~~
~~Milk~~
~~Yogurt~~

Legumes, Nuts, Seeds

Black-eyed peas
Coconut
Flax seeds
Garbanzo beans
Lentils
Lima beans
Water chestnuts

Other

Carob
Coffee
Honey (1 tbsp)
Jellies, jams, preserves (made with low/moderate fruits, 1 tbsp)
Maple syrup (pure, 1 tbsp)
~~Sugar (all kinds)~~
Herbal tea
Vanilla extract
Vinegar
Oils

Dr. Shippy does **not** recommend consuming the foods with a line through them.

Autoimmunity and Fertility: Additional Details

The body of research around the impact of autoimmune processes and fertility continues to grow. Here is some additional information:

Inflammatory Mechanisms Impacting Fertility

- DNA methylation errors affecting gametes
- NK cell overactivation impairing embryo implantation
- Th1/Th17 immune shifts interfering with tolerance needed for pregnancy

Expanded Testing for Subclinical Autoimmunity

- ANA (even low-positive results matter)
- Anti-thyroid antibodies (TPO, Tg)
- Anti-phospholipid antibodies (cardiolipin, beta-2 glyco-protein)
- Complement C3 and C4
- NK cell activity panels
- Cytokine panels (IL-6, TNF-α, IL-1β)
- Zonulin and leaky gut panels
- Gluten and casein sensitivity (even without full-blown celiac disease)

Expanded Immune-Calming Protocols

- High-dose omega-3 (EPA/DHA)
- Liposomal curcumin
- Specialized Pro-Resolving Mediators (SPMs)
- Vitamin D optimization (50–80 ng/mL range)
- Methylation pathway support
- Gut microbiome rebalancing protocols
- Gentle detoxification (mold, heavy metals if indicated)

Chapter 13: Fertility GPS: Navigating Your Reproductive Journey

This whole journey, everything you've been reading and the plan you've been following in this book has been leading up to the moment of conception. So let's just spend a moment going through the specific steps of how a baby is conceived. I find it to be fascinating!

The Oocyte: From Follicle to Egg

The journey to conception begins with the development of the oocyte, or egg. In females, a group of immature oocytes is present in the ovaries from birth, contained within follicles. Each menstrual cycle, hormonal signals (primarily from the hypothalamus and pituitary gland) stimulate several follicles to begin maturation. However, typically only one follicle becomes dominant, undergoing a series of changes that allow it to develop into a mature egg (oocyte).

Follicular Development

The dominant follicle produces increasing amounts of estrogen, which triggers a surge of luteinizing hormone (LH). This surge is crucial for the final maturation of the oocyte and the follicle's transformation into a corpus luteum after ovulation. As the follicle matures, it undergoes structural changes, developing a fluid-filled antrum that allows the egg to be released during ovulation.

Ovulation

When the mature follicle ruptures, it releases the oocyte into the fallopian tube. This process is tightly regulated by hormonal interactions and reflects the importance of a healthy endocrine system.

The Journey of the Sperm

The journey of the sperm is an incredible and complex process, where somewhere between 80 and 300 million sperm are released during ejaculation. Yet only one will successfully fertilize the egg. From the moment of release, the sperm embark on a challenging voyage through the female reproductive system, facing numerous obstacles. The acidic environment of the vagina, the narrowing of the cervix, and the long journey through the uterus and fallopian tubes all reduce the number of viable sperm.

Sperm Capacitation

Sperm undergo a process called *capacitation*, which prepares them to penetrate the egg's outer layer (the *zona pellucida*). This involves biochemical changes in the sperm's membrane and is essential for successful fertilization.

Navigating to the Egg

Sperm are guided by a combination of chemical signals (chemotaxis) and physical structures in the female reproductive tract. Only the healthiest and most motile sperm can reach the egg; of the millions that start the journey, only a few hundred will reach the egg. And with all the work you've been putting into optimizing your health and epigenetics, those few hundred healthy sperm are likely much healthier than they would have been just a few months ago! The ultimate success depends on the sperm's ability to navigate these barriers and penetrate the egg's outer layers, a feat accomplished by just one sperm.

Fertilization

For fertilization to occur, both the egg and sperm undergo critical changes. After sperm is deposited in the vagina, it begins a process called *capacitation*, which increases its motility and metabolism, aiding its journey to the fallopian tube. Capacitation is triggered by the acidic environment of the vagina, which activates ATP enzymes in the sperm's cytosol. This process alters the sperm's plasma membrane by modifying the lipid and glycoprotein composition, preparing it for fertilization.

The second major change occurs when the sperm actually reaches the egg. The sperm's acrosome, which contains lysosomal enzymes, releases these enzymes through exocytosis to penetrate the egg's extracellular matrix. One enzyme, hyaluronidase, digests the cells embedded in hyaluronic acid surrounding the oocyte. This exposes acrosin, an enzyme needed to digest the zona pellucida (the egg's protective layer). Once the acrosome reaction occurs, calcium levels rise, prompting the egg's cortical granules to release enzymes that alter the extracellular matrix. These enzymes digest sperm receptor glycoproteins ZP2 and ZP3, making the zona pellucida impenetrable to additional sperm, thus ensuring proper chromosome pairing and preventing conditions like trisomy.[544]

What is trisomy? This is when a person has three copies of a chromosome instead of the usual two. We usually get two copies of each chromosome—one from each parent. If there is an extra copy, however, the balance of genetic information is disrupted, leading to developmental and health issues, such as Down syndrome (caused by an extra copy of chromosome 21). Most trisomy cases do not last to full term (newborn incidence is about 1 in 5,000).[545]

Epigenetic Markers in Fertility and Reproduction

If you have optimized your epigenetics, it means you're more likely to have a healthier baby. This is the crux of everything we've been working toward—it's where the real gold is. Epigenetics is an awe-inspiring design feature of the human body, and by fine-tuning yours, you're passing down a beautifully equipped toolbox to your child. Inside are the tools their body will use to grow, repair, adapt, and thrive—a gift that will shape not just how they begin life but how they live it.

I'd like to take you on a deeper exploration into the interplay between hormones, reproduction, and epigenetics. Some of this information is repeated from earlier in the book, but I think it's helpful to tie it all together.

Influence of Estrogen on Epigenetic Markers

Estrogen can modulate DNA methylation patterns at genes involved in reproductive processes, such as follicle development, ovulation, and endometrial preparation for implantation. For example, estrogen receptor (ER) genes themselves are subject to DNA methylation and histone modifications, which can influence the sensitivity of cells to estrogen. In conditions like PCOS, abnormal methylation of estrogen receptor genes can impact fertility. Exposure to estrogenic compounds (like endocrine disruptors) in utero can cause epigenetic changes that affect not only the reproductive system of the fetus but also future generations.

Progesterone's Role in Epigenetic Regulation

Progesterone plays a key role in making the uterine lining receptive to the implantation of a fertilized egg. It achieves this partly through epigenetic modifications, including DNA methylation and histone changes in the endometrium. Progesterone influences DNA methylation in genes important for placental development and maternal-fetal signaling. These changes are essential for the proper nourishment of the developing fetus. For example, studies show that abnormal epigenetic regulation of the progesterone receptor can lead to recurrent pregnancy loss or infertility.

Testosterone and Sperm Epigenetics

Testosterone influences DNA methylation patterns and histone modifications during sperm production. Epigenetic regulation is crucial for ensuring that sperm cells have the appropriate gene expression for normal development. For example, abnormal DNA methylation in sperm can lead to male infertility. Environmental factors such as endocrine disruptors or stress can cause changes in the sperm's epigenetic profile, affecting both fertility and the health of the offspring.

Epigenetic markers in sperm can be passed down to the next generation, potentially influencing the development of offspring and their risk for certain diseases.

Human Chorionic Gonadotropin (hCG) and Epigenetic Regulation

The hormone hCG is produced soon after implantation and helps maintain the corpus luteum, which produces progesterone. The influence of hCG on the endometrium includes changes in DNA methylation and histone acetylation patterns that promote a favorable environment for fetal development. Additionally, hCG regulates the expression of genes involved in placental formation, which is crucial for proper nutrient exchange between mother and fetus. Epigenetic markers such as DNA methylation help modulate these genes, ensuring proper placental function.

Epigenetic Markers Influenced by Environmental and Lifestyle Factors

Now let's look at how environmental and lifestyle factors impact and influence specific epigenetic markers. I know this can be dense information to absorb, but I think it serves to motivate couples to adopt changes in their lifestyle because it really shows the deep impact of those changes.

Maternal Diet and Nutrient Availability

Folate (vitamin B9) is a key nutrient for DNA methylation. A folate-deficient diet during pregnancy can lead to improper DNA methylation in the developing embryo, which may increase the risk of neural tube defects and other developmental abnormalities. Obesity has been linked to altered DNA methylation patterns in both the mother and fetus, influencing genes related to metabolism and possibly leading to an increased risk of obesity and metabolic disorders in offspring.

Environmental Exposures (Endocrine Disruptors)

BPA, the endocrine disruptor found in plastics that we discussed in an earlier chapter, can interfere with hormone signaling and lead to abnormal DNA methylation patterns in reproductive tissues. Studies suggest that prenatal exposure to BPA can cause long-term epigenetic changes in both the mother and offspring, potentially affecting fertility and increasing the risk of reproductive disorders. Exposure to phthalates, another class of endocrine disruptors, during pregnancy can modify DNA methylation patterns in the fetus, potentially leading to altered reproductive development and increased risk of diseases later in life.

Stress and Cortisol

High levels of cortisol, the stress hormone, can lead to epigenetic changes that affect fertility. For instance, stress-induced changes in DNA methylation can alter the expression of genes involved in ovulation or sperm production. In mice, prenatal exposure to stress has been shown to cause DNA methylation changes in offspring, leading to altered stress responses and increased susceptibility to anxiety or depression later in life.

Prenatal Hormone Exposure and Developmental Programming

Hormones like estrogen and progesterone influence epigenetic programming in the fetus. For example, in-utero exposure to abnormal hormone levels (e.g., from maternal stress or endocrine disruptors) can affect DNA methylation and histone modification patterns, altering how genes are expressed throughout the life of the child. Some epigenetic changes caused by hormone imbalances can be passed down to future generations, even if the subsequent generations are not directly exposed to the hormonal disturbance.

Key Epigenetic Genes and Processes in Reproduction

Without getting too much in the weeds when it comes to genetic code, I want to share some insights on a few key genes that play a role in reproduction.

IGF2 (Insulin-like Growth Factor 2)

IGF2 is an important gene for fetal growth and placental development. DNA methylation at the IGF2 gene can be influenced by hormonal changes during pregnancy. Abnormal methylation of IGF2 has been associated with poor fetal growth, increased risk of metabolic disorders, and developmental issues.

Hox Genes

Hox genes are involved in determining the body plan of the developing embryo. Hormones like estrogen and progesterone can influence the epigenetic regulation of Hox genes, affecting implantation and placental development. Changes in the methylation status of these genes can lead to pregnancy complications, such as preeclampsia or intrauterine growth restriction (IUGR).

ACKNOWLEDGMENTS

This book would not exist without the remarkable people who have touched my life, each contributing in their own way to the journey that brought these pages to fruition. It is with immense gratitude that I acknowledge those who have walked alongside me, offering wisdom, encouragement, and unwavering support. Whether through research, mentorship, collaboration, or simply believing in this mission, your influence has shaped not just this book but the impact it will have on the world. Thank you for being a part of this extraordinary journey. (And please know this list of amazing people is written in no particular order!)

To Jill Smith, Billie Brownell, Jennifer Gingerich, and Justin Batt, along with the entire, incredibly talented team at Forefront Books: Thank you for believing in this project and helping me shape it into something that can truly impact lives and future generations.

To my patients: Your courage, your trust, and your commitment to healing continue to inspire me every day. The insights gained from working with you have given me such a unique perspective and a front row seat to the transformations that can occur at the intersection of genetics, epigenetics, nutrition, the microbiome, and mitochondrial health. Your willingness to embark on this journey has allowed me to deepen my understanding and share it with others. Without you, this book would remain theoretical; you bring it to life.

To the researchers who dedicate their lives to studying the intricate connections between epigenetics, environmental medicine, preconception health, and fertility: Your work is laying the foundation for a healthier future. Your discoveries illuminate the profound ways in which our choices before conception shape not only our own well-being but also the health of generations to come. I am endlessly grateful for your commitment to advancing this critical field.

To my children, Grant and Reed: You are my heart and my deepest motivation. Thank you for giving me the most precious gift of motherhood.

To Angela and Jim Lennon, my mother and stepfather: As you navigate this season of life, I am grateful for the opportunity to offer my support, just as you have always supported me. Your love and resilience inspire me.

To my father, Phil Nacke, who taught me how to think, not just memorize: Your encouragement shaped my ability to question, learn, and explore. You instilled in me the drive to push boundaries. I know you would have loved to have been part of this book's creation, and I carry your influence with me always.

To my sisters Laura Roberts and Onyay Pheori: Thank you both for teaching me how to love and be loved, and so much more. You are both so special to me, truly bright shining lights in the world.

To my nieces Ava and Ella: It is a dream come true being your aunt and being so close to you. I'm in awe of the women you are becoming.

To Sam Horn: Your expertise in communication and thought leadership has been invaluable in helping me refine and articulate my message with clarity and impact. Your guidance has made a lasting impression on my work, and I am so grateful for your wisdom, friendship, and encouragement.

To Bharti Kher: When I first encountered your artwork on a trip to India, I was instantly captivated. Your work spoke to something deep in my spirit and stayed with me long after I returned home. It has inspired more than just reflection—it stirred a creative energy and boldness that I needed as the final pieces of this book were culminating. Thank you for the beauty and bravery you bring into the world.

To JJ Virgin, Tim Organ, and the Mindshare Collaborative: Your belief in me so early on encouraged me to find my voice and share my message with the world. Your mentorship and friendship have been instrumental in this journey.

Manish Vora, "NISHY": I have so much gratitude for that fateful day we met at the airport on our way to Burning Man in 2022. With our flight canceled and rescheduled for the next day, we had many unexpected hours to share our dreams and passions. Your belief in my mission to help men and women have healthy babies was instrumental in boosting my urgency to complete the book. You are such a dear friend; thank you.

Cynthia and Zak Garcia: Thank you for all the love and encouragement and for helping me to realize the vision for Every Baby Well. You are bright lights on this planet!

To Dave Asprey: You are one of the biggest believers in my work, and no one understands the importance of preconception better than you. You have been such a supporter, not only by aligning with this mission but also by recommending my practice to your friends. Your vision for optimizing human health is inspiring, and I am so grateful for your encouragement.

To Monaica Ledell: You helped me take my vision for helping humanity and transform it into powerful brand names: *Every Life Well* and *Every Baby Well.* Your insistence on helping me articulate my mission was a gift, and I deeply appreciate your vision and guidance.

To Dr. Mark Hyman: Your fearlessness in speaking the truth and your courage in pioneering functional medicine have inspired me beyond words. You have normalized these conversations and empowered countless people to think and practice differently. I am deeply honored by your willingness to write the foreword for this book and to amplify this message. Your trust, confidence, and referrals mean the world to me.

To Dr. Jeffrey Bland, the father of functional medicine: Your pioneering work has transformed the way we understand health. I am profoundly grateful for your wisdom and encouragement.

To Mimi Doe: I'm so grateful to be on this life journey with you! You are truly an angel in human form. Your dear friendship and belief in this soul mission is such a precious gift. Your guidance and your belief in the urgency of this book and its importance for humanity have been a steadying force.

To Dr. Jill Carnahan: You continuously inspire me. Our backgrounds are so similar, both of us engineers who turned to medicine after personal health crises, and our journeys have run parallel in environmental medicine. Your unwavering belief in me and our deep respect for each other's work have made this path so much richer. Your friendship has been a guiding light, not only in medicine but in the spiritual, emotional, and metaphysical aspects of healing as well. I am so grateful you introduced me to Forefront Books.

To Deborah Dunn, MD: You push all the boundaries, taking it upon yourself to investigate topics beyond anyone else I know. The way you hold me accountable for my viewpoints means so much. I love having conversations with you. You embody fearlessness, trusting yourself, and going for it. You've discovered that delicate balance between work and play. On top of all that, I just love having fun with you!

To Beth Shirley: Thank you for believing in my mission and encouraging me to take the leap from traditional internal medicine into practicing medicine in a way that truly helps people heal.

To my medical practice and online team—Susan, Amity, Lisa, Michelle, Juli, Jaimie, Brooke, Michele, Linda, and Jaimie: You are the angels that extend the love I have for my patients into everything we do. This book would not be possible without you.

To Karen Shank, MD; Gabrielle Lyon, MD; David Haase, MD; Todd Lepine, MD; Elisa Song, MD; Deborah Dunn, MD; Amy Myers, MD; Robyn Benson, D.O.M.: I want to thank each of you for the many meaningful conversations we've had about practicing medicine in a way that truly heals. You are true, gifted healers.

To Casey Means, MD: Casey, I don't know you personally yet, but your work has helped me refine my voice and connect more powerfully with my audience. Thank you.

To Whitney Gossett: Your insights in the publishing world validated my decision to go with Forefront Books, and your belief in this book's urgency helped me prioritize it above all else.

To Stephanie Hahn: Thank you for taking time out of your schedule to share such powerful insight on pelvic floor health for this book. And thank you for the thoughtful ways you always help our mutual patients.

To Patricia Kane at Body Bio: Thank you for highlighting the importance of choline, appropriate fatty acids, and phosphatidylcholine.

To Dr. Reiser, my former ethics professor: It has been one of the greatest honors of my career to have you and your wife as patients and to engage in deeply meaningful conversations with you. Your trust in me, coming from an allopathic model into my functional medicine journey, has been profoundly affirming.

To Lisa Clark: You have been the doula of this book, ensuring it was birthed into the world with love, intention, and care. Thank you for believing in this book from day one.

To my teachers on the nature of the universe and how the divine is expressed through humanity's expression of love—Genpo Roshi, Mary Morrisey, Joe Dispenza, and Alison Armstrong: I'm immensely grateful.

To Dawn and Lance: What started as a patient-doctor relationship has turned into family, and I cherish being part of your family now!

To Derek Gulliory, MD: Thank you for your similar vision of the problems in medicine and the best solutions to go from "sick care" to health care and actually helping people be healthy.

To Jason and Jessica Karp: Your unwavering support means more than I can express, and I am grateful to be on this mission with you to create health for humanity. Team Humanity!

To my friends Ping Fu, Thomas Romm, Ricardo Santa Cruz, Ammaji, and the Ganga River at Kumbh Mela in India: Thank you for teaching me about embodying Faith. It truly is an integral thread of life that is transformational.

To Pippa Malmgren: Thank you for exploring and tapping into manifestation and the realms of possibility it holds.

To Bo and Dawn Eason: You've been instrumental in helping me find my voice and embrace the power of storytelling. Thank you for your friendship.

To Andi Pitt, Nick Matzorkis, Brian Nolan, Kay Wicoll, and Liz Hoffmaster: You are all such gifted sounding boards who have validated the need and this mission. Thank you for lending your brilliance, your forward thinking vision, and your hearts to the goal of helping millions of children and parents. You each have a beautiful capacity to dream with me about what's possible for this mission to make a real difference.

To Stacey Livens: My telepathic soul sister, you reach out at the most perfect times to send love, encouragement, and support. I'm so grateful for you.

To Molly Cummings and Willow Dea: We have traversed the joys and trials of the last two decades together with love, generosity, support, and compassion for each of our journeys.

To Shel Lalji: You have taught me and all your friends about soul partnership. Your extraordinary expression of true love amplified by grace and faith is so inspiring.

To my dear patient Suzanne Stratton: You cared enough to listen to your angels and help me and my family get to the root cause when we were so ill from the mold *Chaetomium*. Because of you, I learned how to help my patients heal from toxic mold exposure. You are so generous with your care, intuition, and wisdom.

To David and Leslie Shippy: Thank you for pouring your hearts into the boys. Coparenting with you is an honor. My greatest wish is for them to know how deeply loved they are; you are instrumental in that wish coming true.

To my forever friends, you know who you are: Thank you for enriching my life and this mission in countless ways.

This book is not just mine—it belongs to all of you who have supported, encouraged, and helped me bring it into the world. I am deeply grateful beyond words.

With all my heart,

Dr. Ann Shippy

ENDNOTES

1. Elizabeth Stone. "Why the Decision to Have a Child Is Momentous." *The Village Voice*, January 15, 1985.

2. Institute for Functional Medicine. "What Is Functional Medicine?" Accessed June 16, 2024. https://www.ifm.org/functional-medicine/.

3. Cary Funk and Kim Parker. "Women and Men in STEM Often at Odds over Workplace Equity." January 9, 2018. Accessed June 16, 2024. https://www.pewresearch.org/science/2018/01/09/women-and -men-in-stem-often-at-odds-over-workplace-equity/.

4. I suppose if I had stayed with IBM, I probably would've been recruited by Dell and would be retired by now, with a nice chunk of change because of stock options. But that wasn't my path, and I'm grateful for where life took me instead!

5. Kexin Zhang et al. "Global, Regional, and National Epidemiology of Diabetes in Children from 1990 to 2019." *JAMA Pediatrics* 177, no. 8 (2023): 837–46. https://doi.org/10.1001/jamapediatrics.2023.2029.

6. Centers for Disease Control and Prevention. "Data and Statistics on Autism Spectrum Disorder." May 27, 2025, accessed June 16, 2025. https://www.cdc.gov/autism/data-research/index.html.

7. CDC. "Data and Statistics on Autism Spectrum Disorder."

8. World Health Organization. "Obesity and Overweight." https://www .who.int/news-room/fact-sheets/detail/obesity-and-overweight.

9. Elie Abdelnour et al. "ADHD Diagnostic Trends: Increased Recognition or Overdiagnosis?" *Mo Med* 119, no. 5 (2022): 467–73. https:// pmc.ncbi.nlm.nih.gov/articles/PMC9616454/.

10. Cynthia Reuben and Nazik Elgaddal. *Attention-Deficit/Hyperactivity Disorder in Children Ages 5–17 Years: United States, 2020–2022*, NCHS Data Brief No. 499 (National Center for Health Statistics, March 2024). https://www.cdc.gov/nchs/data/databriefs/db499.pdf.

11. American Childhood Cancer Organization. "US Childhood Cancer Statistics." Accessed March 3, 2025. https://www.acco.org/us-childhood-cancer-statistics/.

12. U.S. Environmental Protection Agency. *NIEHS/EPA Children's Environmental Health and Disease Prevention Research Centers Impact Report: Protecting Children's Health Where They Live, Learn, and Play.* EPA Publication No. EPA/600/R-17/407 (2017). https://www.epa.gov/sites/production/files/2017-10/documents/niehs_epa_childrens_centers_impact_report_2017_0.pdf?pdf=childrens-center-report; Iyad Sultan et al. "Trends in Childhood Cancer: Incidence and Survival Analysis over 45 Years of SEER Data." *PLoS One* 20, no. 1 (2025): e0314592. https://doi.org/10.1371/journal.pone.0314592.

13. National Cancer Institute. "Childhood and Adolescent Cancer Fact Sheet." Updated February 9, 2024, accessed March 3, 2025. https://www.cancer.gov/types/childhood-cancers/child-adolescent-cancers-fact-sheet#r1.

14. Nady Braidy, Maria D. Villalva, and Sam van Eeden. "Sobriety and Satiety: Is NAD+ the Answer?" *Antioxidants* 9, no. 5: 425. https://doi.org/10.3390/antiox9050425.

15. Nady Braidy et al. "Sobriety and Satiety: Is NAD+ the Answer?"

16. David Grotto and Elisa Zied. "The Standard American Diet and Its Relationship to the Health Status of Americans." *Nutrition in Clinical Practice* 25, no. 6 (2010): 603–12. https://doi.org/10.1177/0884533610386234.

17. CDC. "Facts About Radiation from Air Travel." February 20, 2024. https://www.cdc.gov/radiation-health/data-research/facts-stats/air-travel.html.

18. Hanna Pamuła. "Flight Radiation Calculator." Omni Calculator, updated July 24, 2024. https://www.omnicalculator.com/everyday-life/flight-radiation.

19. Amy Blanchett and Laurie Abadie. "Space Radiation Is Risky Business for the Human Body." NASA, September 19, 2017. https://www.nasa.gov/humans-in-space/space-radiation-is-risky-business-for-the-human-body/.

20. Blanchett and Abadie. "Space Radiation Is Risky Business."

21. Fan Zhang et al. "Selenium and Selenoproteins in Health." *Biomolecules* 13, no. 5 (2023): 799. https://doi.org/10.3390/biom13050799.

22. Yang Song et al. "Zinc Deficiency Affects DNA Damage, Oxidative Stress, Antioxidant Defenses, and DNA Repair in Rats." *The Journal of Nutrition* 139, no. 9 (2009): 1626–31. https://doi.org/10.3945/jn.109.106369.

23. Chad Kerksick and Darryn Willoughby. "The Antioxidant Role of Glutathione and N-Acetyl-Cysteine Supplements and Exercise-Induced Oxidative Stress." *Journal of the International Society of Sports Nutrition* 2, no. 2 (2005): 38. https://doi.org/10.1186/1550-2783-2-2-38.

24. Annia Galano et al. "Melatonin: A Versatile Protector Against Oxidative DNA Damage." *Molecules* 23, no. 3 (2018): 530. https://doi.org/10.3390/molecules23030530.

25. Kirushmita Anbualakan et al. "A Scoping Review on the Effects of Carotenoids and Flavonoids on Skin Damage Due to Ultraviolet Radiation." *Nutrients* 15, no. 1 (2022): 92. https://doi.org/10.3390/nu15010092.

26. Ayse L. Mindikoglu et al. "Intermittent Fasting from Dawn to Sunset for 30 Consecutive Days Is Associated with Anticancer Proteomic Signature and Upregulates Key Regulatory Proteins of Glucose and Lipid Metabolism, Circadian Clock, DNA Repair, Cytoskeleton Remodeling, Immune System and Cognitive Function in Healthy Subjects." *Journal of Proteomics* 217 (2020): 103645. https://doi.org/10.1016/j.jprot.2020.103645.

27. Nicole O. Palmer et al. "Impact of Obesity on Male Fertility, Sperm Function and Molecular Composition." *Spermatogenesis* 2, no. 4 (2012): 253–263. https://doi.org/10.4161/spmg.21362.

28. J. K. Lake et al. "Women's Reproductive Health: The Role of Body Mass Index in Early and Adult Life." *International Journal of Obesity* 21 (1997): 432–38. https://doi.org/10.1038/sj.ijo.0800424.

29. Faye Chleilat et al. "Paternal High Protein Diet Modulates Body Composition, Insulin Sensitivity, Epigenetics, and Gut Microbiota Intergenerationally in Rats." *FASEB Journal* 35, no. 9 (2021): e21847. https://doi.org/10.1096/fj.202100198RR.

30. Chelsea Marcho et al. "The Preconception Environment and Sperm Epigenetics." *Andrology* 8, no. 4 (2020): 924–42. https://doi.org/10.1111/andr.12753.

31. Jamie R. Robinson et al. "Quantifying the Phenome-Wide Disease Burden of Obesity Using Electronic Health Records and Genomics." *Obesity* 30, no. 12 (2022): 2477–88. https://doi.org/10.1002/oby.23561.

32. Reuby Staviss et al. "'Be More Positive and More Kind to Your Own Bodies: Adolescent and Young Adult Preferences for How Parents Can Support Their Children with Weight-Related Pressures." *Body Image* 50 (2024): 101725. https://doi.org/10.1016/j.bodyim.2024.101725.

33. Kristin Neff. "Self-Compassion Test." Self-Compassion, accessed June 25, 2024. https://self-compassion.org/self-compassion-test/.

34. Elaine N. Aron, "The Highly Sensitive Person." The Highly Sensitive Person, accessed June 25, 2024. https://hsperson.com/.

35. Byron Katie. "Loving What Is," The Work of Byron Katie. Accessed June 25, 2024. https://thework.com/loving-what-is-revised-edition/.

36. ACEs Aware. "Adverse Childhood Experiences (ACE) Questionnaire for Adults." Identified English version, last revised July 26, 2022, accessed July 5, 2024. https://www.acesaware.org/wp-content/uploads/2022/07/ACE-Questionnaire-for-Adults-Identified-English-rev.7.26.22.pdf.

37. Samson Nivins et al. "Prenatal Exposure to Maternal Hypertension and Higher Body Mass Index and Risks of Neurodevelopmental and Psychiatric Disorders During Childhood." *Acta Obstetricia et Gynecologica Scandinavica* 104, no. 2 (2025): 319–30. https://doi.org/10.1111/aogs.15021.

38. Jorge A. Alegría-Torres et al. "Epigenetics and Lifestyle." *Epigenomics* 3, no. 3 (2011): 267–77. https://doi.org/10.2217/epi.11.22.

39. Hannah L. Morgan and Adam J. Watkins. "Transgenerational Impact of Environmental Change." *Advances in Experimental Medicine and Biology* 1200 (2019): 71–89. https://www.ncbi.nlm.nih.gov/pubmed /31471795.

40. Albert Machado et al. "Chronic Stress as a Risk Factor for Alzheimer's Disease." *Reviews in the Neurosciences* 25, no. 6 (2014): 785–804. https://doi.org/10.1515/revneuro-2014-0035.

41. Saeid Golbidi et al. "Chronic Stress Impacts the Cardiovascular System: Animal Models and Clinical Outcomes." *American Journal of Physiology: Heart and Circulatory Physiology* 308, no. 12 (2015): H1476–98. https://doi.org/10.1152/ajpheart.00859.2014.

42. Stefanie E. Mayer et al. "Cumulative Lifetime Stress Exposure and Leukocyte Telomere Length Attrition: The Unique Role of Stressor Duration and Exposure Timing." *Psychoneuroendocrinology* 104 (2019): 210–18. https://doi.org/10.1016/j.psyneuen.2019.03.002.

43. Carlo Dal Lin et al. "Thoughts Modulate the Expression of Inflammatory Genes and May Improve the Coronary Blood Flow in Patients after a Myocardial Infarction." *Journal of Traditional and Complementary Medicine* 8, no. 1 (2017): 150–63. https://doi.org/10.1016/j.jtcme .2017.04.011.

44. Environmental Working Group. "Body Burden: The Pollution in Newborns." July 14, 2005, accessed June 24, 2024. https://www.ewg .org/research/body-burden-pollution-newborns.

45. Xiaowen Xia et al. "Nontarget Identification of Novel Per- and Polyfluoroalkyl Substances in Cord Blood Samples." *Environmental Science and Technology Journal* 56, no. 23 (2022): 17061–69. https://doi.org/10 .1021/acs.est.2c04820.

46. Karen Chan Barrett et al. "Art and Science: How Musical Training Shapes the Brain." *Frontiers in Psychology* 4 (2013). https://doi.org/10 .3389/fpsyg.2013.00713.

47. Eric E. Nilsson et al. "Multiple Generation Distinct Toxicant Exposures Induce Epigenetic Transgenerational Inheritance of Enhanced

Pathology and Obesity." *Environmental Epigenetics* 9, no. 1 (2023): dvad006. https://doi.org/10.1093/eep/dvad006.

48. Yi-Ping Wang and Qun-Ying Lei. "Metabolic Recoding of Epigentics in Cancer." *Cancer Communications* 38, no. 1 (2018): 1–8. https://doi .org/10.1186/s40880-018-0302-3.

49. Rita Castro et al. "Increased Homocysteine and S-Adenosylhomocysteine Concentrations and DNA Hypomethylation in Vascular Disease." *Clinical Chemistry* 49, no. 8 (2003): 1292–96. https://doi.org/10 .1373/49.8.1292.

50. Cristina M. Lanata et al. "DNA Methylation 101: What Is Important to Know About DNA Methylation and Its Role in SLE Risk and Disease Heterogeneity." *Lupus Science & Medicine* 5, no. 1 (2018): e000285. https://doi.org/10.1136/lupus-2018-000285.

51. Lisa D. Moore et al. "DNA Methylation and Its Basic Function." *Neuropsychopharmacology* 38, no. 1 (2012): 23–38. https://doi.org/10.1038 /npp.2012.112.

52. Zachary D. Smith and Alexander Meissner. "DNA Methylation: Roles in Mammalian Development." *Nature Reviews Genetics* 14, no. 3 (2013): 204–20. https://doi.org/10.1038/nrg3354.

53. Smith and Meissner. "DNA Methylation."

54. Krista S. Crider et al. "Folate and DNA Methylation: A Review of Molecular Mechanisms and the Evidence for Folate's Role." *Advances in Nutrition* 3, no. 1 (2012): 21–38. https://doi.org/10.3945/an.111 .000992.

55. Office of Dietary Supplements. "Folate: Fact Sheet for Health Professionals." National Institutes of Health, updated November 30, 2022. https://ods.od.nih.gov/factsheets/Folate-HealthProfessional/.

56. Dietmar Rösler et al. "The Impact of B Vitamins on Methylations, Regeneration and Epigenetics: Results of a Randomized Double-Blind Study of Synthetic versus Plant-Based Vitamin Complexes." *Integrative Food, Nutrition, and Metabolism* 10 (2023). https://www.oatext .com/the-impact-of-b-vitamins-on-methylations-regeneration-and -epigenetics-results-of-a-randomized-double-blind-study-of-synthetic -versus-plant-based-vitamin-complexes.php.

57. Ilan Weisberg et al. "A Second Genetic Polymorphism in Methylenetetrahydrofolate Reductase (MTHFR) Associated with Decreased Enzyme Activity, Molecular Genetics and Metabolism." *Molecular Genetics and Metabolism* 64, no. 3 (1998): 169–72. https://doi.org/10.1006/mgme.1998.2714.

58. Laura Dean. "Methylenetetrahydrofolate Reductase Deficiency." Eds. Victoria M. Pratt et al. *Medical Genetics Summaries* (National Center for Biotechnology Information, 2012). https://pubmed.ncbi.nlm.nih.gov/28520345/.

59. Diego Scheggia et al. "COMT as a Drug Target for Cognitive Functions and Dysfunctions." *CNS Neurological Disorders—Drug Targets* 11, no. 3 (2012): 209–21. https://doi.org/10.2174/187152712800672481.

60. Guo-Lian Ding et al. "The Effects on Male Fertility and Epigenetic Regulation During Spermatogenesis." *Asian Journal of Andrology* 17, no. 6 (2015): 948–53. https://doi.org/10.4103/1008-682X.150844.

61. Harvard T. H. Chan School of Public Health. "Studying the Link Between the Menstrual Cycle and Blood Sugar." November 30, 2023, accessed July 16, 2024. https://www.hsph.harvard.edu/news/hsph-in-the-news/studying-the-link-between-the-menstrual-cycle-and-blood-sugar/.

62. Lotta S. Holopainen et al. "Pre-Pregnancy Body Surface Area and Risk for Gestational Diabetes Mellitus." *Acta Diabetologica* 60, no. 4 (2023): 527–34. https://doi.org/10.1007/s00592-022-02029-0.

63. Orit Pinhas-Hamiel and Philip Zeitler. "Type 2 Diabetes in Children and Adolescents: A Focus on Diagnosis and Treatment." In *Endotext*, edited by K. R. Feingold et al. (MDText.com, Inc., 2000). https://www.ncbi.nlm.nih.gov/books/NBK597439/.

64. Yanan Duan et al. "Inflammatory Markers in Women with Infertility: A Cross-Sectional Study." *International Journal of General Medicine* 16 (2023): 1113–21. https://doi.org/10.2147/IJGM.S405793.

65. Marc D. Rudolph et al. "Maternal IL-6 During Pregnancy Can Be Estimated from Newborn Brain Connectivity and Predicts Future Working Memory in Offspring." *Nature Neuroscience* 21, no. 5 (2018): 765–72. https://doi.org/10.1038/s41593-018-0128-y.

66. Meredith A. J. Huller and Benjamin C. Fu. "Diet, the Gut Microbiome, and Epigenetics." *The Cancer Journal* vol. 20, 3 (2014): 170–5. https://doi.org/10.1097/PPO.0000000000000053.

67. Kailyn L. Stefan et al. "Commensal Microbiota Modulation of Natural Resistance to Virus Infection." *Cell* 183, no. 5 (2020): 1312–24. https://www.cell.com/cell/fulltext/S0092-8674(20)31454-9?_returnURL=https%3A%2F%2Flinkinghub.elsevier.com%2Fretrieve%2Fpii%2FS0092867420314549%3Fshowall%3Dtrue.

68. Selma P. Wiertsema et al. "The Interplay Between the Gut Microbiome and the Immune System in the Context of Infectious Diseases Throughout Life and the Role of Nutrition in Optimizing Treatment Strategies." *Nutrients* 13, no. 3 (2021): 886. https://doi.org/10.3390/nu13030886.

69. Elakshi Dekaboruah et al. "Human Microbiome: An Academic Update on Human Body Site Specific Surveillance and Its Possible Role." *Archives of Microbiology* 202, no. 8 (2020): 2147–67. https://doi.org/10.1007/s00203-020-01931-x.

70. Jing Xu et al. "New Insights into the Epigenetic Regulation of Inflammatory Bowel Disease." *Frontiers in Pharmacology* 13, no. 813659 (2022). https://doi.org/10.3389/fphar.2022.813659.

71. Comprehensive Gut Health Test from Genova Diagnostics. https://www.gdx.net/products/gi-effects.

72. Xinyu Qi et al. "The Impact of the Gut Microbiota on the Reproductive and Metabolic Endocrine System." *Gut Microbes* 13, no. 1 (2021): 1–21. https://doi.org/10.1080/19490976.

73. Munkhtuya Bataa et al. "Exploring Progesterone Deficiency in First-Trimester Miscarriage and the Impact of Hormone Therapy on Foetal Development: A Scoping Review." *Children* 11, no. 4 (2024): 422. https://doi.org/10.3390/children11040422.

74. Prenuvo. "Put Your Health in Our Hands." Accessed July 18, 2024. https://marketing.prenuvo.com/blog/breaking-it-down-prenuvos-whole-body-mri-screening-explained.

75. Mirela E. Iancu et al. "Prolactin Relationship with Fertility and In Vitro Fertilization Outcomes—A Review of the Literature." *Pharmaceuticals* 16, no. 1 (2023): 122. https://doi.org/10.3390/ph16010122.

76. Zeinab Dabbous and Stephen L. Atkin. "Hyperprolactinaemia in Male Infertility: Clinical Case Scenarios." *Arab Journal of Urology* 16, no. 1 (2017): 44–52. https://doi.org/10.1016/j.aju.2017.10.002.

77. Lauren Thau et al. "Physiology, Cortisol." *StatPearls* (2023). https://www.ncbi.nlm.nih.gov/books/NBK538239/.

78. Bheena Vyshali Karunyam et al. "Infertility and Cortisol: A Systematic Review." *Frontiers in Endocrinology* 14 (2023). https://doi.org/10.3389/fendo.2023.1147306.

79. Spyridoula Maraka et al. "Subclinical Hypothyroidism in Women Planning Conception and During Pregnancy: Who Should Be Treated and How?" *Journal of the Endocrine Society* 2, no. 6 (2018): 533–46. https://doi.org/10.1210/js.2018-00090.

80. Precision Analytical Inc. "DUTCH Complete Provider Info Sheet." Accessed July 16, 2024. https://dutchtest.com/wp-content/uploads/2020/03/Dutch-Complete-Provider-Info-Sheet-Ref032720.pdf.

81. Genova Diagnostics. "Test Menu: Featured Products." Accessed July 16, 2024. https://www.gdx.net/products.

82. Zoya Enakshi Ali et al. "Role, Benefits, and Risks of AMH Testing for Non-ART Related Indications." *Human Reproduction* 39, no. 12 (2024): 2873–77. https://doi.org/10.1093/humrep/deae234.

83. Path Fertility. "Sperm QT Takes a Deep Dive into Sperm Health." July 13, 2024. https://pathfertility.com/.

84. Katherine W. Greeson et al. "Inheritance of Paternal Lifestyles and Exposures Through Sperm DNA Methylation." *Nature Reviews Urology* 20, no. 6 (2023): 356–70. https://doi.org/10.1038/s41585-022-00708-9.

85. Genova Diagnostics. "NutrEval: A Comprehensive Profile for Identifying Nutritional Deficiencies and Insufficiencies." Accessed November 19, 2024, https://www.gdx.net/products/nutreval.

86. Genova Diagnostics. *ION Profile®: Individual, Optimal, Nutritional* (2019), accessed November 19, 2024. https://www.gdx.net/core/sales -sheets/ION-Sales-Sheet.pdf.

87. S. Raghubeer and T. E. Matsha. "Methylenetetrahydrofolate (MTHFR), the One-Carbon Cycle, and Cardiovascular Risks." *Nutrients* 13, no. 12 (2021): 4562. https://doi.org/10.3390/nu13124562.

88. Hervé Robert et al. "Impact of Mycotoxins on the Intestine: Are Mucus and Microbiota New Targets?" *Journal of Toxicology and Environmental Health, Part B: Critical Reviews* 20, no. 5 (2017): 249–75. https://doi.org/10.1080/10937404.2017.1326071.

89. Lulu Li et al. "Role of Epigenetics in Mycotoxin Toxicity: A Review." *Environmental Toxicology and Pharmacology* 100 (2023): 104154. https://doi.org/10.1016/j.etap.2023.104154.

90. El Khoury, Diala, et al. "Updates on the Effect of Mycotoxins on Male Reproductive Efficiency in Mammals." *Toxins* 11, no. 9 (2019): 515. https://doi.org/10.3390/toxins11090515.

91. A. Alavian-Ghavanini and J. Rüegg. "Understanding Epigenetic Effects of Endocrine Disrupting Chemicals: From Mechanisms to Novel Test Methods." *Basic and Clinical Pharmacology and Toxicology* 122, no. 1 (2018): 38–45. https://doi.org/10.1111/bcpt.12878.

92. Alexandra A. Korolenko et al. "Epigenetic Inheritance and Transgenerational Environmental Justice." *The Yale Journal of Biology and Medicine* 96, no. 2 (2023): 241–50. https://doi.org/10.59249/FKWS5176.

93. Joseph Pizzorno. "Environmental Toxins and Infertility." *Integrative Medicine* 17, no. 2 (2018): 8–11.

94. Environmental Working Group. "Body Burden: The Pollution in Newborns." EWG, July 14, 2005. https://www.ewg.org/research/body -burden-pollution-newborns.

95. Vibrant Wellness. "Total Tox Burden." Vibrant Labs, accessed July 18, 2024. https://vibrant-wellness.com/tests/toxins/total-tox-burden.

96. Vibrant Wellness. "Total Tox Burden."

97. Mosaic Diagnostics. "EnviroTOX Suite of Panels." MosaicDX, accessed November 25, 2024. https://mosaicdx.com/test/envirotox -panels/.

98. Sanjana Kurup and Alexander Pozun. "Biochemistry, Autoimmunity." *StatPearls* (2024). https://www.ncbi.nlm.nih.gov/books/NBK576418.

99. Quest Diagnostics. "Thyroid Peroxidase Antibodies (TPO)." Accessed June 25, 2025. https://testdirectory.questdiagnostics.com/test/test-detail/5081/thyroid-peroxidase-antibodies-tpo?q=TPO&cc=MASTER.

100. Vibrant Wellness. "Neural Zoomer Plus Test." Vibrant Labs, accessed July 18, 2024.

101. Mescreen. "Your Health Begins with Me." Accessed July 16, 2024. https://mescreen.com/pages/clinical.

102. Doctor's Data, Inc. "Comprehensive Neurotransmitter Profile: Urine." Accessed July 16, 2024. https://www.doctorsdata.com/Comprehensive-Neurotransmitter-Profile-urine.

103. Gary E. Gibson and John P. Blass. "Nutrition and Functional Neurochemistry." In G. J. Siegel et al., eds. *Basic Neurochemistry: Molecular, Cellular and Medical Aspects.* 6th ed. (Lippincott-Raven, 1999). https://www.ncbi.nlm.nih.gov/books/NBK28242/.

104. Avijit Banik et al. "Maternal Factors That Induce Epigenetic Changes Contribute to Neurological Disorders in Offspring." *Genes* 8, no. 6 (2017): 150. https://doi.org/10.3390/genes8060150.

105. Translational Science and Medical Team. "Breaking New Ground in Revealing the Mechanisms of Inflammation." TLAB, accessed November 20, 2024. https://www.tlabdx.com/.

106. Vittoria D'Alessio. "Clues to Autism's Causes May Lie in the Gut." *Horizon*, January 25, 2024. https://projects.research-and-innovation.ec.europa.eu/en/horizon-magazine/clues-autisms-causes-may-lie-gut.

107. Genova Diagnostics, "Methylation Panel," accessed July 14, 2024. https://www.gdx.net/products/methylation-panel.

108. Swaran J. S. Flora and Vidhu Pachauri. "Chelation in Metal Intoxication." *International Journal of Environmental Research and Public Health* 7, no. 7 (2010): 2745–88. https://doi.org/10.3390/ijerph7072745.

109. Here is the Quicksilver Scientific website where you can purchase this test: https://www.quicksilverscientific.com

110. Lisa V. Farland et al. "Celiac Disease and Reproductive Disorders: Meta-Analysis of Epidemiologic Associations and Potential Pathogenic

Mechanisms." *Nutrients* 12, no. 11 (2020): 3390. https://doi.org/10.3390/nu12113390.

111. University of Texas Health Science Center at San Antonio. "Parental Avoidance of Toxic Exposures Could Help Prevent Autism, ADHD in Children, New Study Shows." March 27, 2024. https://news.uthscsa.edu/parental-avoidance-of-toxic-exposures-could-help-prevent-autism-adhd-in-children-new-study-shows/.

112. U.S. Environmental Protection Agency. "Glyphosate." Last updated May 9, 2025. https://www.epa.gov/ingredients-used-pesticide-products/glyphosate.

113. Juan P. Muñoz et al. "Glyphosate Mimics 17β-Estradiol Effects Promoting Estrogen Receptor Alpha Activity in Breast Cancer Cells." *Chemosphere* 313, no. 137201 (2023). https://doi.org/10.1016/j.chemosphere.2022.137201.

114. María Florencia Rossetti et al. "Epigenetic Changes Associated with Exposure to Glyphosate-Based Herbicides in Mammals." *Frontiers in Endocrinology* 12, no. 671991 (2021). https://doi.org/10.3389/fendo.2021.671991.

115. Galateia Stathori et al. "Endocrine-Disrupting Chemicals, Hypothalamic Inflammation and Reproductive Outcomes: A Review of the Literature." *International Journal of Molecular Sciences* 25, no. 21 (2024): 11344, accessed November 18, 2024. https://doi.org/10.3390/ijms252111344.

116. You can read the full blog here: https://annshippymd.com/dont-raise-glass-may-toxic/.

117. National Institute of Environmental Health Sciences. "Bisphenol A (BPA)." Accessed June 25, 2025. https://www.niehs.nih.gov/health/topics/agents/sya-bpa.

118. National Institute of Environmental Health Sciences. "Bisphenol A (BPA)."

119. Mingzhe Yuan et al. "Estrogenic and Non-Estrogenic Effects of Bisphenol A and Its Action Mechanism in the Zebrafish Model: An

Overview of the Past Two Decades of Work." *Environment International* 176, no. 107976 (2023). https://doi.org/10.1016/j.envint.2023.107976.

120. Federica Cariati et al. "Bisphenol A-Induced Epigenetic Changes and Its Effects on the Male Reproductive System." *Frontiers in Endocrinology* 11 (2020): 453. doi:10.3389/fendo.2020.00453.

121. Galateia Stathori et al. "Endocrine-Disrupting Chemicals, Hypothalamic Inflammation and Reproductive Outcomes: A Review of the Literature." *International Journal of Molecular Sciences* 25, no. 21 (2024): 11344. https://www.mdpi.com/1422-0067/25/21/11344.

122. M. B. Thomas et al. "Demographic and Dietary Risk Factors in Relation to Urinary Metabolites of Organophosphate Flame Retardants in Toddlers." *Chemosphere* 185 (2017): 918–25. https://doi.org/10.1016/j.chemosphere.2017.07.015.

123. Haoxiang Wu and Jonathan Woon Chung Wong. "Temperature Versus Relative Humidity: Which Is More Important for Indoor Mold Prevention?" *Microorganisms* 8, no. 7 (2020): 696. https://www.mdpi.com/2309-608X/8/7/696.

124. U.S. Environmental Protection Agency, "A Brief Guide to Mold, Moisture, and Your Home." Last updated March 27, 2025. https://www.epa.gov/mold/brief-guide-mold-moisture-and-your-home.

125. Bill Walker. "'Erin Brockovich' Carcinogen in Tap Water of More than 200 Million Americans." Environmental Working Group, September 20, 2016. https://www.ewg.org/research/erin-brockovich-carcinogen-tap-water-more-200-million-americans.

126. National Cancer Institute. "Hexavalent Chromium Compounds - Cancer-Causing Substances." *Cancer.gov*. Last modified June 7, 2024. https://www.cancer.gov/about-cancer/causes-prevention/risk/substances/chromium.

127. Tap Score. "Hexavalent Chromium Water Test." Accessed November 18, 2024. https://mytapscore.com/products/hexavalent-chromium-water-test.

128. Charlotte Debras et al. "Artificial Sweeteners and Cancer Risk: Results from the NurtiNet Santé Population-Based Cohort Study." *PLoS*

Medicine 19, no. 3 (2022): e1003950. https://doi.org/10.1371/journal
.pmed.1003950.

129. Iheanyichukwu Wopara et al. "Synthetic Food Dyes Cause Testicular Damage via Up-Regulaion of Pro-Inflammatory Cytokines and Down Regulation of FSH-R and TESK 1 Gene Expression." *JBRA Assisted Reproduction* 25, no. 3 (2021): 341–48. https://doi.org/10.5935/1518-0557.20200097.

130. Bolun Kang et al. "Mercury-Induced Toxicity: Mechanisms, Molecular Pathways, and Gene Regulation." *Science of the Total Environment* 943, no. 173577 (2024). https://doi.org/10.1016/j.scitotenv.2024.173577.

131. U.S. Food and Drug Administration. "Thimerosal and Vaccines." Last updated January 15, 2025. https://www.fda.gov/vaccines-blood-biologics/safety-availability-biologics/thimerosal-and-vaccines.

132. Mayyadah S. Abed et al. "Heavy Metals in Cosmetics and Tattoos: A Review of Historical Background, Health Impact, and Regulatory Limits." *Journal of Hazardous Materials Advances* 13, no. 100390 (2024). https://doi.org/10.1016/j.hazadv.2023.100390.

133. U.S. EPA. "Our Current Understanding of the Human Health and Environmental Risks of PFAS." Last updated November 26, 2024. https://www.epa.gov/pfas/our-current-understanding-human-health-and-environmental-risks-pfas.

134. Kevin Loria. "Dangerous PFAS Chemicals Are in Your Food Packaging." *Consumer Reports*, May 11, 2022. https://www.consumerreports.org/health/food-contaminants/dangerous-pfas-chemicals-are-in-your-food-packaging-a3786252074/.

135. Pheruza Tarapore and Bin Ouyang. "Perfluoroalkyl Chemicals and Male Reproductive Health: Do PFOA and PFOS Increase Risk for Male Infertility?" *International Journal of Environmental Research and Public Health* 18, no. 7, April 5, 2021: 3794. https://doi.org/10.3390/ijerph18073794.

136. Rebekah L. Petroff et al. "Mediation Effects of DNA Methylation and Hydroxymethylation on Birth Outcomes after Prenatal Per- and Polyfluoroalkyl Substances (PFAS) Exposure in the Michigan Mother

Infant Pairs Cohort." *Clinical Epigenetics* 15, no. 49 (2023). https://doi
.org/10.1186/s13148-023-01461-5.

137. Environmental Working Group. "Our Mission." Accessed July 22,
2024. https://www.ewg.org/who-we-are/our-mission.

138. Peter M. Habib et al. "Breast Implant Illness: A Case Series." *Cureus:
Journal of Medical Science* 14, no. 3 (2022): e23680. https://www.ncbi
.nlm.nih.gov/pmc/articles/PMC9060741/.

139. J. Mutter, "Is Dental Amalgam Safe for Humans? The Opinion of
the Scientific Committee of the European Commission." *Journal of
Occupational Medicine and Toxicology* 6, no. 2 (2011). https://doi.org
/10.1186/1745-6673-6-2.

140. U.S. Food and Drug Administration. "Information for Patients About
Dental Amalgam Fillings." Last updated December 5, 2022. https://
www.fda.gov/medical-devices/dental-amalgam-fillings/information
-patients-about-dental-amalgam-fillings.

141. Jaroslaw Sobieszczański et al. "Root Canal Infection and Its Impact
on the Oral Cavity Microenvironment in the Context of Immune
System Disorders in Selected Diseases: A Narrative Review." *Journal
of Clinical Medicine* 12, no. 12 (2023): 4102. https://doi.org/10.3390
/jcm12124102.

142. Rewa E. Zurub et al. "Microplastics Exposure: Implications for Human
Fertility, Pregnancy and Child Health." *Frontiers in Endocrinology* 14,
no. 1330396 (2024). https://doi.org/10.3389/fendo.2023.1330396.

143. Daniel Sol et al. "Contribution of Household Dishwashing to Micro-
plastic Pollution." *Environmental Science and Pollution Research International* 30, no. 15 (2023): 45140–50. https://doi.org/10.1007/s11356
-023-25433-7.

144. Brenda Eskenazi et al. "In Utero and Childhood Polybrominated
Diphenyl Ether (PBDE) Exposures and Neurodevelopment in the
CHAMACOS Study." *Environmental Health Perspectives* 121, no. 2
(2013): 257–62. https://doi.org/10.1289/ehp.1205597.

145. Global Organic Textile Standard. "*Why GOTS: Control of Chemicals in GOTS Goods.*" Version 2, July 3, 2023. chrome-extension://
efaidnbmnnnibpcajpcglclefindmkaj/https://global-standard.org

/images/resource-library/documents/GOTS-fact-sheets/Why_GOTS
_Factsheet_Control_of_Chemicals_in_GOTS_Goods_v2.pdf.

146. Julie Carré et al. "Does Air Pollution Play a Role in Infertility?: A Systematic Review." *Environmental Health* 16, no. 82 (2017). https://doi.org/10.1186/s12940-017-0291-8.

147. For more information on air filtration systems and other healthy home products, here is a list of my favorites: https://annshippymd.com/resources/.

148. For more info on choosing new flooring, here is the Environmental Working Group's Healthy Living Home Guide on Flooring: https://www.ewg.org/healthyhomeguide/flooring/.

149. For more information on purchasing paint, here is the Environmental Working Group's Healthy Living Home Guide on Paint: https://www.ewg.org/healthyhomeguide/paint/.

150. Farhan Jamil Emon et al. "Bioaccumulation and Bioremediation of Heavy Metals in Fishes—A Review." *Toxics* 11, no. 6 (2023): 510. https://doi.org/10.3390/toxics11060510.

151. Hyun-Wook Ryu et al. "Influence of Toxicologically Relevant Metals on Human Epigenetic Regulation." *Toxicological Research* 31, no. 1 (2015): 1–9. https://doi.org/10.5487/TR.2015.31.1.001.

152. Nadia Barbo et al. "Locally Caught Freshwater Fish Across the United States Are Likely a Significant Source of Exposure to PFOS and Other Perfluorinated Compounds." *Environmental Research* 220, no. 115165 (2023). https://doi.org/10.1016/j.envres.2022.115165.

153. National Toxicology Program. "Per- and Polyfluoroalkyl Substances (PFAS)." U.S. Department of Health and Human Services, last updated June 23, 2025. https://ntp.niehs.nih.gov/go/PFAS. https://ntp.niehs.nih.gov/whatwestudy/topics/pfas.

154. Samara Geller. "BPA Update: Tracking the Canned Food Phaseout." Environmental Working Group, November 2, 2020. https://www.ewg.org/news-insights/news/bpa-update-tracking-canned-food-phaseout.

155. U.S. Food and Drug Administration. "Code of Federal Regulations Title 21, Part 177.1520." Last updated December 24, 2024. https://

www.accessdata.fda.gov/scripts/cdrh/cfdocs/cfCFR/CFRSearch.cfm
?fr=177.1520.

156. Caroline Silveira Martinez et al. "Aluminum Exposure for 60 Days at Human Dietary Levels Impairs Spermatogenesis and Sperm Quality in Rats." *Reproductive Toxicology* 73 (2017): 128–41. https://doi.org/10.1016/j.reprotox.2017.08.008.

157. Maha Lokman et al. "Aluminum Chloride-Induced Reproductive Toxicity in Rats: The Protective Role of Zinc Oxide Nanoparticles." *Biological Trace Elemement Research* 200, no. 9 (2022): 4035–44. https://doi.org/10.1007/s12011-021-03010-8.

158. Sang-Hee Jeong et al. "Effects of Butylated Hydroxyanisole on the Development and Functions of Reproductive System in Rats." *Toxicology* 208, no. 1 (2005): 49–62. https://doi.org/10.1016/j.tox.2004.11.014.

159. Itsuki Kageyama et al. "Differential Effects of Excess High Fructose Corn Syrup on the DNA Methylation of Hippocampal Neurotrophic Factor in Childhood and Adolescence." *PLoS One* 17, no. 6 (2022): e0270144. https://doi.org/10.1371/journal.pone.0270144.

160. Kavindra Kumar Kesari et al. "Radiations and Male Fertility." *Reproductive Biology and Endocrinology,* 16 (2018): 118. https://doi: 10.1186/s12958–018-0431-1. PMID: 30445985; PMCID: PMC6240172.

161. Geoffrey N. De Iuliis et al. "Mobile Phone Radiation Induces Reactive Oxygen Species Production and DNA Damage in Human Spermatozoa in Vitro." *PloS One* 4, no. 7 (2009): e6446. https://doi.org/10.1371/journal.pone.0006446.

162. Gregory Zajac. "Toxic Fashion: Evaluation of Chemicals in Clothing and Recommendations for the Amended TSCA." *Master's Projects and Capstones,* University of San Francisco (School of Nursing and Health Professionals, 2023). https://repository.usfca.edu/capstone/1624.

163. For specific ideas on clothing brands that offer nontoxic fabrics, check out this website: https://www.thegoodtrade.com/features/organic-clothing-brands/.

164. Erica Chung. "Killer Looks: Getting Toxics Out of Jewelry." *Center for Environmental Health*, April 5, 2019. https://ceh.org/stories/killer-looks-getting-toxics-out-of-jewelry/.

165. California Office of Environmental Health Hazard Assessment. "Cadmium and Cadmium Compounds." Proposition 65 Fact Sheets. Accessed November 18, 2024. https://www.p65warnings.ca.gov/fact-sheets/cadmium-and-cadmium-compounds.

166. Scott Faber, "The Toxic Twelve Chemicals and Contaminants in Cosmetics." Environmental Working Group, updated May 5, 2020. https://www.ewg.org/the-toxic-twelve-chemicals-and-contaminants-in-cosmetics.

167. Environmental Working Group. "Personal Care Products." Accessed July 22, 2024. https://www.ewg.org/areas-focus/personal-care-products.

168. L. G. Lebin and A. M. Novick. "Selective Serotonin Reuptake Inhibitors (SSRIs) in Pregnancy: An Updated Review on Risks to Mother, Fetus, and Child." *Current Psychiatry Reports* 24, no. 11 (2022): 687–95. https://doi.org/10.1007/s11920-022-01372-x.

169. O. Watanabe. "Current Evaluation of Teratogenic and Fetotoxic Effects of Psychotropic Drugs." *Seishin Shinkeigaku Zasshi* 116, no. 12 (2014): 996–1004. PMID: 25823351.

170. R. Ogelman et al. "Serotonin Modulates Excitatory Synapse Maturation in the Developing Prefrontal Cortex." *Nature Communications* 15 (2024): 1368. https://doi.org/10.1038/s41467-024-45734-w.

171. A. Mezzacappa et al. "Risk for Autism Spectrum Disorders According to Period of Prenatal Antidepressant Exposure: A Systematic Review and Meta-Analysis." *JAMA Pediatrics* 171, no. 6 (2017): 555–563. https://doi.org/10.1001/jamapediatrics.2017.0124.

172. S. E. Maloney et al. "Antidepressants, Pregnancy, and Autism: Setting the Record(s) Straight." *American Journal of Psychiatry* 177, no. 6 (2020): 479–481. https://doi.org/10.1176/appi.ajp.2020.20040418.

173. Maloney et al. "Antidepressants, Pregnancy, and Autism."

174. Merck & Co., Inc. *MMR® II: Highlights of Prescribing Information.* Accessed November 27, 2024. https://www.merck.com/product/usa/pi_circulars/m/mmr_ii/mmr_ii_pi.pdf.

175. Merck & Co., Inc. *MMR II*.

176. U.S. Food and Drug Administration. 450/477 *Fluzone Quadrivalent: Highlights of Prescribing Information*. Sanofi Pasteur, revised July 2022. https://www.fda.gov/media/119856/download, 17.

177. Sara Ilnitsky and Stan Van Uum. "Marijuana and Fertility." *Canadian Medical Association Journal* 191, no. 23 (2019): E638. https://doi.org/10.1503/cmaj.181577.

178. Kristin van Heertum and Brooke Rossi. "Alcohol and Fertility: How Much Is Too Much?" *Fertility Research and Practice* 3, no. 10 (2017). https://doi.org/10.1186/s40738-017-0037-x.

179. Office of the Surgeon General (US); Office on Smoking and Health (US). "Reproductive Effects." Chapter 5 in *The Health Consequences of Smoking: A Report of the Surgeon General* (CDC, 2004). https://www.ncbi.nlm.nih.gov/books/NBK44697/.

180. N. T. Kitaba et al. "Fathers' Preconception Smoking and Offspring DNA Methylation." *Clinical Epigenetics* 15, 131 (2023). https://doi.org/10.1186/s13148-023-01540-7.

181. Carol Potera. "Marine and Coastal Science: Red Tide Chokehold." *Environmental Health Perspectives* 115, no. 4 (2007): A188. https://doi.org/10.1289/ehp.115-a188.

182. If you'd like to find out how much galactic radiation you received in flight, you can use this calculator provided by the Federal Aviation Administration Office of Aerospace Medicine: https://jag.cami.jccbi.gov/cariprofile.asp.

183. Environmental Working Group. "New Study Confirms BPA in Receipts." Last modified July 29, 2010. https://www.ewg.org/research/new-study-confirms-bpa-receipts.

184. Occupational Safety and Health Administration. "Chemical Hazards." U. S. Department of Labor, accessed June 25, 2025. https://www.osha.gov/nail-salons/chemical-hazards.

185. Kristen Bole. "Hot Tubs Hurt Fertility, UCSF Study Shows." University of California San Francisco. March 2, 2007. https://www.ucsf.edu/news/2007/03/97970/hot-tubs-hurt-fertility-ucsf-study-shows.

186. Andrea Garolla et al. "Seminal and Molecular Evidence That Sauna Affects Human Spermatogenesis." *Human Reproduction* 28, no. 4 (2013): 877–85. https://doi.org/10.1093/humrep/det020.

187. Mary D. Willis et al. "Residential Proximity to Oil and Gas Development and Mental Health in a North American Preconception Cohort Study: 2013–2023." *American Journal of Public Health* 114, no. 9 (2024): 923–34. https://doi.org/10.2105/ajph.2024.307730.

188. National Institute for Occupational Safety and Health. "Examples of Jobs and Reproductive Health." CDC, April 3, 2024. https://www.cdc.gov/niosh/reproductive-health/risk-factors/index.html.

189. Joseph Pizzorno. "Environmental Toxins and Infertility." *Integrative Medicine: A Clinician's Journal* 17, no. 2 (2018): 8–11. PMCID: PMC6396757.

190. Environmental Working Group. "Body Burden: The Pollution in Newborns." July 14, 2005. https://www.ewg.org/research/body-burden-pollution-newborns.

191. Yuexin Cao and Carla Ng. "Absorption, Distribution, and Toxicity of Per- and Polyfluoroalkyl Substances (PFAS) in the Brain: A Review." *Environmental Science & Impacts* 23, no. 11 (2021): 1623–40. https://doi.org/10.1039/D1EM00228G.

192. Harvard T. H. Chan School of Public Health. "Breastfeeding May Expose Infants to Toxic Chemicals." *The Harvard Gazette*, August 20, 2015. https://news.harvard.edu/gazette/story/newsplus/breastfeeding-may-expose-infants-to-toxic-chemicals/.

193. Cao and Ng. "Absorption, Distribution, and Toxicity."

194. Arjun Kalra et al. "Physiology, Liver." *StatPearls* (2024). http://www.ncbi.nlm.nih.gov/books/NBK535438/.

195. Ifeanyichukwu Ogobuiro and Faiz Tuma. "Physiology, Renal." *StatPearls* (2024). http://www.ncbi.nlm.nih.gov/books/NBK538339/.

196. D. Olivieri and E. Scoditti. "Impact of Environmental Factors on Lung Defences." *European Respiratory Review* 14, no. 95 (2005): 51–56. https://doi.org/10.1183/09059180.05.00009502.

197. Scott Frothingham. "Sweating Benefits: Beyond Body Temperature Regulation." Healthline, April 25, 2019. https://www.healthline.com /health/sweating-benefits.

198. Ian Rowland et al. "Gut Microbiota Functions: Metabolism of Nutrients and Other Food Components." *European Journal of Nutrition* 57, no. 1 (2018): 1–24. https://doi.org/10.1007/s00394-017-1445-8.

199. Shelly C. Lu. "Glutathione Synthesis." *Biochimica et Biophysica Acta (BBA) - General Subjects* 1830, no. 5 (2013): 3143–3153. https://doi.org /10.1016/j.bbagen.2012.09.008.

200. Paul Talalay and Julianne W. Fahey. "Phytochemicals from Cruciferous Plants Protect Against Cancer by Modulating Carcinogen Metabolism." *Journal of Nutrition* 131, no. 11 Suppl (2001): 3027S–3033S. https://doi.org/10.1093/jn/131.11.3027S.

201. Robert Clark et al. "Folate, Vitamin B12, and Serum Total Homocysteine Levels in Confirmed Alzheimer Disease." *Archives of Neurology* 55, no. 11 (1998): 1449–1455. https://doi.org/10.1001/archneur.55.11 .1449.

202. James M. Lattimer and Mark D. Haub. "Effects of Dietary Fiber and Its Components on Metabolic Health." *Nutrients* 2, no. 12 (2010): 1266–89. https://doi.org/10.3390/nu2121266.

203. Erica T. Perrier et al. "Hydration for Health Hypothesis: A Narrative Review of Supporting Evidence." *European Journal of Nutrition* 60, no. 3 (2021): 1167–80. https://doi.org/10.1007/s00394-020-02296-z.

204. Geoffrey E. Hespe et al. "Exercise Training Improves Obesity-Related Lymphatic Dysfunction." *The Journal of Physiology* 594, no. 15 (2016): 4267–82. https://doi.org/10.1113/JP271757.

205. Lauren Thau et al. "Physiology, Cortisol." *StatPearls* (2024). http:// www.ncbi.nlm.nih.gov/books/NBK538239/.

206. V. Lobo et al. "Free Radicals, Antioxidants and Functional Foods: Impact on Human Health." *Pharmacognosy Reviews* 4, no. 8 (2010): 118–26. https://doi.org/10.4103/0973-7847.70902.

207. Lobo et al. "Free Radicals, Antioxidants and Functional Foods."

208. Martin L. Pall and Stephen Levine. "Nrf2, a Master Regulator of Detoxification and Also Antioxidant, Anti-Inflammatory, and Other

Cytoprotective Mechanisms, Is Raised by Health-Promoting Factors." *Sheng Li Xue Bao* 67, no. 1 (2015): 1–18. PMID: 25672622.

209. A. A. A. Ismail et al. "Chronic Magnesium Deficiency and Human Disease; Time for Reappraisal?" *QJM: An International Journal of Medicine* 111, no. 11 (2018): 759–63. https://doi.org/10.1093/qjmed /hcx186.

210. Mary P. Guerrera et al. "Therapeutic Uses of Magnesium." *American Family Physician* 80, no. 2 (2009): 157–62. PMID: 19621856.

211. Anna Pastore et al. "Analysis of Glutathione: Implication in Redox and Detoxification." *Clinica Chimica Acta* 333, no. 1 (2003): 19–39. https://doi.org/10.1016/S0009-8981(03)00200-6.

212. R. Sinha et al. "Oral Supplementation with Liposomal Glutathione Elevates Body Stores of Glutathione and Markers of Immune Function." *European Journal of Clinical Nutrition* 72, no. 1 (2018): 105–11. https://doi.org/10.1038/ejcn.2017.132.

213. Mona M. Haemmerle et al. "Adsorption and Release Characteristics of Purified and Non-Purified Clinoptilolite Tuffs Towards Health-Relevant Heavy Metals." *Crystals* 11 (2021): 1343. https:// doi.org/10.3390/cryst11111343.

214. Karolina Samekova et al. "Concomitant Oral Intake of Purified Clinoptilolite Tuff (G-PUR) Reduces Enteral Lead Uptake in Healthy Humans." *Scientific Reports* 11 (2021): 14796. https://doi.org/10.1038 /s41598-021-94245-x.

215. Carlos Carrasco-Gallardo et al. "Shilajit: A Natural Phytocomplex with Potential Procognitive Activity." *International Journal of Alzheimer's Disease* 2012, no. 1 (2012): 674142. https://doi.org/10.1155/2012 /674142.

216. You can find a complete list of protein powders here: https://shop .annshippymd.com/collections/protein-powders/Protein-Powders.

217. Laura S. Bleker et al. "Cohort Profile: The Dutch Famine Birth Cohort (DFBC)—A Prospective Birth Cohort Study in the Netherlands." *BMJ Open* 11 (2021): e042078. https://doi.org/10.1136/bmjopen-2020 -042078.

218. Peter D. Gluckman and Mark A. Hanson. *Developmental Origins of Health and Disease* (Cambridge University Press, 2006).

219. David J. P. Barker. "The Developmental Origins of Adult Disease." *Journal of the American College of Nutrition* 23, no. 6 Supp. (2004): 588S–95S. https://doi.org/10.1080/07315724.2004.10719428.

220. Leena Hilakivi-Clarke and Sonia de Assis. "Fetal Origins of Breast Cancer." *Trends in Endocrinology & Metabolism* 17, no. 9 (2006): 340–48. https://doi.org/10.1016/j.tem.2006.09.002.

221. Robert A. Waterland and Randy L. Jirtle. "Early Nutrition, Epigenetic Changes at Transposons and Imprinted Genes, and Enhanced Susceptibility to Adult Chronic Diseases." *Nutrition* 20, no. 1 (2004): 63–68. https://doi.org/10.1016/j.nut.2003.09.011.

222. Evdoxia Gitsi et al. "Nutritional and Exercise Interventions to Improve Conception in Women Suffering from Obesity and Distinct Nosological Entities." *Frontiers in Endocrinology* 15 (2024): 1426542. https://doi.org/10.3389/fendo.2024.1426542.

223. Adelheid Soubry et al. "Paternal Obesity Is Associated with *IGF2* hypomethylation in Newborns: Results from a Newborn Epigenetics Study (NEST) Cohort." *BMC Medicine* 11, no. 29 (2013). https://doi.org/10.1186/1741-7015-11-29.

224. Soubry et al. "Paternal Obesity Is Associated with *IGF2* hypomethylation in Newborns."

225. Romain Lambrot et al. "Low Paternal Dietary Folate Alters the Mouse Sperm Epigenome and Is Associated with Negative Pregnancy Outcomes." *Nature Communications* 4, no. 2889 (2013). https://doi.org/10.1038/ncomms3889.

226. Romain Barrés et al. "DNA Methylation and Differential Allele-Specific Expression in Human Skeletal Muscle after Acute Exercise." *Nature Communications* 4, no. 2068 (2013), https://doi.org/10.1038/ncomms3068.

227. Kinga Skoracka et al. "Diet and Nutritional Factors in Male(In)fertility—Underestimated Factors." *Journal of Clinical Medicine* 9, no. 5 (2020): 1400. https://doi.org/10.3390/jcm9051400.

228. Klaudia Lakoma et al. "The Influence of Metabolic Factors and Diet on Fertility." *Nutrients* 15, no. 5 (2023). https://doi.org/10.3390/nu15051180.

229. Ella Schaefer and Deborah Nock. "The Impact of Preconceptional Multiple-Micronutrient Supplementation on Female Fertility." *Clinical Medicine Insights: Women's Health* 12 (2019): 1179562X19843868. https://doi.org/10.1177/1179562X19843868.

230. Nicolas Monjotin et al. "Clinical Evidence of the Benefits of Phytonutrients in Human Healthcare." *Nutrients* 14, no. 9 (2022): 1712. https://doi.org/10.3390/nu14091712.

231. Sujan Banik and Mohammad Salim Hossain. "A Comparative Overview on Good Fats and Bad Fats: Guide to Control Healthy Body." *International Journal of Health* 2, no. 2 (2014): 41–44. https://doi.org/10.14419/ijh.v2i2.2903.

232. Jacqueline K. Innes and Philip C. Calder. "Omega-6 Fatty Acids and Inflammation." *Prostaglandins, Leukotrienes and Essential Fatty Acids* 132 (2018): 41–48. https://doi.org/10.1016/j.plefa.2018.03.004.

233. Robert H. Shmerling. "Does Inflammation Contribute to Infertility?" Harvard Health Publishing, February 10, 2023. https://www.health.harvard.edu/blog/does-inflammation-contribute-to-infertility-202302102888.

234. Hadith Rastad et al. "Dairy Consumption and Its Association with Anthropometric Measurements, Blood Glucose Status, Insulin Levels, and Testosterone Levels in Women with Polycystic Ovary Syndrome: A Comprehensive Systematic Review and Meta-Analysis." *Frontiers in Endocrinology* 15 (2024): 1334496. https://doi.org/10.3389/fendo.2024.1334496.

235. Rastad et al. "Dairy Consumption."

236. Kerri M. Gillespie et al. "The Impact of Free Sugar on Human Health—A Narrative Review." *Nutrients* 15, no. 4 (2023): 889. https://doi.org/10.3390/nu15040889.

237. Imran Aziz et al. "The Rise and Fall of Gluten!." *Proceedings of the Nutrition Society* 74, no. 3 (2015): 221–26. https://doi.org/10.1017/S0029665115000038.

238. Artemis Dona and Ioannis S. Arvanitoyannis. "Health Risks of Genetically Modified Foods." *Critical Reviews in Food Science and Nutrition* 49, no. 2 (2009): 164–75. https://doi.org/10.1080/10408390701855993.

239. Joanna Kapusta-Duch et al. "The Beneficial Effects of Brassica Vegetables on Human Health." *Roczniki Państwowego Zakładu Higieny* 63, no. 4 (2012): 389–95. https://pubmed.ncbi.nlm.nih.gov/23631258/.

240. Hatav Ghasemi et al. "Healthy Eating Index and Risk of Diminished Ovarian Reserve: A Case-Control Study." *Scientific Reports* 14, no. 1 (2024): 16861. https://doi.org/10.1038/s41598-024-67734-y.

241. Paul M. Lorenzo et al. "Epigenetic Effects of Healthy Foods and Lifestyle Habits from the Southern European Atlantic Diet Pattern: A Narrative Review." *Advances in Nutrition* 13, no. 5 (2022): 1725–47. https://doi.org/10.1093/advances/nmac038.

242. Selin Sergin et al. "Fatty Acid and Antioxidant Profile of Eggs from Pasture-Raised Hens Fed a Corn- and Soy-Free Diet and Supplemented with Grass-Fed Beef Suet and Liver." *Foods* 11, no. 21 (2022): 3404. https://doi.org/10.3390/foods11213404.

243. Lorenzo et al. "Epigenetic Effects of Healthy Foods and Lifestyle Habits."

244. Lorenzo et al. "Epigenetic Effects of Healthy Foods and Lifestyle Habits."

245. Lorenzo et al. "Epigenetic Effects of Healthy Foods and Lifestyle Habits."

246. Deanna M. Minich. "A Review of the Science of Colorful, Plant-Based Food and Practical Strategies for 'Eating the Rainbow.'" *Journal of Nutrition and Metabolism* 2019 (2019): 1–19. https://doi.org/10.1155/2019/2125070.

247. Sonia Sadeghpour et al. "Associations of Dietary Inflammatory Indices (DII and E-DII) with Sperm Parameters." *Clinical and Experimental Reproductive Medicine*, 52, no. 1 (2025): 79–86. https://doi.org/10.5653/cerm.2024.06982.

248. Simon Alesi et al. "Anti-Inflammatory Diets in Fertility: An Evidence Review." *Nutrients* 14, no. 19 (2022): 3914. https://doi.org/10.3390/nu14193914.

249. Ajaikumar B. Kunnumakkara et al. "Chronic Diseases, Inflammation, and Spices: How Are They Linked?" *Journal of Translational Medicine* 16, no. 14 (2018). https://doi.org/10.1186/s12967-018-1381-2.

250. Berrak Basturk et al. "Evaluation of the Effect of Macronutrients Combination on Blood Sugar Levels in Healthy Individuals." *Iranian Journal of Public Health* 50, no. 2 (2021): 280–87. https://doi.org/10.18502/ijph.v50i2.5340.

251. Alonzo Brody. "Take Control of Your Blood Sugar Levels with Targeted Nutrient Compounds." *Life Extension* (2011). https://go.gale.com/ps/i.do?p=HRCA&sw=w&issn=1524198X&v=2.1&it=r&id=GALE%7CA251955221&sid=googleScholar&linkaccess=abs.

252. Brody. "Take Control of Your Blood Sugar Levels."

253. Stephanie K. Nishi et al. "Impact of Nut Consumption on Cognition Across the Lifespan." *Nutrients* 15, no. 4 (2023): 1000. https://doi.org/10.3390/nu15041000.

254. Ilka M. Vasconcelos and Jose T. Oliveira. "Antinutritional Properties of Plant Lectins." *Toxicon* 44, no. 4 (2004): 385–403. https://doi.org/10.1016/j.toxicon.2004.05.005.

255. Bodo C. Melnik et al. "The Role of Cow's Milk Consumption in Breast Cancer Initiation and Progression." *Current Nutrition Reports* 12 (2023): 122–40. https://doi.org/10.1007/s13668-023-00457-0.

256. Bodo C. Melnik. "Milk Consumption: Aggravating Factor of Acne and Promoter of Chronic Diseases of Western Societies." *Journal der Deutschen Dermatologischen Gesellschaft* 7, no. 4 (2009): 364–70. https://doi.org/10.1111/j.1610-0387.2009.07019.x.

257. Bodo C. Melnik. "Lifetime Impact of Cow's Milk on Overactivation of mTORC1: From Fetal to Childhood Overgrowth, Acne, Diabetes, Cancers, and Neurodegeneration." *Biomolecules* 11, no. 3 (2021): 404. https://doi.org/10.3390/biom11030404.

258. Melnik. "Lifetime Impact of Cow's Milk on Overactivation of mTORC1."

259. Jeff S. Volek et al. "Carbohydrate Restriction Has a More Favorable Impact on the Metabolic Syndrome Than a Low Fat Diet." *Lipids* 44, no. 4 (2009): 297–309. https://doi.org/10.1007/s11745-008-3274-2.

260. Loren Cordain et al. "Origins and Evolution of the Western Diet: Health Implications for the 21st Century." *The American Journal of Clinical Nutrition* 81, no. 2 (2005): 341–54. https://doi.org/10.1093/ajcn.81.2.341.

261. S. Boyd Eaton et al. "Paleolithic Nutrition Revisited: A Twelve-Year Retrospective on Its Nature and Implications." *European Journal of Clinical Nutrition* 51, no. 4 (1997): 207-16. https://doi.org/10.1038/sj.ejcn.1600389.

262. Erica D. Sonnenburg and Justin L. Sonnenburg. "Starving Our Microbial Self: The Deleterious Consequences of a Diet Deficient in Microbiota-Accessible Carbohydrates." *Cell Metabolism* 20, no. 5 (2014): 779–86. https://doi.org/10.1016/j.cmet.2014.07.003.

263. Nicola M. McKeown et al. "Carbohydrate Nutrition, Insulin Resistance, and the Prevalence of the Metabolic Syndrome in the Framingham Offspring Cohort." *Diabetes Care* 27, no. 2 (2004): 538–46. https://doi.org/10.2337/diacare.27.2.538.

264. Bradfield, Christopher A., and M. Marcia Bjeldanes. "Role of Dietary Indoles in the Regulation of Xenobiotic-Metabolizing Enzymes." *The Journal of Nutrition* 121, no. 5 (1991): 597–603.

265. C. Rolf et al. "Zinc and Selenium in Infertility." *Current Opinion in Obstetrics & Gynecology* 14, no. 3 (2002): 275–282.

266. Julie E. Flood-Obbagy and Barbara J. Rolls. "The Effect of Fruit in Different Forms on Energy Intake and Satiety at a Meal." *Appetite* 52, no. 2 (2009): 416–22. https://doi.org/10.1016/j.appet.2008.12.001.

267. Christopher S. Baird. "Is Fruit Juice Healthier Than Whole Fruit?" Science Questions with Surprising Answers, December 2, 2013, accessed September 2, 2024. https://wtamu.edu/~cbaird/sq/2013/12/02/is-fruit-juice-healthier-than-whole-fruit/.

268. Isao Muraki et al. "Fruit Consumption and Risk of Type 2 Diabetes: Results from Three Prospective Longitudinal Cohort Studies." *The BMJ* 347 (2013): f5001. https://doi.org/10.1136/bmj.f5001.

269. Kirsty Anderson et al. "Lifestyle Factors in People Seeking Infertility Treatment—A Review." *Australian and New Zealand Journal of Obstetrics and Gynaecology* 50, no. 1 (2010): 8–20. https://doi.org/10.1111/j.1479-828x.2009.01119.x.

270. Alessando Ilacqua et al. "Lifestyle and Fertility: The Influence of Stress and Quality of Life on Male Fertility." *Reproductive Biology and Endocrinology* 16, no. 1 (2018): 115. https://doi.org/10.1186/s12958-018-0436-9.

271. Ilacqua et al. "Lifestyle and Fertility."

272. Ilacqua et al. "Lifestyle and Fertility."

273. Miriam Arnold et al. "Dealing with Information Overload: A Comprehensive Review." *Frontiers in Psychology* 14 (2023): 1122200. https://doi.org/10.3389/fpsyg.2023.1122200.

274. Marcia P. Jimenez et al. "Associations Between Nature Exposure and Health: A Review of the Evidence." *International Journal of Environmental Research and Public Health* 18, no. 9 (2021): 4790. https://doi.org/10.3390/ijerph18094790.

275. Kaye K. Brownlee et al. "Relationship Between Circulating Cortisol and Testosterone: Influence of Physical Exercise." *Journal of Sports Science & Medicine* 4, no. 1 (2005): 76–83. https://www.ncbi.nlm.nih.gov/pmc/articles/PMC3880087/.

276. Harvard Health Publishing. "A 20-Minute Nature Break Relieves Stress." July 1, 2019. https://www.health.harvard.edu/mind-and-mood/a-20-minute-nature-break-relieves-stress.

277. Kai Triebner et al. "Lifelong Exposure to Residential Greenspace and the Premenstrual Syndrome: A Population-Based Study of Northern European Women." *Environment International* 158 (2022): 106975. https://doi.org/10.1016/j.envint.2021.106975.

278. Kristin L. Rooney and Alice D. Domar. "The Relationship Between Stress and Infertility." *Dialogues in Clinical Neuroscience* 20, no. 1 (2018): 41–47. https://doi.org/10.31887/DCNS.2018.20.1/klrooney.

279. M. Kuo and A. Taylor. "Nature's Impact on Psychological and Physiological Stress: Forest Bathing and Its Effects on Mental Health and Epigenetics." *Frontiers in Psychology* 12 (2021): 737.

280. Q. Li. "Effect of Forest Bathing Trips on Human Immune Function." *Environmental Health and Preventative Medicine* 15 (2010): 9–17. https://doi.org/10.1007/s12199-008-0068-3.

281. Rashida Brown et al. "Neighborhood Social Environment and Changes in Leukocyte Telomere Length: The Multi-Ethnic Study of Atherosclerosis (MESA)." *Health & Place* 67 (2021): 102488. https://doi.org/10.1016/j.healthplace.2020.102488.

282. Alessandro Ilacqua et al. "Lifestyle and Fertility: The Influence of Stress and Quality of Life on Male Fertility." *Reproductive Biology & Endocrinology* 16, no. 115 (2018). https://doi.org/10.1186/s12958-018-0436-9.

283. Ilacqua et al. "Lifestyle and Fertility."

284. Joe Dispenza. "The Role of Brainwaves in Meditation: Part I." *Dr. Joe Dispenza Unlimited* (blog), May 5, 2017. https://drjoedispenza.com/dr-joes-blog/the-role-of-brainwaves-in-meditation-part-i.

285. Rooney and Domar. "The Relationship Between Stress and Infertility."

286. Aanchal Sharma and Deepti Shrivastava. "Psychological Problems Related to Infertility." *Cureus* 14, no. 10 (2022): e30320. https://doi.org/10.7759/cureus.30320.

287. American Pyschological Association. "Stress." Accessed September 4, 2024. https://www.apa.org/topics/stress.

288. Arash Emamzadeh. "How Stress Disrupts a Couple's Support for Each Other . . . and Three Ways to Restore a Supportive Connection." *Psychology Today*, December 10, 2021, accessed September 17, 2024. https://www.psychologytoday.com/intl/blog/finding-new-home/202112/how-stress-disrupts-couples-support-each-other.

289. National Institutes of Health. "Circadian Rhythms." Last updated May 20, 2025. https://www.nigms.nih.gov/education/fact-sheets/Pages/circadian-rhythms.aspx.

290. Francesca Sciarra et al. "Disruption of Circadian Rhythms: A Crucial Factor in the Etiology of Infertility." *International Journal of Molecular Sciences* 21, no. 11 (2020): 3943. https://doi.org/10.3390/ijms21113943.

291. Sciarra et al. "Disruption of Circadian Rhythms."

292. Sciarra et al. "Disruption of Circadian Rhythms."

293. Jane Blood-Siegfried and Elizabeth K. Rende. "The Long-Term Effects of Perinatal Nicotine Exposure on Neurologic Development." *Journal of Midwifery & Women's Health* 55, no. 2 (2010): 143. https://doi.org/10.1016/j.jmwh.2009.05.006.

294. George L. Wehby et al. "The Impact of Maternal Smoking During Pregnancy on Early Child Neurodevelopment." *Journal of Human Capital* 5, no. 2 (Summer 2011): 207. https://doi.org/10.1086/660885.

295. Debbie Montjean et al. "An Overview of E-Cigarette Impact on Reproductive Health." *Life* 13, no. 3 (2023): 827. https://doi.org/10.3390/life13030827.

296. T. S. Omolaoye et al. "The Mutagenic Effect of Tobacco Smoke on Male Fertility." *Environmental Science and Pollution Research International* 29, no. 41 (2022): 62055–66. https://doi.org/10.1007/s11356-021-16331-x.

297. Lead Analysts, and MoTrPAC Study Group. "Temporal Dynamics of the Multi-Omic Response to Endurance Exercise Training." *Nature* 629 (2024): 174–83. https://doi.org/10.1038/s41586-023-06877-w.

298. Rebecca A. Maher et al. "The Current Landscape of Exercise and Female Fertility Research: A Narrative Review." *Reproduction* 168, no. 1 (2024): e220317. https://doi.org/10.1530/REP-22-0317.

299. Maher et al. "The Current Landscape of Exercise and Female Fertility Research."

300. Anjali Yadav et al. "Yoga and Lifestyle Changes: A Path to Improved Fertility—A Narrative Review." *International Journal of Yoga* 17, no. 1 (2024): 10–19. https://doi.org/10.4103/ijoy.ijoy_211_23.

301. Hunter W. Korsmo et al. "Choline: Exploring the Growing Science on Its Benefits for Moms and Babies." *Nutrients* 11, no. 8 (2019): 1823. https://doi.org/10.3390/nu11081823.

302. Office of Dietary Supplements. "Choline: Fact Sheet for Health Professionals." National Institutes of Health, last updated March 29, 2023. https://ods.od.nih.gov/factsheets/Choline-HealthProfessional/.

303. Hyo Kyozuka et al. "Preconception Vitamin D Intake and Obstetric Outcomes in Women Using Assisted Reproductive Technology:

The Japan Environment and Children's Study." *BMC Pregnancy and Childbirth* 22, no. 1 (2022): 542. https://doi.org/10.1186/s12884-022 -04861-2.

304. Kyozuka et al. "Preconception Vitamin D Intake and Obstetric Outcomes in Women."

305. Aiyong Cui et al. "Prevalence, Trend, and Predictor Analyses of Vitamin D Deficiency in the US Population, 2001–2018." *Frontiers in Nutrition* 9 (2022): 965376. https://doi.org/10.3389/fnut.2022 .965376.

306. Office of Dietary Supplements. "Calcium: Fact Sheet for Health Professionals." National Institutes of Health, last updated July 24, 2024. https://ods.od.nih.gov/factsheets/Calcium-HealthProfessional/.

307. Sergi Puig et al. "The Elemental Role of Iron in DNA Synthesis and Repair." *Metallomics: Integrated Biometal Science* 9, no. 11 (2017): 1483–500. https://doi.org/10.1039/c7mt00116a.

308. Mohammad S. Akhter et al. "Iron Deficiency Anemia as a Factor in Male Infertility: Awareness in Health College Students in the Jazan Region of Saudi Arabia." *International Journal of Environmental Research and Public Health* 18, no. 24 (2021): 12866. https://doi.org /10.3390/ijerph182412866.

309. Mayo Clinic. "Iron Deficiency During Pregnancy: Prevention Tips." January 31, 2025. https://www.mayoclinic.org/healthy-lifestyle /pregnancy-week-by-week/in-depth/anemia-during-pregnancy/art -20114455.

310. James J. DiNicolantonio et al. "Subclinical Magnesium Deficiency: A Principal Driver of Cardiovascular Disease and a Public Health Crisis." *Open Heart* 5, no. 1 (2018): e000668. https://doi.org/10.1136 /openhrt-2017-000668.

311. Daniela Fannie et al. "The Role of Magnesium in Pregnancy and in Fetal Programming of Adult Diseases." *Biological Trace Element Research* 199, no. 10 (2021): 3647–57. https://doi.org/10.1007/s12011 -020-02513-0.

312. Fanni et al. "The Role of Magnesium."

313. Fanni et al. "The Role of Magnesium."

314. Salvatore Sciacchitano et al. "Galectin-3: One Molecule for an Alphabet of Diseases, from A to Z." *International Journal of Molecular Sciences* 19, no. 2 (2018): 379. https://doi.org/10.3390/ijms19020379.

315. Deanna M. Minich and Benjamin I. Brown. "A Review of Dietary (Phyto)Nutrients for Glutathione Support." *Nutrients*, 11, no. 9, (2019): 2073. PubMed Central, https://doi.org/10.3390/nu11092073.

316. Alessandra Fraternale et al. "Glutathione and Glutathione Derivatives in Immunotherapy." *Biological Chemistry* 398, no. 2 (2017): 261–75. https://doi.org/10.1515/hsz-2016-0202.

317. Garth L. Nicolson. "Mitochondrial Dysfunction and Chronic Disease: Treatment with Natural Supplements." *Integrative Medicine: A Clinician's Journal* 13, no. 4 (2014): 35–43. https://www.ncbi.nlm.nih.gov/pmc/articles/PMC4566449/.

318. Guneet Gandhi et al. "Glutathione: The Master Antioxidant—Beyond Skin Lightening Agent." *Pigment International* 8, no. 3 (2021): 144–52. https://doi.org/10.4103/pigmentinternational.pigmentinternational_29_21.

319. Jinghan Jenny Chen et al. "Altered Central and Blood Glutathione in Alzheimer's Disease and Mild Cognitive Impairment: A Meta-Analysis." *Alzheimer's Research & Therapy* 14, no. 1 (2022): 23. https://doi.org/10.1186/s13195-022-00961-5.

320. Luca Valgimigli. "Lipid Peroxidation and Antioxidant Protection." *Biomolecules* 13, no. 9 (2023): 1291. https://doi.org/10.3390/biom13091291.

321. Usama Al-Zubaidi et al. "Mitochondria-Targeted Therapeutics, MitoQ and BGP-15, Reverse Aging–Associated Meiotic Spindle Defects in Mouse and Human Oocytes." *Human Reproduction* 36, no. 3 (2021): 771–84. https://doi.org/10.1093/humrep/deaa300.

322. M. Hosseinzadeh Shirzeyli et al. "Exposing Mouse Oocytes to MitoQ During *In Vitro* Maturation Improves Maturation and Developmental Competence." *Iranian Journal of Biotechnology* 18, no. 3 (2020): e2454. https://doi.org/10.30498/ijb.2020.154641.2454.

323. Gema Marín-Royo et al. "The Role of Mitochondrial Oxidative Stress in the Metabolic Alterations in Diet-Induced Obesity in Rats."

FASEB Journal 33, no. 11 (2019): 12060–72. https://doi.org/10.1096/fj
.201900347RR.

324. E. Salahi et al. "The Effect of Mitochondria-Targeted Antioxidant
MitoQ10 on Redox Signaling Pathway Components in PCOS Mouse
Model." *Archives of Gynecology and Obstetrics* 305, no. 4 (2022): 985–
94. https://doi.org/10.1007/s00404-021-06230-4.

325. Mais M. Aljunaidy et al. "Maternal Treatment with a Placental-Targeted
Antioxidant (MitoQ) Impacts Offspring Cardiovascular Function in a
Rat Model of Prenatal Hypoxia." *Pharmacological Research* 134 (2018):
332–42. https://doi.org/10.1016/j.phrs.2018.05.006.

326. Aljunaidy et al. "Maternal Treatment with a Placental-Targeted Antioxidant (MitoQ)."

327. Waleed F. A. Marei et al. "Mitochondria-Targeted Therapy Rescues Development and Quality of Embryos Derived from Oocytes
Matured Under Oxidative Stress Conditions: A Bovine in Vitro
Model." *Human Reproduction* 34, no. 10 (2019): 1984–98. https://doi
.org/10.1093/humrep/dez161.

328. Sabina Bastos Maia et al. "Vitamin A and Pregnancy: A Narrative
Review." *Nutrients* 11, no. 3 (2019): 681. https://doi.org/10.3390
/nu11030681.

329. Bastos Maia et al. "Vitamin A and Pregnancy."

330. Manuela Strobel et al. "The Importance of Beta-Carotene as a Source
of Vitamin A with Special Regard to Pregnant and Breastfeeding
Women." *European Journal of Nutrition* 46, no. 1 Supp. (2007): 1–20.
https://doi.org/10.1007/s00394-007-1001-z.

331. Strobel et al. "The Importance of Beta-Carotene."

332. Cathryn A. Hogarth and Michael D. Griswold. "The Key Role of
Vitamin A in Spermatogenesis." *The Journal of Clinical Investigation*
120, no. 4 (2010): 956–62. https://doi.org/10.1172/JCI41303.

333. Hogarth and Griswold. "The Key Role of Vitamin A in Spermatogenesis."

334. Hogarth and Griswold. "The Key Role of Vitamin A in Spermatogenesis."

335. Afshin Mohammadi-Bardbori et al. "Protective Effects of Astaxanthin on Post-Thaw Sperm Quality in Normozoospermic Men." *Andrologia*, March 20, 2024. https://doi.org/10.1155/2024/2332443.

336. Y. Li et al. "Astaxanthin Improves the Development of the Follicles and Oocytes Through Alleviating Oxidative Stress Induced by BPA in Cultured Follicles." *Scientific Reports* 12, no. 7853 (2022). https://doi.org/10.1038/s41598-022-11566-1.

337. Riccardo Gambioli et al. "Myo-Inositol as a Key Supporter of Fertility and Physiological Gestation." *Pharmaceuticals* 14, no. 6 (2021): 504. https://doi.org/10.3390/ph14060504.

338. Gambioli et al. "Myo-Inositol as a Key Supporter of Fertility and Physiological Gestation."

339. Ashok Agarwal et al. "Role of L-Carnitine in Female Infertility." *Reproductive Biology and Endocrinology* 16, no. 1 (2018): 5. https://doi.org/10.1186/s12958-018-0323-4.

340. Leila Kooshesh et al. "Evaluation of L-Carnitine Potential in Improvement of Male Fertility." *Journal of Reproduction & Infertility* 24, no. 2 (2023): 69–84. https://doi.org/10.18502/jri.v24i2.12491.

341. Majid S. Koozehchian et al. "Effects of Nine Weeks L-Carnitine Supplementation on Exercise Performance, Anaerobic Power, and Exercise-Induced Oxidative Stress in Resistance-Trained Males." *Journal of Exercise Nutrition & Biochemistry* 22, no. 4 (2018): 7. https://doi.org/10.20463/jenb.2018.0026.

342. Kooshesh et al. "Evaluation of L-Carnitine Potential in Improvement of Male Fertility."

343. Myrthe A. J. Smits et al. "Human Ovarian Aging Is Characterized by Oxidative Damage and Mitochondrial Dysfunction." *Human Reproduction* 38, no. 11 (2023): 2208–20. https://doi.org/10.1093/humrep/dead177.

344. Smits et al. "Human Ovarian Aging."

345. Charley-Lea Pollard et al. "NAD⁺, Sirtuins, and PARPs: Enhancing Oocyte Developmental Competence." *Journal of Reproduction and Development* 68, no. 6 (2022): 345–54. https://doi.org/10.1262/jrd.2022-052.

346. Kingsley C. Anukam et al. "Probiotic Lactobacillus Rhamnosus GR-1 and Lactobacillus Reuteri RC-14 May Help Downregulate TNF-Alpha, IL-6, IL-8, IL-10 and IL-12 (P70) in the Neurogenic Bladder of Spinal Cord Injured Patient with Urinary Tract Infections: A Two-Case Study." *Advances in Urology* (2009): 680363. https://doi.org/10.1155/2009/680363.

347. Elahe Abedi and Seyed Mohammad Bagher Hashemi. "Lactic Acid Production—Producing Microorganisms and Substrates Sources—State of Art." *Heliyon* 6, no. 10 (2020): e04974. https://doi.org/10.1016/j.heliyon.2020.e04974.

348. Anukam et al. "Probiotic Lactobacillus Rhamnous GR-1 and Lactobacillus Reuteri RC-14."

349. Eva Tvrdá et al. "The Role of Selected Natural Biomolecules in Sperm Production and Functionality." *Molecules* 26, no. 17 (2021): 5196. https://doi.org/10.3390/molecules26175196.

350. ScienceDirect. "Naringenin." Accessed November 15, 2024. https://www.sciencedirect.com/topics/biochemistry-genetics-and-molecular-biology/naringenin.

351. ScienceDirect. "Naringenin."

352. Aleksandra Duda-Chodak and Tomasz Tarko. "Possible Side Effects of Polyphenols and Their Interactions with Medicines." *Molecules* 28, no. 6 (2023): 2536. https://doi.org/10.3390/molecules28062536.

353. Tvrdá et al. "The Role of Selected Natural Biomolecules in Sperm Production and Functionality."

354. L. J. Ignarro et al. "Endothelium-Derived Relaxing Factor Produced and Released from Artery and Vein Is Nitric Oxide." *Proceedings of the National Academy of Sciences of the United States of America* 84, no. 24 (1987): 9265–69. https://doi.org/10.1073/pnas.84.24.9265.

355. G. Wu et al. "Role of L-Arginine in Nitric Oxide Synthesis and Health in Humans." *Advances in Experimental Medicine and Biology* 1332 (2021): 167–87. https://doi.org/10.1007/978-3-030-74180-8_10.

356. S. Dutta and P. Sengupta. "The Role of Nitric Oxide on Male and Female Reproduction." *Malaysian Journal of Medical Sciences* 29, no. 2 (2022): 18–30. https://doi.org/10.21315/mjms2022.29.2.3.

357. Dutta and Sengupta. "The Role of Nitric Oxide on Male and Female Reproduction."

358. HumanN. "Neo40® - Blood Pressure Support and Nitric Oxide Restoration." Accessed November 15, 2024. https://humann.com/pages/get_neo40-2.

359. Mark Hyman. "How 'Getting an Oil Change' Fixed My Brain Fog and Fatigue." *Dr. Mark Hyman, MD*, August 1, 2024, accessed November 13, 2024. https://drhyman.com/blogs/content/how-i-fixed-my-brain-fog-and-fatigue.

360. M. J. Bertoldo et al. "NAD+ Repletion Rescues Female Fertility During Reproductive Aging." *Cell Reports* 30, no. 6 (2020): 1670–81. https://doi.org/10.1016/j.celrep.2020.01.058.

361. J. Liang et al. "Impact of NAD+ Metabolism on Ovarian Aging." *Immunity & Ageing* 20, no. 70 (2023). https://doi.org/10.1186/s12979-023-00398-w.

362. Andrew P. Shoubridge et al. "The Gut Microbiome and Mental Health: Advances in Research and Emerging Priorities." *Molecular Psychiatry* 27, no. 4 (2022): 1908–19. https://doi.org/10.1038/s41380-022-01479-w.

363. Zuzanna Lewandowska-Pietruszka et al. "The History of the Intestinal Microbiota and the Gut-Brain Axis." *Pathogens* 11, no. 12 (2022): 1540. https://doi.org/10.3390/pathogens11121540.

364. Lewandowska-Pietruszka et al. "The History of the Intestinal Microbiota and the Gut-Brain Axis."

365. The Human Microbiome Project Consortium. "Structure, Function and Diversity of the Healthy Human Microbiome." *Nature* 486, no. 7402 (2012): 207–214. https://doi.org/10.1038/nature11234.

366. Timothy G. Dinan et al. "Psychobiotics: A Novel Class of Psychotropic." *Biological Psychiatry* 74, no. 10 (2013): 720–726. https://doi.org/10.1016/j.biopsych.2013.05.001.

367. P. Shobeiri et al. "Shedding Light on Biological Sex Differences and Microbiota-Gut-Brain Axis: A Comprehensive Review of Its Roles in Neuropsychiatric Disorders." *Biology of Sex Differences* 13, no. 12 (2022). https://doi.org/10.1186/s13293-022-00422-6.

368. Taiwo Bankole et al. "Dietary Impacts on Gestational Diabetes: Connection Between Gut Microbiome and Epigenetic Mechanisms." *Nutrients* 14, no. 24 (2022): 5269. https://doi.org/10.3390/nu14245269.

369. Bankole et al. "Dietary Impacts on Gestational Diabetes."

370. Research and Markets. "Microbiome Therapeutics Market Forecast at $21.5 Billion by 2030, Witnessing a 56.9% CAGR—Rising Prevalence of Gastrointestinal Disorders Driving Demand." GlobeNewswire, September 30, 2024. https://www.globenewswire.com/news-release/2024/09/30/2954992/28124/en/Microbiome-Therapeutics-Market-Forecast-at-21-5-Billion-by-2030-Witnessing-a-56-9-CAGR-Rising-Prevalence-of-Gastrointestinal-Disorders-Driving-Demand.html.

371. Microbiotica. "Microbiotica Raises £50 Million ($67 Million) to Advance Pipeline of Microbiome-Based Therapeutics." March 7, 2022. https://microbiotica.com/microbiotica-raises-50-million-67-million-to-advance-pipeline-of-microbiome-based-therapeutics/.

372. *Microbiome Times.* "EIB Has Signed €20 Million in Venture Debt Financing with Microbiome Health Company the Akkermansia Company." December 14, 2023. https://www.microbiometimes.com/eib-has-signed-e20-million-in-venture-debt-financing-with-microbiome-health-company-the-akkermansia-company/.

373. National Institutes of Health. "Human Microbiome (HMP)." Accessed October 28, 2024. https://commonfund.nih.gov/hmp.

374. Susana Camacho. "Microbiome Research for Human, Animal and Planetary Health." University of Cambridge School of the Biological Sciences, October 30, 2023. https://www.bio.cam.ac.uk/research/research-themes/microbiome-research-human-animal-and-planetary-health.

375. Maria D. Zambrano and Graham A. Colditz. "The Microbiome, Estrogen Metabolism, and Breast Cancer Risk." *JNCI: Journal of the National Cancer Institute* 108, no. 8 (2016): djw130. https://pmc.ncbi.nlm.nih.gov/articles/PMC10416750/#s0006.

376. Xinyu Qi et al. "The Impact of the Gut Microbiota on the Reproductive and Metabolic Endocrine System." *Abstract* 13, no. 1 (2021): 1894070. https://www.ncbi.nlm.nih.gov/pmc/articles/PMC7971312/.

377. Qi et al. "The Impact of the Gut Microbiota."

378. Runpei Deng et al. "Association Between Gut Microbiota and Male Infertility: A Two-Sample Mendelian Randomization Study." *International Microbiology* 27 (2024): 1655–63. https://doi.org/10.1007/s10123-024-00512-y.

379. Shuya Lv et al. "Gut Microbiota Is Involved in Male Reproductive Function: A Review." *Frontiers in Microbiology* 15 (2024). https://doi.org/10.3389/fmicb.2024.1371667.

380. Lv et al. "Gut Microbiota."

381. Lv et al. "Gut Microbiota."

382. Michael J. Martin et al. "Antibiotics Overuse in Animal Agriculture: A Call to Action for Health Care Providers." *American Journal of Public Health* 105, no. 12 (2015): 2409. https://doi.org/10.2105/AJPH.2015.302870.

383. The Detox Project. "Glyphosate Residue Free." The Detox Project. Accessed October 31, 2024. https://detoxproject.org/.

384. Alexandria Turner et al. "Intense Sweeteners, Taste Receptors and the Gut Microbiome: A Metabolic Health Perspective." *International Journal of Environmental Research and Public Health* 17, no. 11 (2020): 4094. https://doi.org/10.3390/ijerph17114094.

385. Columbia University Mailman School of Public Health. "Low-Level Lead Poisoning Is Still Pervasive in the U.S. and Globally." October 30, 2024. https://www.publichealth.columbia.edu/news/low-level-lead-poisoning-still-pervasive-u-s-globally.

386. *Medical News Today.* "Over 400,000 U.S. Deaths per Year Caused by Lead Exposure." March 13, 2018. https://www.thelancet.com/journals/lanonc/article/PIIS2468-2667(18)30025-2/fulltext.

387. U.S. Geological Survey. "Widespread Mercury Contamination Across Western North America." September 14, 2016, accessed October 31, 2024. https://www.usgs.gov/news/featured-story/comprehensive-study-finds-widespread-mercury-contamination-across-western-north.

388. Vaccine Safety. "Thimerosal and Vaccines." CDC, December 19, 2024. https://www.cdc.gov/vaccine-safety/about/thimerosal.html.

389. National Institute of Environmental Health Sciences. "Bisphenol A (BPA)." Accessed October 26, 2024. https://www.niehs.nih.gov/health/topics/agents/sya-bpa.

390. Leonardo Trasande et al. "Association Between Urinary Bisphenol A Concentration and Obesity Prevalence in Children and Adolescents." *JAMA* 308, no. 11 (2012): 1113–21. https://doi.org/10.1001/2012.jama.11461.

391. Environmental Working Group. "EWG's 2025 Shopper's Guide to Pesticides in Produce." June 11, 2025. https://www.ewg.org/foodnews/summary.php.

392. Lana Barhum. "Are Ultra-Processed Foods Bad for You?" Verywell Health, January 24, 2025. https://www.verywellhealth.com/ultra-processed-foods-ibd-risk-5194645.

393. Paul A. Engen et al. "The Gastrointestinal Microbiome: Alcohol Effects on the Composition of Intestinal Microbiota." *Alcohol Research* 37, no. 2 (2015): 223–36. https://pmc.ncbi.nlm.nih.gov/articles/PMC4590619/.

394. U.S. Environmental Protection Agency. *America's Children and the Environment, Third Edition; Biomonitoring: Phthalates* (2017). https://www.epa.gov/sites/default/files/2017-08/documents/phthalates_updates_live_file_508_0.pdf.

395. Katherine Z. Sanidad et al. "Triclosan, a Common Antimicrobial Ingredient, on Gut Microbiota and Gut Health." *Gut Microbes* 10, no. 3 (2019): 434–37. https://doi.org/10.1080/19490976.2018.1546521.

396. Xuewei Zhou et al. "The Impact of Food Additives on the Abundance and Composition of Gut Microbiota." *Molecules* 28, no. 2 (2023): 631. https://doi.org/10.3390/molecules28020631.

397. Sherri A. Mason et al. "Synthetic Polymer Contamination in Bottled Water." *Frontiers in Chemistry* 6 (2018): 407. https://doi.org/10.3389/fchem.2018.00407.

398. Zara Abrams. "USC Study Finds Link Between PFAS, Kidney Function and Gut Health." Press release, Keck School of Medicine of USC, October

17, 2024. https://keck.usc.edu/news/usc-study-finds-link-between-pfas
-kidney-function-and-gut-health/.

399. Abrams. "USC Study Finds Link Between PFAS, Kidney Function and Gut Health."

400. Abigail P. Bline et al. "Public Health Risks of PFAS-Related Immunotoxicity Are Real." *Current Environmental Health Reports* 11, no. 2 (2024): 118–27. https://doi.org/10.1007/s40572-024-00441-y.

401. Federica Di Vincenzo et al. "Gut Microbiota, Intestinal Permeability, and Systemic Inflammation: A Narrative Review." *Internal and Emergency Medicine* 19, no. 2 (2024): 275–93. https://doi.org/10.1007/s11739-023-03374-w.

402. Di Vincenzo et al. "Gut Microbiota, Intestinal Permeability, and Systemic Inflammation."

403. Menna Teffera et al. "Diverse Mechanisms by Which Chemical Pollutant Exposure Alters Gut Microbiota Metabolism and Inflammation." *Environment International* 190 (2024): 108805. https://doi.org/10.1016/j.envint.2024.108805.

404. Partho Sen et al. "Exposure to Environmental Toxicants Is Associated with Gut Microbiome Dysbiosis, Insulin Resistance and Obesity." *Environment International* 186 (2024): 108569. https://doi.org/10.1016/j.envint.2024.108569.

405. Scott Belcher. "PFAS Chemicals: EDCs Contaminating Our Water and Food Supply." Endocrine Society. Accessed November 12, 2024. https://www.endocrine.org/topics/edc/what-edcs-are/common-edcs/pfas.

406. R. K. Singh et al. "Influence of Diet on the Gut Microbiome and Implications for Human Health." *Journal of Translational Medicine* 15, no. 1 (2017): 73. https://doi.org/10.1186/s12967-017-1175-y.

407. Maris Fessenden. "Microbe Cells Don't Outnumber Your Own." *Smithsonian Magazine.* January 11, 2016, accessed October 28, 2024. https://www.smithsonianmag.com/smart-news/microbe-cells-dont-outnumber-your-own-180957762/.

408. Rachel Nuwer. "Your Microbes Get Jet Lagged, Too." *Smithsonian Magazine.* October 17, 2014, accessed October 28, 2024. https://www

.smithsonianmag.com/smart-news/your-microbes-get-jet-lagged-too
-180953076/.

409. Yiding Chen et al. "The Microbiota: A Crucial Mediator in Gut
Homeostasis and Colonization Resistance." *Frontiers in Microbiology*
15 (2024). https://doi.org/10.3389/fmicb.2024.1417864.

410. Robert G. Nichols and Emily R. Davenport. "The Relationship
Between the Gut Microbiome and Host Gene Expression: A Review."
Human Genetics 140, no. 5 (2021): 747–60. https://doi.org/10.1007
/s00439-020-02237-0.

411. Joy Yang. "The Human Microbiome Project: Extending the Definition
of What Constitutes a Human." The Human Microbiome Project.
July 16, 2012, accessed October 28, 2024. https://www.genome.gov
/27549400/the-human-microbiome-project-extending-the-definition
-of-what-constitutes-a-human.

412. Joan Miro-Blanch and Oscar Yanes. "Epigenetic Regulation at the
Interplay Between Gut Microbiota and Host Metabolism." *Frontiers
in Genetics* 10 (2019). https://doi.org/10.3389/fgene.2019.00638.

413. Brunella Zizolfi et al. "Endometriosis and Dysbiosis: State of Art."
Frontiers in Endocrinology 14 (2023): 1140774. https://doi.org/10.3389
/fendo.2023.1140774.

414. Remco Kort et al. "Shaping the Oral Microbiota Through Intimate
Kissing." *Microbiome* 2, no. (2014): 41. https://doi.org/10.1186/2049
-2618-2-41.

415. Ann Shippy, MD. "Pucker Up! Can Kissing Change Your Microbiome?" Every Life Well, February 6, 2019. https://annshippymd.com
/pucker-up-can-kissing-change-your-microbiome/.

416. Antonio Barrientos-Durán et al. "Reviewing the Composition of Vaginal Microbiota: Inclusion of Nutrition and Probiotic Factors in the
Maintenance of Eubiosis." *Nutrients* 12, no. 2 (2020): 419. https://doi
.org/10.3390/nu12020419.

417. Jacques Ravel et al. "Bacterial Vaginosis and Its Association with
Infertility, Endometritis, and Pelvic Inflammatory Disease." *American
Journal of Obstetrics & Gynecology* 224, no. 3 (2021): 251–257. https://
doi.org/10.1016/j.ajog.2020.10.019.

418. Resa G. Magill and Susan M. MacDonald. "Male Infertility and the Human Microbiome." *Frontiers in Reproductive Health* 5 (2023): 116201. https://doi.org/10.3389/frph.2023.1166201.

419. Mario Caldarelli et al. "Gut-Brain Axis: Focus on Sex Differences in Neuroinflammation." *International Journal of Molecular Sciences* 25, no. 10 (2024): 5377. https://doi.org/10.3390/ijms25105377.

420. Caldarelli et al. "Gut-Brain Axis."

421. Katarzyna Zych-Krekora et al. "Potential Impact of a Pregnant Woman's Microbiota on the Development of Fetal Heart Defects: A Review of the Literature." *Biomedicines* 12, no. 3 (2024): 654. https://doi.org/10.3390/biomedicines12030654.

422. Stephen T. Holgate et al. "Asthma." *Nature Reviews Disease Primers* 1, no. 1 (2015): 1–22. https://doi.org/10.1038/nrdp.2015.25.

423. Yuanyuan Li. "Epigenetic Mechanisms Link Maternal Diets and Gut Microbiome to Obesity in the Offspring." *Frontiers in Genetics* 9 (2018): 342. https://doi.org/10.3389/fgene.2018.00342.

424. Patti Verbanas. "The Hidden Reason Children Born by C-Section Are More Likely to Develop Asthma." Rutgers. November 11, 2021, accessed November 1, 2024. https://www.rutgers.edu/news/hidden-reason-children-born-c-section-are-more-likely-develop-asthma.

425. Taylor K. Soderborg et al. "Microbial Transmission from Mothers with Obesity or Diabetes to Infants: An Innovative Opportunity to Interrupt a Vicious Cycle." *Diabetologia* 59, no. 5 (2016): 895. https://doi.org/10.1007/s00125-016-3880-0.

426. Francesco Petrillo et al. "Current Evidence on the Ocular Surface Microbiota and Related Diseases." *Microorganisms* 8, no. 7 (2020): 1033. https://doi.org/10.3390/microorganisms8071033.

427. Nicole O. Palmer et al. "Impact of Obesity on Male Fertility, Sperm Function and Molecular Composition." *Spermatogenesis* 2, no. 4 (2012): 253–63. https://doi.org/10.4161/spmg.21362.

428. Palmer et al. "Impact of Obesity on Male Fertility, Sperm Function, and Molecular Composition."

429. University of Oxford. "Global Study Shows the Experience of Endometriosis Is Rooted in Genetics." March 14, 2023. https://www.ox.ac

.uk/news/2023-03-14-global-study-shows-experience-endometriosis
-rooted-genetics.

430. Thomas T. Tapmeier et al. "Neuropeptide S Receptor 1 Is a Non-hormonal Treatment Target in Endometriosis." *Science Translational Medicine* 13, no. 608 (2021): eabd6469. https://doi.org/10.1126/scitranslmed.abd6469.

431. Shay M. Freger and Warren G. Foster. "The Link Between Environmental Toxicant Exposure and Endometriosis Re-Examined." *Endometriosis* (2020). https://doi.org/10.5772/intechopen.91002.

432. Ayako Muraoka et al. "*Fusobacterium* Infection Facilitates the Development of Endometriosis Through the Phenotypic Transition of Endometrial Fibroblasts." *Science Translational Medicine* 15, no. 700 (2023): eadd1531. https://doi.org/10.1126/scitranslmed.add1531.

433. Endometriosis.org. "Inflammation Gene May Be Possible Drug Target for Endometriosis." Last updated August 26, 2021, accessed October 14, 2024. https://endometriosis.org/news/research/inflammation-gene-may-be-possible-drug-target-for-endometriosis/.

434. Thomas T. Tapmeier et al. "Neuropeptide S Receptor 1 Is a Non-hormonal Treatment Target in Endometriosis."

435. World Health Organization. "Polycystic Ovary Syndrome." February 7, 2025. https://www.who.int/news-room/fact-sheets/detail/polycystic-ovary-syndrome.

436. Evanthia Diamanti-Kandarakis and Andrea Dunaif. "Insulin Resistance and the Polycystic Ovary Syndrome Revisited: An Update on Mechanisms and Implications," *Endocrine Reviews* 33, no. 6 (2012): 981–1030. https://doi.org/10.1210/er.2011-1034.

437. CDC. "Childhood Obesity Facts." April 2, 2024. https://www.cdc.gov/obesity/childhood-obesity-facts/childhood-obesity-facts.html.

438. CDC. "Childhood Obesity Facts."

439. Orit Pinhas-Hamiel and Philip Zeitler. "Type 2 Diabetes in Children and Adolescents: A Focus on Diagnosis and Treatment." *Endotext* (2023). https://www.ncbi.nlm.nih.gov/books/NBK597439/.

440. Pinhas-Hamiel and Zeitler. "Type 2 Diabetes in Children and Adolescents."

441. Pinhas-Hamiel and Zeitler. "Type 2 Diabetes in Children and Adolescents."

442. Harald Lehnen et al. "Epigenetics of Gestational Diabetes Mellitus and Offspring Health: The Time for Action Is in Early Stages of Life." *Molecular Human Reproduction* 19, no. 7 (2013): 415–22. https://doi.org/10.1093/molehr/gat020.

443. Xia Li et al. "Inflammation and Aging: Signaling Pathways and Intervention Therapies." *Signal Transduction and Targeted Therapy* 8, no. 1 (2023): 1–29. https://doi.org/10.1038/s41392-023-01502-8.

444. Stephen Ameho and Michael Klutstein. "The Effect of Chronic Inflammation on Female Fertility." *Reproduction* 169, no. 4 (2025): e240197. https://doi.org/10.1530/REP-24-0197.

445. National Center for Health Statistics. "U.S. Fertility Rate Drops to Another Historic Low." CDC, April 24, 2024. https://www.cdc.gov/nchs/pressroom/nchs_press_releases/2024/20240525.htm.

446. Laura Maintz and Novak Natalija. "Histamine and Histamine Intolerance," *The American Journal of Clinical Nutrition* 85, no. 5 (2007): 1185–1196. https://doi.org/10.1093/ajcn/85.5.1185.

447. F. M. Menzies et al. "The Role of Mast Cells and Their Mediators in Reproduction, Pregnancy and Labour." *Human Reproduction Update* 17, no. 3 (2011): 383–96. https://doi.org/10.1093/humupd/dmq053.

448. Jarrod. "Oxalate Sensitivity: Is Yeast or Candida Overgrowth the Underlying Cause?" *Advanced Functional Medicine* (blog), July 11, 2021. https://advancedfunctionalmedicine.com.au/oxalates-and-candida-overgrowth/.

449. Vinay Kumar et al. "Manipulation of Oxalate Metabolism in Plants for Improving Food Quality and Productivity." *Phytochemistry* 158 (2019): 103–9. https://doi.org/10.1016/j.phytochem.2018.10.029.

450. Isabel Cuadrado-Torroglosa et al. "The Impacts of Inflammatory and Autoimmune Conditions on the Endometrium and Reproductive Outcomes." *Journal of Clinical Medicine* 13, no. 13 (2024): 3724. https://doi.org/10.3390/jcm13133724.

451. Carolyn Serraino. "Examining Pre-Autoimmunity: Can Autoimmune Disease Be Prevented?" Global Autoimmune Institute, December 22,

2023. https://www.autoimmuneinstitute.org/articles/examining-pre
-autoimmunity-can-autoimmune-disease-be-prevented.

452. Kamila Tańska et al. "Thyroid Autoimmunity and Its Negative Impact on Female Fertility and Maternal Pregnancy Outcomes." *Frontiers in Endocrinology* 13 (2023). https://doi.org/10.3389/fendo.2022.1049665.

453. Cuadrado-Torroglosa et al. "The Impacts of Inflammatory and Auto-immune Conditions."

454. Valeriy A. Chereshnev et al. "Pathogenesis of Autoimmune Male Infertility: Juxtacrine, Paracrine, and Endocrine Dysregulation." *Pathophysiology* 28, no. 4 (2021): 471–88. https://doi.org/10.3390/pathophysiology28040030.

455. Cuadrado-Torroglosa et al. "The Impacts of Inflammatory and Auto-immune Conditions."

456. Tańska et al. "Thyroid Autoimmunity."

457. Shiju Chen et al. "Association Between Antinuclear Antibody and Female Infertility: A Meta-analysis." *Scandinavian Journal of Immunology* 98, no. 1 (2023): e13285. https://doi.org/10.1111/sji.13285.

458. Xiaoqing Zheng and Amr H. Sawalha "The Role of Oxidative Stress in Epigenetic Changes Underlying Autoimmunity." *Antioxidants & Redox Signaling* 36, nos. 7–9 (2022): 423–40. https://doi.org/10.1089/ars.2021.0066.

459. Zheng and Sawalha. "The Role of Oxidative Stress."

460. Zheng and Sawalha. "The Role of Oxidative Stress."

461. World Health Organization. *Infertility Prevalence Estimates, 1990–2021* (2023). https://www.who.int/publications/i/item/978920068315.

462. World Health Organization. *Infertility Prevalence Estimates, 1990–2021.*

463. U.S. Department of Health and Human Services. "Fact Sheet: In Vitro Fertilization (IVF) Use Across the United States." HHS.gov, March 13, 2024. https://www.hhs.gov/about/news/2024/03/13/fact-sheet-in -vitro-fertilization-ivf-use-across-united-states.html.

464. Anne O'Rourke et al. "Employer Funded Egg Freezing: An Advance for Women in the Workplace or a Return to the Unencumbered

Employee?" *Women's Studies International Forum* 98 (2023): 102698. https://doi.org/10.1016/j.wsif.2023.102698.

465. O'Rourke et al. "Employer Funded Egg Freezing."

466. O'Rourke et al. "Employer Funded Egg Freezing."

467. Max Roser. "Until the Late 1960s, the Total Fertility Rate Was Five—Since Then It Has Halved." *Our World in Data* (2019). https://ourworldindata.org/global-fertility-has-halved.

468. Jasmine L. Chiang et al. "Mitochondria in Ovarian Aging and Reproductive Longevity." *Ageing Research Reviews* 63 (2020): 101168. https://doi.org/10.1016/j.arr.2020.101168.

469. Chiang et al. "Mitochondria in Ovarian Aging."

470. National Institutes of Health. "Chronic Hypertension in Pregnancy Doubled in U.S. from 2007 to 2021." June 17, 2024. https://www.nih.gov/news-events/news-releases/chronic-hypertension-pregnancy-doubled-us-2007-2021.

471. Cande V. Ananth et al. "Pre-Eclampsia Rates in the United States, 1980–2010: Age-Period-Cohort Analysis." *The BMJ* 347 (2013): f6564. https://doi.org/10.1136/bmj.f6564.

472. Centers for Disease Control and Prevention. "Data from the Prenancy Mortality Surveillance System." January 30, 2025. https://www.cdc.gov/maternal-mortality/php/pregnancy-mortality-surveillance-data/?CDC_AAref_Val=https://www.cdc.gov/maternal-mortality/php/pregnancy-mortality-surveillance/index.html.

473. Hagai Levine et al. "Temporal Trends in Sperm Count: A Systematic Review and Meta-Regression Analysis of Samples Collected Globally in the 20th and 21st Centuries." *Human Reproduction Update* 29, no. 2 (2023): 157–76. https://doi.org/10.1093/humupd/dmac035.

474. Levine et al. "Temporal Trends in Sperm Count."

475. Levine et al. "Temporal Trends in Sperm Count."

476. *Environmental Health News*. "Keep PFAS out of Your Sex Life." February 7, 2024. https://www.ehn.org/pfas-condoms-2667132759.html.

477. You can go to this website for a list of safer condoms: https://millionmarker.com/blogs/blog/pfas-condoms-study.

478. Oova. "Fertility Technology." Accessed October 14, 2024. https://www.oova.life/fertility-technology.

479. Path Fertility. "SpermQT." Accessed October 14, 2024, https://pathfertility.com/product/.

480. American Society for Reproductive Medicine. "IVF-Assisted Pregnancies Constitute 2.5% of All U.S. Births in 2022." Last modified October 11, 2023. https://www.asrm.org/news-and-events/asrm-news/press-releasesbulletins/ivf-assisted-pregnancies-constitute/.

481. American Society for Reproductive Medicine. "IVF-Assisted Pregnancies."

482. T. Wainstock et al. "Fertility Treatments and Pediatric Neoplasms of the Offspring: Results of a Population-Based Cohort with a Median Follow-Up of 10 Years." *American Journal of Obstetrics and Gynecology* 216, no. 3 (2017): 314.e1–314.e14. https://doi.org/10.1016/j.ajog.2017.01.015.

483. Wainstock et al. "Fertility Treatments and Pediatric Neoplasms of the Offspring."

484. N. Shachor et al. "Fertility Treatments and Gastrointestinal Morbidity of the Offspring." *Early Human Development* 144 (2020): 195921. https://doi.org/10.1016/j.earlhumdev.2020.105021.

485. Shachor et al. "Fertility Treatments and Gastrointestinal Morbidity of the Offspring."

486. Hamid Ahmadi et al. "Long-Term Effects of ART on the Health of the Offspring." *International Journal of Molecular Sciences* 24, no. 17 (2023): 13564. https://doi.org/10.3390/ijms241713564.

487. Srdjan Saso et al. "An Umbrella Review of Meta-Analyses Regarding the Incidence of Female-Specific Malignancies after Fertility Treatment." *Fertility and Sterility* 123, no. 3 (2025): 506–19. https://doi.org/10.1016/j.earlhumdev.2020.105021.

488. Saso et al. "An Umbrella Review of Meta-Analyses."

489. Saso et al. "An Umbrella Review of Meta-Analyses."

490. It's worth noting that the cost per live birth via IVF can be higher than $60,000 in some parts of the country, as of 2024. More cost information is at Rachel Gurevich. "How Much Does IVF Really Cost?"

Parents, July 25, 2024. https://www.parents.com/how-much-ivf-costs-8622386.

491. Azer Scientific, Inc. "Glucose Drinks Ingredient List." Accessed June 30, 2025. https://www.azerscientific.com/glucose-drink-resources.

492. Learn more about this alternative version of a diagnostic glucose beverage at www.thefreshtest.com.

493. James M. Rippe. "Lifestyle Medicine: The Health Promoting Power of Daily Habits and Practices." *American Journal of Lifestyle Medicine* 12, no. 6 (2018): 499–512. https://doi.org/10.1177/1559827618785554.

494. Genomic Diagnostics. "Genetic Carrier Screening." Accessed June 30, 2025. https://www.genomicdiagnostics.com.au/tests/genetic-carrier-screening.

495. DNA Life. "GrowBaby." Accessed November 18, 2024. https://www.dnalife.healthcare/products/dna/growbaby.

496. Ajurani Siddesh et al. "Platelet-Specific Collagen Receptor *Glycoprotein VI* Gene Variants Affect Recurrent Pregnancy Loss." *Fertility and Sterility* 102, no. 4 (2014): 1078–84.e3. https://doi.org/10.1016/j.fertnstert.2014.07.002.

497. A. F. Amin et al. "N-Acetyl Cysteine for Treatment of Recurrent Unexplained Pregnancy Loss." *Reproductive BioMedicine Online* 17, no. 5 (2008): 722–26. https://doi.org/10.1016/S1472-6483(10)60322-7.

498. RealTime Labs. "Clinical Test Panel for Mycotoxins." January 31, 2023. https://realtimelab.com/clinical-test-panel/.

499. Mosaic Diagnostics. "MycoTOX Profile." Accessed July 18, 2024. https://mosaicdx.com/test/mycotox-profile/.

500. Nader Salari et al. "Aflatoxin M1 in Milk Worldwide from 1988 to 2020: A Systematic Review and Meta-Analysis." *Journal of Food Quality* 2020 (2020): 1–14. https://doi.org/10.1155/2020/8862738.

501. Janette H. Hope and Bradley E. Hope. "A Review of the Diagnosis and Treatment of Ochratoxin A Inhalational Exposure Associated with Human Illness and Kidney Disease Including Focal Segmental Glomerulosclerosis." *Journal of Environmental and Public Health* (2012): 835059. https://doi.org/10.1155/2012/835059.

502. A. Rogowska et al. "Zearalenone and Its Metabolites: Effect on Human Health, Metabolism and Neutralisation Methods." *Toxicon: Official Journal of the International Society on Toxinology* 162 (2019): 46–56. https://doi.org/10.1016/j.toxicon.2019.03.004.

503. Moldpedia. "Trichothecene Mycotoxins, Symptoms, T-2." Accessed August 9, 2024. https://moldpedia.com/trichothecene-mycotoxins.

504. Quest Diagnostics. "Test Directory." Accessed August 9, 2024. https://testdirectory.questdiagnostics.com/test/test-detail/19492/sperm-antibody-iga-igg?cc=MASTER.

505. Gül Kadan and Neriman Aral. "Effects of Mycotoxins on Child Development." *Current Molecular Pharmacology* 14, no. 5 (2021): 770–781. https://doi.org/10.2174/1874467213999201214225531.

506. Kadan and Aral, "Effects of Mycotoxins."

507. Dimitrios Braun et al. "The Presence of Mycotoxins in Human Amniotic Fluid." *Toxins* 13, no. 6 (2021): 409. https://doi.org/10.3390/toxins13060409.

508. Braun et al. "The Presence of Mycotoxins in Human Amniotic Fluid."

509. İlknur Münevver Gönenç et al. "Mycotoxin Exposure and Pregnancy." *Environmental Toxicology and Pharmacology* 78 (2020): 10408444. https://www.tandfonline.com/doi/full/10.1080/10408444.2020.1803791.

510. F. Peter Guengerich. "Common and Uncommon Cytochrome P450 Reactions Related to Metabolism and Chemical Toxicity." *Chemical Research in Toxicology,* 14, no. 6 (2001): 611–50. https://doi.org/10.1021/tx0002583.

511. G. Gordon Gibson and Peter Skett. *Introduction to Drug Metabolism* (Nelson Thornes, 2001).

512. Henry Jay Forman et al. "Glutathione: Overview of Its Protective Roles, Measurement, and Biosynthesis." *Molecular Aspects of Medicine,* 77, nos. 1–2 (2021): 1–12. https://doi.org/10.1016/j.mam.2008.08.006.

513. Petra Jancova et al. "Phase II Drug Metabolizing Enzymes." *Biomedical Papers of the Medical Faculty of the University Palacky, Olomouc,*

Czechoslovakia 154, no. 2 (2010): 103–116. https://doi.org/10.5507/bp
.2010.017.

514. Joseph Pizzorno. "Glutathione." *Integrative Medicine: A Clinician's
Journal* 13, no. 1 (2014): 8–12. https://pubmed.ncbi.nlm.nih.gov
/26770075/.

515. Jancova et al. "Phase II Drug Metabolizing Enzymes."

516. Jancova et al. "Phase II Drug Metabolizing Enzymes."

517. Jancova et al. "Phase II Drug Metabolizing Enzymes."

518. Susan J. Duthie et al. "Impact of Folate Deficiency on DNA Stability."
Journal of Nutrition 132, no. 8 (2002): 2444S–49S. https://doi.org/10
.1093/jn/132.8.2444S.

519. Elaine M. Leslie et al. "Multidrug Resistance Proteins: Role of
P-Glycoprotein, MRP1, MRP2, and BCRP (ABCG2) in Tissue
Defense." *Toxicology and Applied Pharmacology* 204, no. 3 (2005):
216–237 https://doi.org/10.1016/j.taap.2004.10.012.

520. ScienceDirect. "Renal Excretion." Accessed August 21, 2024.
https://www.sciencedirect.com/topics/pharmacology-toxicology-and
-pharmaceutical-science/renal-excretion.

521. Michael Schieber and Navdeep S. Chandel. "ROS Function in Redox
Signaling and Oxidative Stress." *Current Biology* 24, no. 10 (2014):
R453–62. https://doi.org/10.1016/j.cub.2014.03.034.

522. John D. Hayes et al. "Glutathione Transferases." *Annual Review of
Pharmacology and Toxicology* 45 (2005): 51–88 https://doi.org/10.1146
/annurev.pharmtox.45.120403.095857.

523. Bernard Ketterer. "Glutathione S Transferases: A Review." *Molecular
Aspects of Medicine* 10, no. 2 (1988): 73–83.

524. Mercedes Alfonso-Prieto et al. "The Molecular Mechanism of the Catalase Reaction." *Journal of the American Chemical Society* 131, no. 33
(2009): 11751–61. https://doi.org/10.1021/ja9018572.

525. Nazzareno Ballatori et al. "Glutathione Dysregulation and the Etiology and Progression of Human Diseases." *Biological Chemistry* 390,
no. 3 (2009): 191–214. https://doi.org/10.1515/BC.2009.033.

526. Paul Talalay and Jed W. Fahey. "Phytochemicals from Cruciferous Plants Protect Against Cancer by Modulating Carcinogen

Metabolism." *Journal of Nutrition* 131, no. 11 Supp. (2001): 3027S–33S. https://doi.org/10.1093/jn/131.11.3027S.

527. James M. Lattimer and Mark D. Haub. "Effects of Dietary Fiber and Its Components on Metabolic Health." *Nutrients* 2, no. 12 (2010): 1266–89. https://doi.org/10.3390/nu2121266.

528. Daniel W. Nebert and Thomas P. Dalton, "The Role of Cytochrome P450 Enzymes in Endogenous Signalling Pathways and Environmental Carcinogenesis." *Nature Reviews Cancer* 6, no. 12 (2006): 947–60. https://doi.org/10.1038/nrc2015.

529. Nebert and Dalton. "The Role of Cytochrome P450 Enzymes."

530. Nebert and Dalton. "The Role of Cytochrome P450 Enzymes."

531. John D. Hayes et al. "Glutathione Transferases." *Annual Review of Pharmacology and Toxicology* 45 (2005): 51–88. https://doi.org/10.1146/annurev.pharmtox.45.120403.095857.

532. Hayes et al. "Glutathione Transferases."

533. Petra Jancova et al. "Phase II Drug Metabolizing Enzymes." *Biomedical Papers of the Medical Faculty of the University Palacky, Olomouc, Czechoslovakia* 154, no. 2 (2010): 103–116. https://doi.org/10.5507/bp.2010.017.

534. Jancova et al. "Phase II Drug Metabolizing Enzymes."

535. Changjian Xu et al. "Induction of Phase I, II, and III Drug Metabolism/Transport by Xenobiotics." *Archives of Pharmacal Research* 28, no. 3 (2005): 249–268. https://doi.org/10.1007/BF02977789.

536. Jancova et al. "Phase II Drug Metabolizing Enzymes."

537. Jancova et al. "Phase II Drug Metabolizing Enzymes."

538. Jancova et al. "Phase II Drug Metabolizing Enzymes."

539. Despina Komninou et al. "S-Adenosylmethionine and Transmethylation Pathways in Cancer Prevention and Treatment." *Advances in Experimental Medicine and Biology* 566 (2005): 79–96.

540. Lindsay B. Baker. "Physiology of Sweat Gland Function: The Roles of Sweating and Sweat Composition in Human Health." *Temperature: Multidisciplinary Biomedical Journal* 6, no. 3 (2019): 211–59. https://doi.org/10.1080/23328940.2019.1632145.

541. Michael Schieber and Navdeep S. Chandel. "ROS Function in Redox Signaling and Oxidative Stress." *Current Biology* 24, no. 10 (2014): R453–62. https://doi.org/10.1016/j.cub.2014.03.034.

542. Danyelle M. Townsend et al. "The Importance of Glutathione in Human Disease." *Biomedicine & Pharmacotherapy* 57, nos. 3–4 (2003): 145–155. https://doi.org/10.1016/s0753-3322(03)00043-x.

543. ScienceDirect. "Transcription Factor Nrf2." accessed August 19, 2024. https://www.sciencedirect.com/topics/biochemistry-genetics-and-molecular-biology/transcription-factor-nrf2.

544. R. Oliver and H. Basit. "Embryology, Fertilization." *StatPearls* (2023). https://www.ncbi.nlm.nih.gov/books/NBK542186/.

545. ScienceDirect. "Trisomy." Accessed October 10, 2024.

INDEX

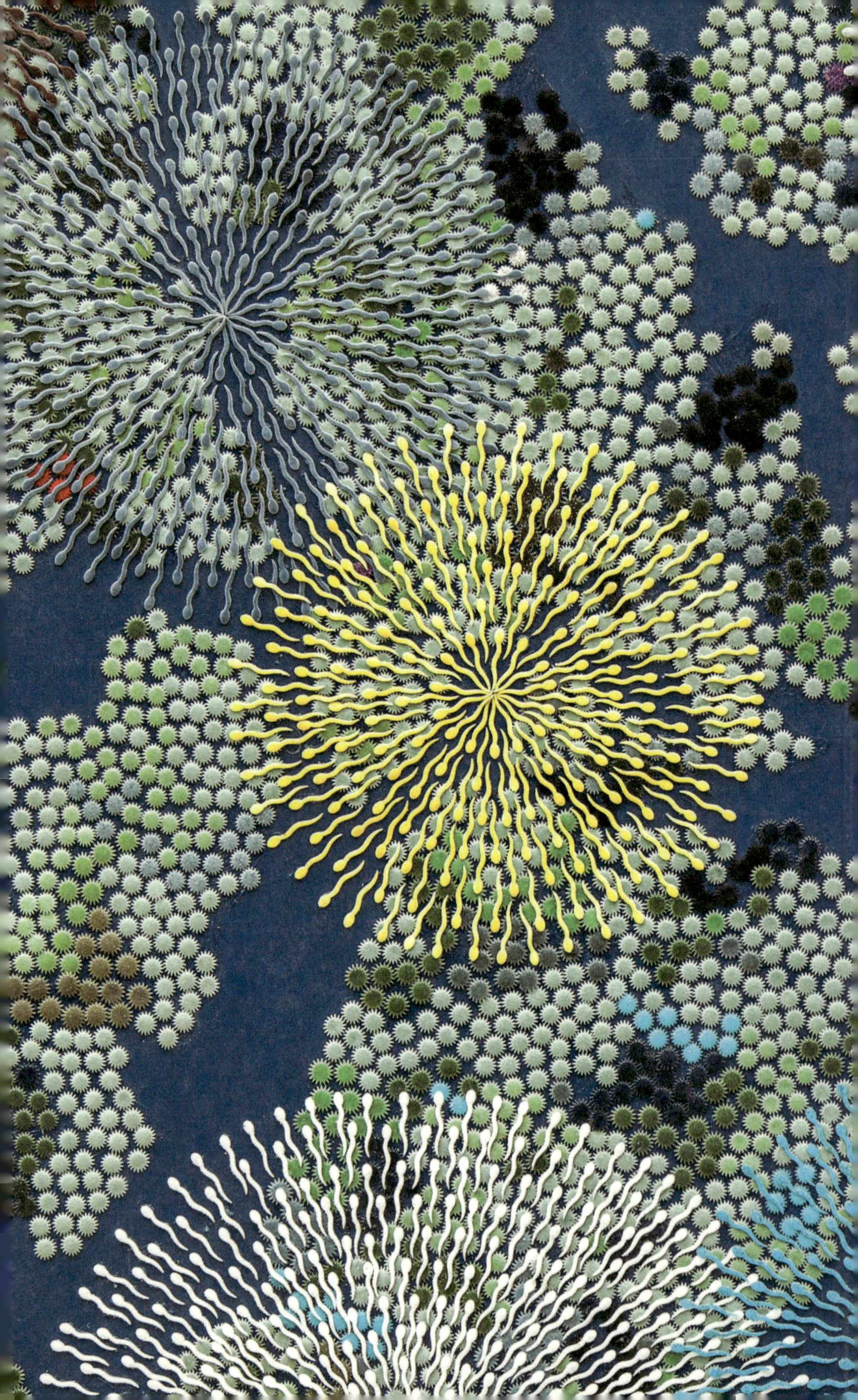